# Disease Prevention and Health Promotion in Developing Countries

Abdesslam Boutayeb
Editor

# Disease Prevention and Health Promotion in Developing Countries

Springer

*Editor*
Abdesslam Boutayeb
Emirates Aviation University
Dubai, United Arab Emirates

ISBN 978-3-030-34701-7 ISBN 978-3-030-34702-4 (eBook)
https://doi.org/10.1007/978-3-030-34702-4



This Springer imprint is published by the registered company Springer Nature Switzerland AG
The registered company address is: Gewerbestrasse 11, 6330 Cham, Switzerland

# Foreword

Inspired by research papers, refereed conference proceedings and other books published during the last 15 years, the parts of this book bring together two important features.

The first part is devoted to the burden of disease, health equity and social determinants of health, and the second part presents bio-mathematical models and epidemiological studies.

The chapters of the first part are dedicated to public health in developing countries with emphasis on the African and Eastern Mediterranean Regions of the World Health Organisation.

The book places emphasis on health equity and social determinants. It provides readers with updated research which shows that recognition of, and acting on, social determinants of health is crucial in order to improve the health of people in developing countries and also (and mostly) to reduce the growing unfairness of remediable health inequalities. Further neglect of these factors, it is argued, will, in some countries, increase infant mortality rates, the spread of parasitic diseases such as malaria, and the growing trend of non-communicable diseases due to obesity and physical inactivity. Elsewhere in the first part of the book, contributing authors cover such topics as environmental impact, the use of herbal medicines in treating chronic diseases and artificial intelligence in oncology—a likely feature of cancer research in the years ahead.

Arguably the most compelling problem facing humanity in the next decades is the changing epidemiological environment of infectious and other diseases. Accordingly, opportunities to prevent disease and promote health in developing countries with high burden of disease and limited resources must not be overlooked. The second part of the book presents mathematical models and epidemiological studies, all relevant to countries with high burden of disease and limited resources. Such countries need cost-effective strategies and cost–benefit analyses in their plans to prevent disease and promote health for their citizens.

For example, planning and scheduling of the operating rooms play an important part in providing appropriate services in hospitals. Uncertainty is one of the major problems associated with the development of accurate operating room schedules or capacity planning strategies. One chapter of the book examines how fuzzy logic can be a good solution to the uncertainty problems within the operating theatre.

There is a review of compartmental models used in the clinical science of diabetes mellitus, its diagnosis, treatment and follow-up, and a mathematical model of glucose homeostasis in Type I diabetes mellitus. Other topics addressed in the second part of the book include global properties of a diffusive HBV infection model, discrete mathematical modelling of tumour therapy, an optimal control approach to the modelling of dengue fever and numerical treatment of multidimensional stochastic, competitive and evolutionary models.

This present book illustrates the challenges countries face in health equity and social determinants of health, and also the diversity of the mathematical approaches that will be available to help in addressing them.

July 2019

E. H. Twizell
Brunel University London, London, UK

# Acknowledgements

The editor of this book would like to thank all the authors who were committed to contribute a chapter in the fixed deadline.

A special acknowledgement is dedicated to Dr. Mohamed E. N. Lamlili for the great effort devoted to the technical production, including transforming all chapters written in format word doc to Latex and uniformizing references of all chapters following Basic Style.

# Contents

# Contributors

**Mohammed Abdu** Department of Health Information & Research Evidence, Federal Ministry of Health, Khartoum, Sudan

**Nabil Azouagh** Laboratory of Stochastic and Deterministic Modelling (LaSDM), Faculty of Sciences, University Mohamed Ier, Oujda, Morocco

**Souad Ben El Mostafa** Higher Institute of Health Nursing and Technical Professions (ISPITS), Ministry of Health, Nador, Morocco

**Souad Benaich** Faculty of Sciences, Laboratory of Animal Physiology, Research Centre of Human Pathologies Genomics, Mohammed V University, Rabat, Morocco

**Nezha Bouhaddou** Faculty of Sciences, Laboratory of Animal Physiology, Research Centre of Human Pathologies Genomics, Mohammed V University, Rabat, Morocco

**Abdesslam Boutayeb** Emirates Aviation University, Dubai, UAE;
University Mohamed Ier, Oujda, Morocco

**Saber Boutayeb** Faculty of Medicine and Pharmacy, Medical Oncology, Mohammed V University, Rabat, Morocco

**Wiam Boutayeb** School of High Studies in Engineering, Oujda, Morocco

**Abdelaziz Chetouani** Team of Operational Research and Applied Statistics, National School of Commerce and Management, University Mohamed Ier, Oujda, Morocco

**Mohamed Derouich** Laboratory of Stochastic and Deterministic Modelling (LaSDM), National School Applied Sciences (ENSA), University Mohamed Ier, Oujda, Morocco

**Khalid Hattaf** Centre Régional des Métiers de l'Education et de la Formation (CRMEF), Casablanca, Morocco

**Marwa Khalfalli** HF-LAB, HIGHFI, Paris, France

**Mohamed E. N. Lamlili** Laboratory of Stochastic and Deterministic Modelling (LaSDM), Faculty of Sciences, University Mohamed Ier, Oujda, Morocco

**Abdellatif Maamri** Department of Biology, Faculty of Sciences, University Mohamed Ier, Oujda, Morocco

**Anass Majbar** National Oncology Institute, Mohammed V University, Rabat, Morocco

**Slimane Mehdad** Faculty of Sciences, Laboratory of Animal Physiology, Research Centre of Human Pathologies Genomics, Mohammed V University, Rabat, Morocco

**Ahmed Ouazza** Laboratory of Stochastic and Deterministic Modelling (LaSDM), Faculty of Sciences, University Mohamed Ier, Oujda, Morocco

**Jerome Verny** NEOMA Business School, Mont-Saint-Aignan, France

**Noura Yousfi** Laboratory of Analysis, Modelling and simulation (LAMS), Faculty of Sciences Ben M'sik, Hassan II University of Casablanca, Sidi Othman, Casablanca, Morocco

**Mostafa Zahri** College of Sciences, University of Sharjah, Sharjah, UAE

**Naoual Zitouni** Higher Institute of Health Nursing and Technical Professions Oujda (ISPITSO), Oujda, Morocco

# Chapter 1
# Introduction

**Abdesslam Boutayeb**

**Abstract** In this book, a pragmatic deal with disease prevention and health promotion is proposed by different authors through safe environment and healthy lifestyle, physical activity and weight control, herbal medicine and mathematical modelling for communicable and non communicable diseases. Authors showed that reducing health inequalities and ensuring wellbeing for the whole population needs efficient action on social determinants of health such as income, education, gender, marital status, employment, ethnicity, milieu of residence, territorial context and general environment conditions.

## 1.1 Health Equity and Social Determinants of Health

The World Health Organization (WHO) stressed the need for health promotion in 1946. Indeed, the World Health Constitution states that "Health is a state of complete physical, mental and social well-being and not merely the absence of disease or infirmity". Similarly, health equity and health as a fundamental human right are clearly defined in the Constitution which highlights that "the enjoyment of the highest attainable standard of health is one of the fundamental rights of every human being without distinction of race, religion, political belief, economic or social condition" [11]. Unfortunately, economic globalization, structural adjustment programmes, financial crises and other political and technological aspects all contributed to the delay or the eclipse of a real promotion of an equitable health. Consequently, more than 70 years later, many health systems in the world are still dealing with disease and infirmity rather than with health and well-being of their populations. Moreover, health gaps are persisting if not widening, making health far away from being a fundamental human right for all.

The need for intersectoral coordination to act on social determinants of health was a principal axis in the health for All call and its pragmatic importance was reaffirmed

A. Boutayeb (✉)
Emirates Aviation University, Dubai, United Arab Emirates
e-mail: x.boutayeb@gmail.com

University Mohamed Ier, Oujda, Morocco



A. Boutayeb (ed.), *Disease Prevention and Health Promotion in Developing Countries*,
https://doi.org/10.1007/978-3-030-34702-4_1

in the 1978 Alma Ata Declaration which stressed that "Health is a fundamental human right and that the attainment of the highest possible level of health is a most important worldwide social goal whose realization requires the action of many other social and economic sectors in addition to the health sector" [12].

The Commission on Social Determinants of Health (CSDH) launched by the World Health Organization in 2005, defined the social determinants of health as the conditions in which people are born, grow, live, work and age, including the health system. The commission stressed that these circumstances are shaped by the distribution of money, power and resources at global, national and local levels. The social determinants of health are mostly responsible for health inequities—the unfair and avoidable- differences in health status seen within and between countries [8]. For closing the gaps and promoting health equity, the CSDH recommended action on social determinants of health through three main streams: (1) Improve daily living conditions, (2) Tackle the inequitable distribution of power, money and resources, and (3) Measure and understand the problem and assess the impact of Action.

Following the 2011 Rio Political Declaration on Social Determinants of Health [16] and in order to foster pragmatic action on SDH by national governments, civil society and international organizations, and considering the needs of key indicator users, the World Health Organisation proposed in 2016 a framework and basket of core indicators for a global monitoring of action on the social determinants of health [9, 14]. Pragmatically, the WHO's Health Equity Monitor is an initiative that should improve understanding of action on SDH and health equity in every country and at the global level [2].

Authors contributing to this book have clearly proved that reducing health inequalities and ensuring wellbeing for the whole population needs action on social determinants such as income, education, gender, employment, marital status, ethnicity, milieu (rural-urban), territorial context and general environmental conditions (Chaps. 2–7).

## 1.2 Health Promotion

From 1986 to 2016, the World Health Organisation held nine Global Conferences on Health Promotion (GCHP) [15].

1. The first GCHP was held in Ottawa, Canada in 1986. The main objective of the conference was to identify and clarify actions needed to achieve "Health for all". The prerequisites identified were social justice and equity, peace, a stable ecosystem, and resources like food, income and education. Creating supportive environments, strengthening community actions, developing personal skills, building healthy public policy, and reorienting health services were the key recommendations of the conference
2. The Second GCHP was held in Adelaide, Australia in 1988. Highlighting the need for a political commitment to health by all sectors, it urged policy makers at local, national and international levels to increase investments in health. Four

priority areas for action were identified: (1) supporting the health of women; (2) improving food security, safety and nutrition; (3) reducing tobacco and alcohol use; and (4) creating supportive environments for health.
3. The third GCHP was held in Sundsvall, Sweden, in 1991. The Sundsvall Statement on Supportive Environments for Health stressed the importance of sustainable development and urged social action at the community level. It also contributed to the development of Agenda 21 adopted at the Rio Earth Summit in 1992.
4. The fourth GCHP was held in Jakarta, Indonesia in 1997. It ended up with the Jakarta Declaration on "Leading Health Promotion into the 21st Century", proposing five priorities which will be officially stated in the Resolution on Health Promotion adopted by the World Health Assembly in 1998, namely: (1) Promoting Social Responsibility for Health, (2) Increasing Community Capacity and Empowering the Individual, (3) Expanding and Consolidating Partnerships for Health, (4) Increasing Investment for Health Development, and (5) Securing an Infrastructure for Health Promotion.
5. The fifth GCHP was held in Mexico city, Mexico in 2000. Considering that equity is a cornerstone of health promotion and that persisting socioeconomic inequalities and territorial disparities deteriorate and erode the conditions for good health, the conference was held under the title "Health Promotion: Bridging the Equity Gap".
6. The sixth GCHP was held in Bangkok, Thailand in 2005. Endorsing the principles and recommendations of the previous five global conferences on health promotion, the GCHP6 aimed to place reduction of health inequalities and health improvement in the core of global and national development agendas. Consequently, it highlighted the commitments and actions needed by all stakeholders to address the determinants of health.
7. The seventh GCHP was held in Nairobi, Kenya in 2009. Stressing that developing and developed countries are facing a surge of preventable diseases that threatens to undermine their future economic development, the Nairobi acting together call addresses five urgent responsibilities for government and stakeholders: (1) Strengthen leadership and workforce, (2) Build and apply knowledge, (3) Enhance participatory process, (4) Empower communities and individuals, and (5) Mainstream health promotion.
8. The eighth GCHP was held in Helsinki, Finland in 2013. The GCHP8 (re)identified intersectoral action and healthy public policy as essential prerequisites for the promotion of health (as a human right) and the achievement of health equity. For this, it used the heritage provided by Alma Ata Declaration and the previous seven global conferences on health promotion as well as the 2011 Rio Political Declaration on Social Determinants of Health, the 2011 Political Declaration of the UN High-level Meeting of the General Assembly on the Prevention and Control of Noncommunicable Diseases, and finally, the 2012 Rio+20 (the Future We Want).
9. The ninth GCHP was held in Shanghai, China in 2016. Recognizing that health and wellbeing are essential to achieving sustainable development, the GCHP9, reaffirmed health as a universal right, an essential resource for everyday living, a shared social goal and a political priority for all countries. In line with the UN

Sustainable Development Goals (SDGs), investment in health is stated as a duty, especially to ensure universal health coverage and to reduce health inequities for people of all ages and categories by leaving no one behind.

As indicated in the quasi totality of the chapters of this book, a pragmatic deal with disease prevention and health promotion is proposed through safe environment and healthy lifestyle (Chap. 4); physical activity and weight control (Chap. 6); herbal medicine (Chap. 7), global properties of a diffusive HBV infection (Chap. 10); discrete mathematical modelling of tumour therapy (Chap. 11), a model for dengue fever with optimal control (Chap. 12) and mathematical modelling for diabetes (Chaps. 14 and 15).

## 1.3 Noncommunicable Diseases

One of the biggest challenges currently facing humanity is noncommunicable diseases (NCDs) which are sweeping the entire globe, with an increasing trend in developing countries [1]. During the last decades, industrialization, urbanization, economic development and market globalization have accelerated changes in diet and lifestyles, especially in developing countries in transition. A report of the joint WHO/FAO Expert Consultation on Diet, Nutrition and the Prevention of Chronic Diseases was published in 2003. The report stressed that "population-based epidemiological evidence has helped to clarify the role of diet in preventing and controlling morbidity and premature mortality resulting from noncommunicable diseases (NCDs)". Interestingly, the expert report indicated how diet and lifestyle can affect health of people throughout the life course, starting from fetal development and ending at old age, passing by infancy, childhood/adolescence and adulthood [10]. More generally, a large part of the burden of noncommunicable diseases can be avoided by acting on four particular behaviours (tobacco use, physical inactivity, unhealthy diet, and the harmful use of alcohol) and four key metabolic/physiological changes (overweight/obesity, raised blood pressure, raised blood glucose and raised cholesterol) [13].

The United Nations General Assembly in 2011 addressed the prevention and control of non-communicable diseases worldwide, with a particular focus on developmental and other challenges and social and economic impacts, particularly for developing countries. The Political Declaration on the Prevention and Control of NCDs (resolution A/RES/66/2) was adopted [5]. Following this and recognizing the primary role and responsibility of Governments in responding to the challenge of NCDs, the Sixty-Sixth World Health Assembly (WHA66.10) adopted the Global NCD Action Plan for the Prevention and Control of NCDs 2013–2020 developed by WHO and partners [17].

One of the principal axes of this book is the theme of noncommunicable diseases which was dealt with in chapters under different forms such as epidemiology of NCDs in Arab countries (Chap. 5); the role of environment and healthy lifestyle in reducing

NCDs (Chap. 4); artificial intelligence in oncology (Chap. 8); overweight and physical inactivity as risks of NCDs in North Africa (Chap. 6); herbal medicine and chronic disease (Chap. 7); global properties of a diffusive HBV infection (Chap. 10); discrete mathematical modelling of tumour therapy (Chap. 11) and mathematical modelling for diabetes (Chaps. 14 and 15).

## 1.4 Health and Development

### *1.4.1 The Rio Declaration on Environment (1992)*

Health was explicitly and implicitly underlined in the principles of the Rio Declaration on environment (1992) as indicated by principles 1 and 5 [4]:

**Principle 1 Stipulates that:** Humans beings are at the centre of concerns for sustainable development. They are entitled to a healthy and productive life in harmony with nature.

**Principle 5 stipulates that:** All States and all people shall co-operate in the essential task of eradicating poverty as an indispensable requirement for sustainable development, in order to decrease the disparities in standards of living and better meet the needs of the majority of the people of the world.

### *1.4.2 The Millennium Development Goals (2000)*

In 2000, 189 countries of the world came together to face the future. The meeting gave birth to the Millennium Development Goals (MDGs) to be reached by 2015. Three out of eight goals were explicitly dedicated to health: reducing child mortality (MDG4), improving maternal health (MDG5) and combating HIV/AIDS, malaria and other diseases (MDG6), while the remaining goals were indirectly related to health [7].

### *1.4.3 The Sustainable Development Goals (2016): End Poverty and Hunger by 2030*

In 2015, building on the successes and or limitations of MDGs, and hoping to go further, countries adopted the 2030 Agenda for Sustainable Development and its 17 Sustainable Development Goals. The third sustainable development goal is directly devoted to heath: ensure healthy lives and promote well-being for all at all ages (SDG3). However, the remaining 16 SDGs are also indirectly linked to health through poverty reduction (SDG1), zero hunger (SDG2), quality education (SDG4), gender equality (SDG5), clean water and sanitation (SDG6) and others [6].

### *1.4.4 Inequality Adjusted Human Development*

Another illustration of growing interest in inequalities and disparities is provided by the 2010 human development report, introducing a new human development index (HDI) which captures the losses in human development due to inequality in health, education and income, namely: Inequality-adjusted HDI (IHDI) [3]. In 2017, the global loss in the three dimensions varied across countries, ranging from 3.6% in Japan to 45.3% in Comoros. It is sad to notice that the percent loss due to inequality is much higher in countries with the lowest level of human development than in other countries, thus accumulating two dissatisfactions with their populations.

The relationship between Health and Development in its different forms (economic, social, human, sustainable) was treated directly or indirectly by different authors (Chaps. 2–10, 12–13 and 16).

## References

1. Boutayeb A, Boutayeb S (2005) The burden of non communicable diseases in developing countries. Int J Equity Health 4(1):2
2. Hosseinpoor AR, Bergen N, Schlotheuber A, Victora C, Boerma T, Barros AJ (2016) Data resource profile: WHO health equity monitor (HEM). Int J Epidemiol 45(5):1404–1405e
3. UNDP (2015) Inequality-adjusted human development index (IHDI). http://hdr.undp.org/en/content/inequality-adjusted-human-development-index-ihdi
4. United Nations (1992) The declaration on environment and development. http://www.unesco.org/education/pdf/RIO_E.PDF
5. United Nations (2012) Political declaration of the high-level meeting of the general assembly on the prevention and control of non-communicable diseases. https://digitallibrary.un.org/record/720106/files/A_RES_66_2-EN.pdf
6. United Nations General Assembly (2015) Transforming our world: the 2030 agenda for sustainable development. https://www.un.org/sustainabledevelopment/development-agenda/
7. United Nations Statistics Division (2006) Millennium development goal indicators database. http://millenniumindicators.un.org/unsd/mi/mi_goals.asp. Accessed 18 Mar 2018
8. WHO Commission on Social Determinants of Health and World Health Organization (2008) Closing the gap in a generation: health equity through action on the social determinants of health: commission on social determinants of health final report. World Health Organization
9. Working Group for Monitoring Action on the Social Determinants of Health (2018) Towards a global monitoring system for implementing the rio political declaration on social determinants of health: developing a core set of indicators for government action on the social determinants of health to improve health equity. Int J Equity Health 17:1–27
10. World Health Organisation (2003) Diet, nutrition and the prevention of chronic diseases. Report of a joint WHO/FAO expert consultation, WHO Technical report series, p 916
11. World Health Organisation (1946) Constitution of the World Health organisation. In: International health conference. WHO Geneva, New York

12. World Health Organisation (1978) The Declaration of Alma-Ata. In: International conference on primary health care, Alma-Ata
13. World Health Organization (2019) Global health observatory data: risk factors. https://www.who.int/gho/ncd/risk_factors/en/
14. World Health Organization (2016) Global monitoring of action on the social determinants of health: a proposed framework and basket of core indicators. https://www.who.int/social_determinants/consultation-paper-SDH-Action-Monitoring.pdf
15. World Health Organization (2019) Global health promotion conferences. https://www.who.int/healthpromotion/conferences/en/
16. World Health Organization and others (2011) Rio political declaration on social determinants of health. In: World conference on social determinants of health, Rio de Janeiro, pp 19–21
17. World Health Organization and others (2013) Global action plan for the prevention and control of noncommunicable diseases 2013–2020. http://www.who.int/nmh/events/ncd_action_plan/en/

# Part I
# Burden of Disease, Health Equity and Social Determinants of Health

# Chapter 2
# Social Determinants of Health and Health Equity in the WHO African Region

**Abdesslam Boutayeb**

**Abstract** The African Region is one of the six regions of the World Health Organization grouping 47 countries with a total population over one billion inhabitants. The WHO African region is known to have a large number of low-income countries with low human development. In terms of health indicators, this region has many critical average indicators compared with other WHO regions, with large inequalities and disparities between and within countries. This chapter describes and analyses some gaps in health indicators, trying to see how action on social determinants of health can reduce health inequities and improve health and well-being of African population, leaving no one behind. With a life expectancy average of around 60 years, African people are expected to live 17 years less than their counterparts in Europe and the gap between the highest and the lowest level of life expectancy in WHO African countries (76.3–52.2) is nearly a quarter of a century (24 years). Similarly, the under-five mortality rate in the WHO African region is much higher than in other WHO regions with huge gaps between WHO African countries. Within each country, inequalities in under-five mortality rate are described and analysed through social determinants of health like economic status, education level, residence (urban-rural) and geographic context. Health inequality and territorial disparity are also illustrated by huge gaps in maternal mortality ratio and other health indicators.

## 2.1 Introduction

The African Region is one of the six regions of the World Health Organization. In 2015, it's total population was more than one billion inhabitants spread across 47 countries [19]. The population is relatively young with about 95% under age 60 years and the under 15 class of age representing more than 40% of the population in 30 countries (Table 2.1).

A. Boutayeb (✉)
Emirates Aviation University, Dubai, United Arab Emirates
e-mail: x.boutayeb@gmail.com

University Mohamed Ier, Oujda, Morocco



A. Boutayeb (ed.), *Disease Prevention and Health Promotion in Developing Countries*,
https://doi.org/10.1007/978-3-030-34702-4_2

According to the 2017 Human Development Index (HDI) [10] and the 2016 World Bank classification for income, [8], two-third countries in the region are in the low human development class and nearly 60% are low-income countries (Table 2.1).

The African region has worrying health indicators compared with other regions (see Table 2.2). For instance, the average maternal mortality ratio (MMR) in Africa (542 deaths per 100 000 live births) is around 3.3 times the MMR in Eastern Mediterranean region (166) and South-East Asia (164), nearly 10.5 times the MMR in Americas (52), more than 13 times the MMR in Western pacific (41), and nearly 34 times the MMR in Europe (16). Moreover, the ratio 542 is an average that hides huge gaps between maternal mortality in African countries, ranging from the lowest level in Mauritius (53 deaths in 100 000) to the highest level in Sierra Leone (1360 deaths in 100 000). Similarly, the average under-five mortality rate in Africa (76.8 deaths per 1000 live births) is more than 5 times higher than in Americas (76.8 deaths per 1000 live births), 6 times higher than in Western Pacific (12.9 deaths per 1000 live births) and 8 times higher than in Europe (9.6 deaths per 1000 live births). Moreover, a huge gap is seen between African countries ranging from 13.5 per 1000 live births in Mauritius to 156.9 per 1000 live births in Angola.

Other health indicators like health expenditure, out-of-pocket expenditure, vaccination, antenatal care, assisted deliveries show significant differences between the African region and other regions as well as between and within African countries.

In this chapter, we concentrate on social determinants of health and health equity in the WHO African region. Most of disaggregated data used are obtained from well-known international surveys like demographic health surveys (DHS) [15] and Mixed Indicator Cluster Surveys (MICS) [12] carried out in different African countries during the last 10 years.

## 2.2 Social Determinants of Health and Health Equity in Africa

### *2.2.1 A Brief Recall on Social Determinants of Health and Health Equity*

The Pan American Health Organisation (PAHO) defines equity in health as "a cardinal expression of social justice, attained when every individual has the opportunity to reach his full health potential and no one is excluded or hindered from reaching that potential because of his social status or other socially determined circumstances". An example of health inequity is illustrated by inequality gradient in maternal mortality in the Americas, by human development quartiles in the Millennium Development Goals period (1990–2015) (Fig. 2.1) [7]. This figure indicates that some countries may have reached the fifth MDG stipulating an average reduction of MMR by three quarters, between 1990 and 2015, but in the meantime, inequalities persisted or could be even increased.

**Table 2.1** WHO African countries: population, age structure, income and human development

| Country | Population (×1000) | Aged under 15 years (%) | Aged under 15–59 (%) | Aged over 60 years (%) | Income level | HDI level |
|---|---|---|---|---|---|---|
| Algeria | 40376 | 29 | 63 | 8 | U.M.I | H.H.D |
| Angola | 25831 | 48 | 48 | 4 | L.M.I | M.H.D |
| Benin | 11167 | 42 | 53 | 5 | L.I | L.H |
| Botswana | 2304 | 32 | 62 | 6 | U.M.I | H.H.D |
| Burkina Faso | 18634 | 46 | 51 | 4 | L.I | L.H |
| Burundi | 11553 | 45 | 50 | 5 | L.I | L.H |
| Cabo Verde | 527 | | | | L.M.I | M.H.D |
| Cameroon | 23924 | 43 | 53 | 5 | L.M.I | M.H.D |
| C. African R. | 4998 | 39 | 55 | 5 | L.I | L.H |
| Chad | 14497 | 48 | 48 | 4 | L.I | L.H |
| Comoros | 807 | 40 | 55 | 5 | L.I | L.H |
| Congo | 4741 | 43 | 52 | 6 | L.M.I | M.H.D |
| Côte d'Ivoire | 23254 | 43 | 53 | 5 | L.M.I | L.H |
| D. Rep Congo | 79722 | | | | L.I | L.H |
| Equat Guinea | 870 | 39 | 56 | 5 | U.M.I | M.H.D |
| Eritrea | 5352 | 43 | 53 | 4 | L.I | L.H |
| Ethiopia | 101853 | 41 | 53 | 5 | L.I | L.H |
| Gabon | 1763 | 37 | 56 | 7 | U.M.I | H.H.D |
| Gambia | 2055 | 46 | 50 | 4 | L.I | L.H |
| Ghana | 28033 | 39 | 56 | 5 | L.M.I | M.H.D |
| Guinea | 12947 | 43 | 52 | 5 | L.I | L.H |
| Guinea-Bissau | 1888 | 41 | 54 | 5 | L.I | L.H |
| Kenya | 4725 | 42 | 54 | 5 | L.M.I | M.H.D |
| Lesotho | 2160 | 36 | 58 | 6 | L.M.I | L.H |
| Liberia | 4615 | 42 | 53 | 5 | L.I | L.H |
| Madagascar | 24916 | 42 | 53 | 5 | L.I | L.H |
| Malawi | 17750 | 45 | 50 | 5 | L.I | L.H |
| Mali | 18134 | 48 | 48 | 4 | L.I | L.H |
| Mauritania | 4166 | 40 | 55 | 5 | L.M.I | L.H |
| Mauritius | 1277 | 19 | 66 | 15 | U.M.I | H.H.D |
| Mozambique | 28751 | 45 | 50 | 5 | L.I | L.H |
| Namibia | 2514 | 37 | 58 | 6 | U.M.I | M.H.D |
| Niger | 20715 | 51 | 45 | 4 | L.I | L.H |
| Nigeria | 186988 | 44 | 52 | 5 | L.M.I | L.H |
| Rwanda | 11882 | 41 | 54 | 5 | L.I | L.H |
| Sao Tome & P | 194 | | | | L.M.I | L.H |
| Seychelles | 97 | 23 | 66 | 11 | H.I | H.H.D |
| Senegal | 15589 | 44 | 52 | 5 | L.I | L.H |

(continued)

**Table 2.1** (continued)

| Country | Population (×1000) | Aged under 15 years (%) | Aged under 15–59 (%) | Aged over 60 years (%) | Income level | HDI level |
|---|---|---|---|---|---|---|
| Sierra Leone | 6592 | 42 | 53 | 4 | L.I | L.H |
| South Africa | 54979 | | | | U.M.I | M.H.D |
| South Sudan | 12733 | | | | L.I | L.H |
| Swaziland | 1304 | 37 | 57 | 6 | L.M.I | L.H |
| Togo | 7497 | | | | L.I | L.H |
| Uganda | 40323 | 48 | 48 | 4 | L.I | L.H |
| Tanzania | 55155 | 45 | 50 | 5 | L.I | L.H |
| Zambia | 16717 | 46 | 50 | 4 | L.M.I | M.H.D |
| Zimbabwe | 15967 | 42 | 54 | 4 | L.I | L.H |
| Region | 1015368 | | | | | |

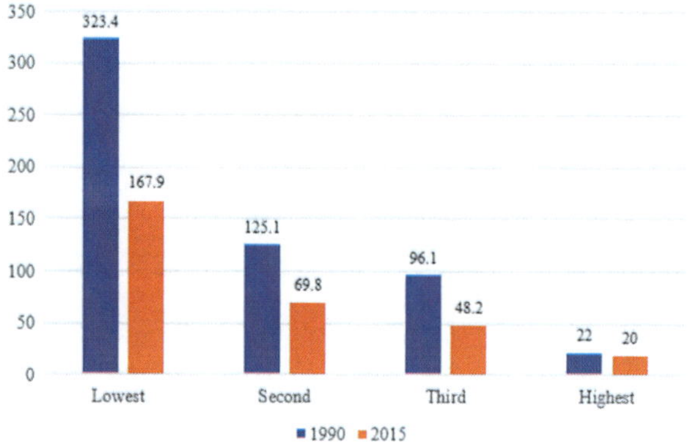


**Fig. 2.1** Maternal Mortality gradient in the Americas by human development *Source* PAHO [7]

During the last two decades, social determinants of health and health equity have known an important development [4]. In 2005, the World Health Organization launched the WHO Commission on Social Determinants of Health which delivered its well-known report in 2008 under the title "Closing the gap in a generation: health equity through action on the social determinants of health". Defined as the conditions in which people are born, grow, live, work and age, including the health system, social determinants of health are seen to be responsible for unfair and avoidable health inequalities within and between countries [16]. Income is seen to be a social determinant of health yielding a clear gradient for many health indicators. An illustration is given by maternal mortality in all countries of the world in 2015, showing that worldwide, women from the poorest quintile are nearly 50 times more exposed to maternal mortality than their counterparts in the richest quintile (Fig. 2.2).

**Table 2.2** Health indicators in WHO African countries

| Country | LE (2017) | U5MR (2015) | MMR (2015) | Births ASP | ANC 4Visitis+ | Over weight | Stunting | DM % | Cholesterol | BP % | HIV |
|---|---|---|---|---|---|---|---|---|---|---|---|
| Algeria | 76.3 | 25.5 | 140 | 97 | 67.4 | 62 | 11.7 | 10.5 | 39 | 25 | 0.5 |
| Angola | 61.8 | 156.9 | 477 | 47 | 61.4 | 27.5 | 37.6 | 5.6 | 31 | 30 | 42.5 |
| Benin | 61.2 | 99.5 | 405 | 77 | 58.7 | 29.5 | 34 | 5.7 | 20.3 | 27 | 21.5 |
| Botswana | 67.6 | 43.6 | 129 | 100 | 73.3 | 43.4 | 31.4 | 6 | 38 | 29 | 169 |
| Burkina Faso | 60.8 | 88.6 | 371 | 66 | 47.2 | 23.2 | 27.3 | 4.2 | 18 | 32 | 16.6 |
| Burundi | 57.9 | 81.7 | 712 | 60 | 49.3 | 22.2 | 55.9 | 2.6 | 19 | 29 | 25.1 |
| Cabo Verde | 73 | 24.5 | 42 | 92 | 58.8 | 33.6 | 6.8 | 22 | 25 | 121 | |
| Cameroon | 58.6 | 87.9 | 596 | 65 | 38.1 | 34.8 | 31.7 | 4.7 | 24 | 29 | 18.9 |
| C. African R. | 52.9 | 130.1 | 882 | 40 | 31 | 26.2 | 40.7 | 5.7 | 22 | 31 | 146 |
| Chad | 53.2 | 138.7 | 856 | 24 | 48.9 | 23.1 | 39.9 | 4.6 | 18 | 32 | 19.3 |
| Comoros | 63.9 | 73.5 | 335 | 82 | 79 | 27.1 | 32.1 | 5.9 | 24 | 28 | 12.3 |
| Congo | 65.1 | 45 | 442 | 94 | 44.2 | 30 | 21.2 | 5.7 | 29 | 26 | 60.1 |
| Côte d'Ivoire | 54.1 | 92.6 | 645 | 56 | 72.3 | 31.6 | 29.6 | 5 | 21 | 27 | 107 |
| D. Rep Congo | 60 | 98.3 | 693 | 80 | 48 | 25.3 | 42.6 | 4.3 | 16 | 28 | 23.8 |
| Equat Guinea | 57.9 | 94.1 | 342 | 68 | 66.9 | 26.7 | 26.2 | 7.6 | 41 | 29 | 115 |
| Eritrea | 65.5 | 46.5 | 501 | 34 | 57.4 | 22 | 50.3 | 3.4 | 21 | 29 | 18.6 |
| Ethiopia | 65.9 | 59.2 | 353 | 16 | 31.8 | 20.9 | 38.4 | 3.8 | 21 | 30 | 19.6 |
| Gabon | 66.5 | 50.8 | 291 | 89 | 77.6 | 40.2 | 17.5 | 8.1 | 42 | 25 | 85 |
| Gambia | 61.4 | 68.9 | 706 | 57 | 77.6 | 31.9 | 25 | 5.8 | 20 | 29 | 53.5 |
| Ghana | 63 | 61.6 | 319 | 71 | 87.3 | 32 | 18.8 | 4.8 | 18 | 24 | 53.5 |
| Guinea | 60.6 | 93.7 | 679 | 45 | 56.6 | 26.6 | 31.3 | 4.7 | 19 | 30 | 44.8 |
| Guinea-Bissa | 57.8 | 92.5 | 549 | 45 | 64.9 | 29.9 | 27.6 | 5.2 | 17 | 30 | 106 |
| Kenya | 67.3 | 49.4 | 510 | 62 | 57.6 | 25.5 | 26 | 4 | 27 | 26 | 76.1 |
| Lesotho | 54.6 | 90.3 | 487 | 78 | 74.4 | 38.7 | 33.2 | 6 | 23 | 28 | 458 |

(continued)

**Table 2.2** (continued)

| Country | LE (2017) | U5MR (2015) | MMR (2015) | Births ASP | ANC 4Visitis+ | Over weight | Stunting | DM % | Cholesterol | BP % | HIV |
|---|---|---|---|---|---|---|---|---|---|---|---|
| Liberia | 63 | 69.9 | 725 | 61 | 78.1 | 30.9 | 32.1 | 5.6 | 16 | 28 | 60.6 |
| Madagascar | 66.3 | 49.6 | 353 | 44 | 51.1 | 23.9 | 49.2 | 3.9 | 24 | 28 | 6.4 |
| Malawi | 63.7 | 64 | 634 | 87 | 50.6 | 23.4 | 37.1 | 4.3 | 24 | 28 | 135 |
| Mali | 58.5 | 114.7 | 587 | 57 | 38 | 28.1 | 30.4 | 5 | 19 | 32 | 33.6 |
| Mauritania | 63.4 | 84.7 | 602 | 65 | 63 | 34.4 | 27.9 | 6.7 | 22 | 32 | 24 |
| Mauritius | 74.9 | 13.5 | 53 | 99 | 90 | 32.3 | | 14.2 | 47 | 25 | |
| Mozambique | 58.9 | 78.5 | 489 | 54 | 50.6 | 26.4 | 43.1 | 4.6 | 36 | 29 | 216 |
| Namibia | 64.9 | 45.4 | 265 | 88 | 62.5 | 40.6 | 23.1 | 5.4 | 33 | 28 | 171 |
| Niger | 60.4 | 95.5 | 553 | 29 | 38 | 22 | 42.2 | 4.1 | 15 | 34 | 16.4 |
| Nigeria | 53.9 | 108.8 | 814 | 35 | 51.1 | 28.9 | 32.9 | 4.3 | 17 | 24 | 85.5 |
| Rwanda | 67.5 | 41.7 | 290 | 91 | 43.9 | 25.1 | 36.7 | 2.8 | 23 | 26 | 27.7 |
| Senegal | 67 | 47.2 | 315 | 59 | 46.7 | 28.4 | 17 | 5.1 | 21 | 30 | 12.1 |
| Sierra Leone | 52.2 | 120.4 | 1360 | 60 | 76 | 27.7 | 37.9 | 4.8 | 58 | 30 | 52 |
| South Africa | 63.4 | 40.5 | 138 | 94 | 75.5 | 53.8 | 27.4 | 9.8 | 36 | 27 | 200 |
| Swaziland | | 60.7 | 389 | 88 | 76.1 | 38.4 | 25.5 | 6.6 | 31 | 29 | 299 |
| Togo | 60.5 | 78.4 | 368 | 29 | 57.2 | 28.1 | 27.5 | 4.9 | 17 | 29 | 68 |
| Uganda | 60.2 | 54.6 | 343 | 58 | 59.9 | 22.4 | 28.9 | 2.8 | 22 | 27 | 69.4 |
| Tanzania | 66.3 | 48.7 | 398 | 49 | 50.7 | 27.7 | 34.4 | 4.3 | 24 | 27 | 99.8 |
| Zambia | 62.3 | 64 | 224 | 64 | 55.5 | 27.8 | 40 | 4.2 | 28 | 27 | 126 |
| Zimbabwe | 61.7 | 70.7 | 443 | 80 | 75.7 | 38.2 | 26.8 | 4.6 | 24 | 28 | 188 |

*U5MR* Under-five mortality rate (number of deaths per 1000 live births)
*MMR* Maternal Mortality Ratio (number of deaths per 100 000 live births)
*HIVMR* HIV Mortality Rate (number of deaths per 100 000 population)
*LE* Life expectancy at birth (in years)
*BASP* Births Assisted by Skilled Personnel (%)
*ANC* Antenatal Care (% of women aged 15–45 who had 4 visits or more during pregnancy)
*Stunting* low weight-for-age
*DM* diabetes mellitus (%)
*BP* Blood Pressure (%)

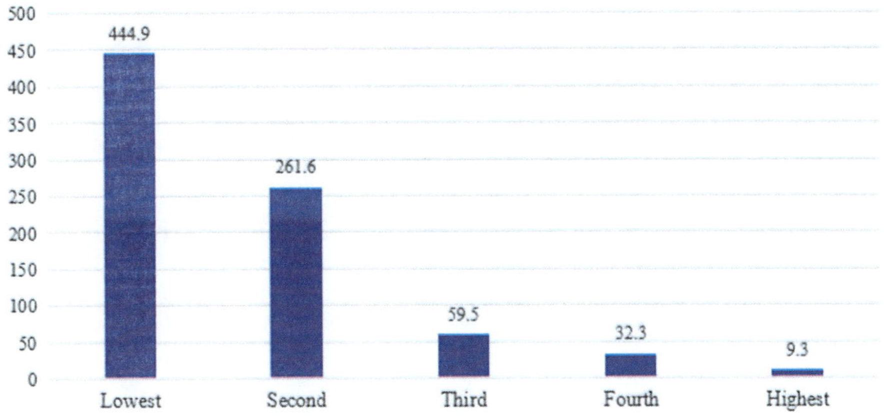


**Fig. 2.2** Maternal Mortality gradient worldwide by income *Source* PAHO [7]

**Table 2.3** The 2011 Rio Political Declaration: five Action areas on SDH

| | |
|---|---|
| 1 | Adopt better governance for health and development |
| 2 | Promote participation in policymaking and implementation |
| 3 | Further reorient the health sector towards promoting health and reducing health inequities |
| 4 | Strengthen global governance and collaboration |
| 5 | Monitor progress and increase accountability |

*Source* WHO Rio Political Declaration [18]

In 2011, the Rio Political Declaration on Social Determinants of health adopted by heads of government, ministers and government representatives, stressed that health equity should become part of a government's social and health agenda [18]. For pragmatic strategies in countries, five action areas on social determinants of health were proposed (Table 2.3).

In 2014, a technical report of the WHO Eastern Mediterranean region analysed health iniquities in selected countries of the region. Inequalities were described and analysed between and within selected countries according to many health indicators, including life expectancy, infant and under-five mortality, stunting, coverage of skilled birth attendance, antenatal visits and place of birth. An important finding was that socioeconomic factors together contributed to 60–75% in inequities in skilled birth attendance at delivery [1] (Fig. 2.3).

The World Health Organisation HQ and the six regions' offices are struggling to improve Health sector monitoring and health inequity analysis within countries. The WHO's Health Equity Monitor is an initiative that should improve understanding of action on SDH and health equity in every country and at the global level [5].

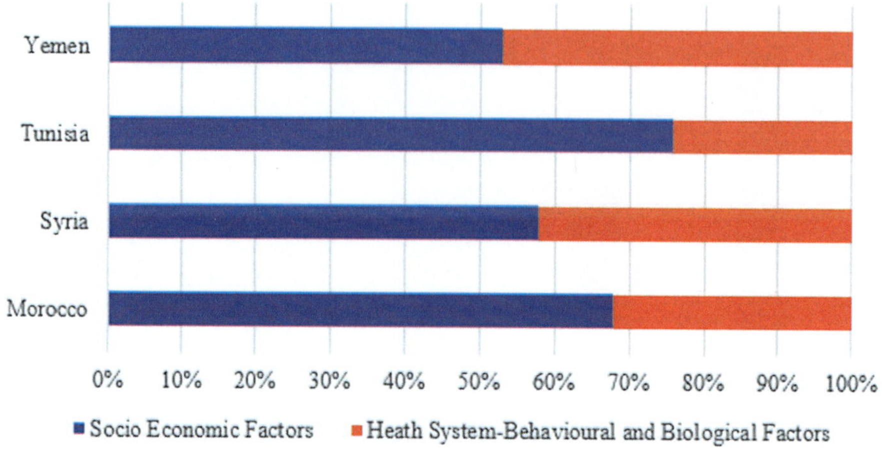


**Fig. 2.3** Contribution of socioeconomic factors in skilled birth attendance *Source* WHO-EMRO [1]

In order to foster pragmatic action on SDH by national governments, international organizations, and civil society and considering the needs of key indicator users, an interdisciplinary working group (WG) was established by WHO and its Canadian partners, the Public Health Agency of Canada (PHAC), and the Canadian Institutes of Health Research—Institute of Population and Public Health (CIHR–IPPH) in 2016. The working group proposed a core set of the 15–20 selected indicators [17].

Another illustration of growing interest in inequalities and disparities is provided by the 2010 human development report, introducing a new human development index (HDI) which captures the losses in human development due to inequality in health, education and income, namely: Inequality-adjusted HDI (IHDI) [10]. In 2017, the global loss in the three dimensions varied across countries, ranging from 3.6% in Japan to 45.3% in Comoros [9].

Recalling and stressing that in all societies, long-standing forms of inequality persist while gaps are opening in new aspects of life, the Human Development Report 2019 is expected to focus on understanding the dimensions of inequality most important to people's wellbeing, and what is behind them. The UNDP is aiming to produce a new kind of Human Development Report, going beyond the usual analysis of disparities due to income to deal with inequalities in other dimensions such as health, education, access to technologies and others. "It will use new data and methods to highlight how inequality affects people's lives in a way that measures based on averages cannot; and it will take a long-term view towards 2030 and the achievement of the Sustainable Development Goals and beyond" [11].

The Millennium Development Goals (MDGs) has significantly proved that reducing poverty and enhancing health and well-being of populations worldwide needs to go beyond average indicators to consider disaggregated data needed for equity analysis [14]. Building on that, the Sustainable Development Goals are aiming to "leave no one behind" [13].

### *2.2.2 Life Expectancy and Healthy Life Expectancy at Birth in the WHO African Region*

According to the WHO estimates in 2015, the average life expectancy at birth in the African Region was 60 years (61.8 for females and 58.3 for males), slowly increasing (57 years in 2010). However, the average hides large gaps between countries. Indeed, the difference is more than 24 years between the highest life expectancy at birth in Algeria (76.3 years) and the lowest life expectancy at birth in Sierra Leone (52.2 years) (Table 2.2). Significant differences can also be seen within each African country. Globally, the average life expectancy at birth in the African Region is much lower than in the other regions. People in the African region are expected to live in average 9 years less than people in the Eastern Mediterranean Region and about 17 years less than their counterparts in Europe, Western Pacific and the Americas. Moreover, the number of years an African person is expected to live in a healthy state (healthy life expectancy at birth) decreases by nearly 15% compared with life expectancy in birth. Again, healthy life expectancy at birth shows that, in average, the African region has the lowest level compared to the other regions with substantial differences between and within African countries (Fig. 2.4).

Life expectancy is one of the three Human Development components and consequently, a large number of African countries are experiencing a low human development partly due to low life expectancy at birth (Table 2.4). As stressed in the introduction section, more than 30 African countries are in the low level of human development representing 82% of all the countries with low Human Development Index. Taking into account the effect of inequalities on the Human Development

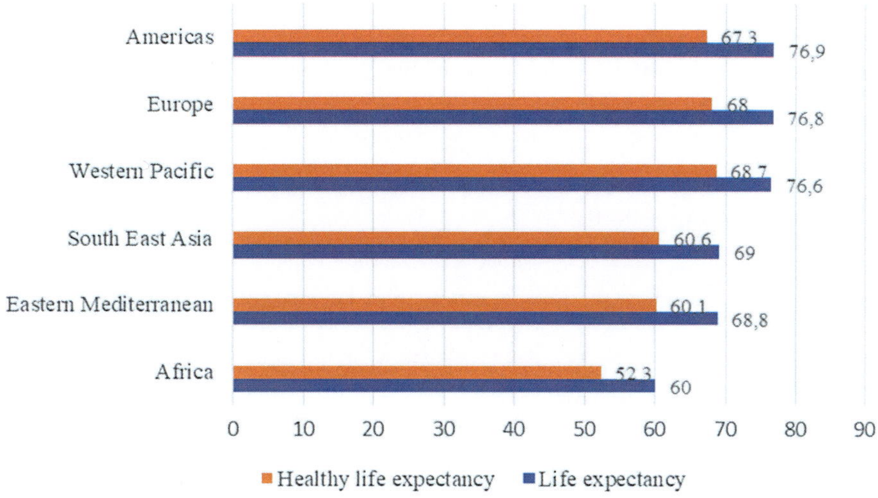


**Fig. 2.4** Life expectancy and healthy life expectancy in WHO regions, 2015 *Source* WHO Regional Office Africa Atlas [19]

Index and considering the Inequality-adjusted Human Development (IHDI) in the African region, nearly 90% of African countries loose more than 25% of their HDI. For instance, being already at the tail of countries in term of HDI, Chad looses 42.4% in life expectancy and 38.3% of its HDI due to inequality, dropping from 0.404 (HDI) to 0.249 (IHDI). Meanwhile, life expectancy at birth is only one among a multitude of health indicators all showing inadmissible levels of inequalities and disparities between and within African countries.

### *2.2.3 Early Childhood Mortality Rates in the WHO African Region*

#### 2.2.3.1 Differences Between WHO Regions

Neonatal mortality rate, infant mortality rate and under-five mortality rate in Africa are much higher than in other WHO regions. Many reasons may explain these differences, including the high burden of communicable diseases, the low universal health coverage and the accessibility to health care in general. Figure 2.5 below shows that the probability for a child to die before his/her fifth birthday is much higher in the WHO African region than in any other WHO region.

#### 2.2.3.2 Differences Between Countries of the WHO African Region

Neonatal mortality, infant mortality and under-five mortality are important indicators reflecting the real level of development in countries worldwide. Reducing infant mortality rate by two-third between 1990 and 2015 was one of the eight Millennium Development Goals (MDGs) while Sustainable Development Goals (SDGs) aim to

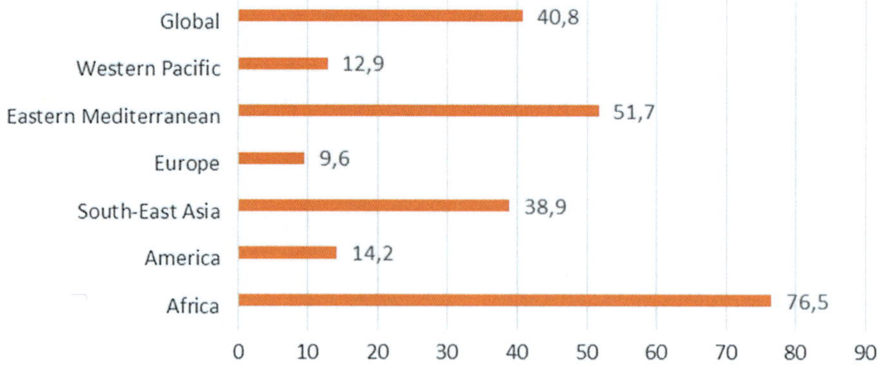


**Fig. 2.5** Under-five mortality rate in WHO regions, 2016

**Table 2.4** Human Development and Inequality-adjusted Human Development in the WHO African region

| Country | HD level | HDI | IHDI | Overallloss (%) | Loss in life expectancy |
|---|---|---|---|---|---|
| High HD | | | | | |
| Seychelles | High HD | 0.797 | | | 7.7 |
| Mauritus | High HD | 0.790 | 0.683 | 13.5 | 8.9 |
| Algeria | High HD | 0.754 | 0.598 | 20.7 | 15.1 |
| Bostwana | High HD | 0.717 | | | |
| Gabon | High HD | 0.702 | 0.545 | 22.3 | 23.1 |
| Medium HD | | | | | |
| South Africa | Medium HD | 0.699 | 0.467 | 33.2 | |
| Capo Verde | Medium HD | 0.654 | | | |
| Namibia | Medium HD | 0.647 | 0.422 | 34.8 | 20.2 |
| Congo | Medium HD | 0.606 | 0.469 | 22.6 | 25.1 |
| Ghana | Medium HD | 0.592 | 0.420 | 28.9 | 23.2 |
| Kenya | Medium HD | 0.590 | 0.434 | 26.4 | 22.8 |
| Sao Tome | Medium HD | 0.589 | 0.473 | 19.8 | 25.9 |
| Zambia | Medium HD | 0.588 | 0.388 | 34.1 | 28.8 |
| Angola | Medium HD | 0.581 | 0.3893 | 32.4 | 33.8 |
| Cameroon | Medium HD | 0.556 | 0.366 | 36.2 | 33.7 |
| Low HD | | | | | |
| Tanzania | Low HD | 0.538 | 0.404 | 24.8 | 24.9 |
| Nigeria | Low HD | 0.532 | 0.347 | 34.7 | |
| Zimbabwe | Low HD | 0.535 | | | 23.6 |
| Nigeria | Low HD | 0.532 | 0.347 | 34.7 | 37.4 |
| Rwanda | Low HD | 0.524 | 0.367 | 30 | 23.8 |
| Lesotho | Low HD | 0.520 | 0.359 | 31 | 28.5 |
| Mauritania | Low HD | 0.520 | 0.348 | 33 | 32.6 |
| Madagascar | Low HD | 0.519 | 0.385 | 25.9 | 21.3 |
| Uganda | Low HD | 0.516 | 0.37 | 28.3 | 32.5 |
| Senegal | Low HD | 0.505 | 0.34 | 32.6 | 21.1 |
| Togo | Low HD | 0.503 | 0.344 | 31.7 | 30.5 |
| Cote Ivoire | Low HD | 0.492 | 0.311 | 36.9 | 34.2 |
| Malawi | Low HD | 0.477 | 0.332 | 30.4 | 30.2 |
| Ethiopia | Low HD | 0.463 | 0.331 | 28.4 | 24.9 |
| Gambia | Low HD | 0.460 | 0.289 | 37.2 | 28.5 |
| Guinea | Low HD | 0.459 | 0.306 | 33.4 | 31.2 |
| C Africa | Low HD | 0.367 | 0.21 | 42.1 | 41.7 |
| Niger | Low HD | 0.354 | 0.250 | 29.3 | 34.9 |
| Benin | Low HD | 0.515 | 0.3255 | 36.6 | 35 |
| Comoros | Low HD | 0.503 | 0.275 | 45.3 | 26.9 |
| Mali | Low HD | 0.427 | 0.282 | 34 | 36.8 |
| Chad | Low HD | 0.404 | 0.249 | 38.3 | 42.4 |

*Source* UNDP Human Development Index [9]

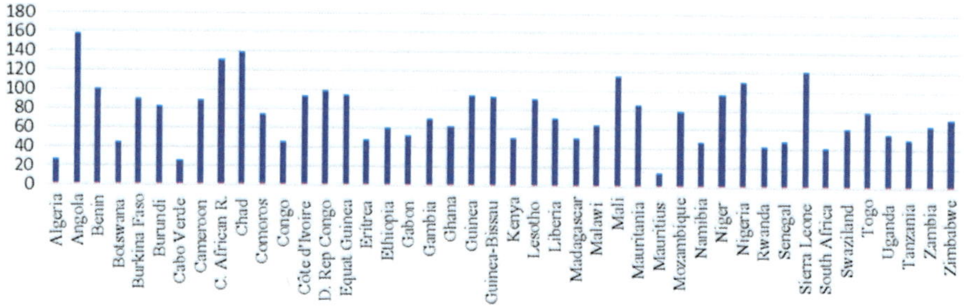


**Fig. 2.6** Under-five mortality rate in the WHO African countries, 2016

reduce neonatal mortality rate (NNR) to 12 deaths per 1000 live births and under-five mortality rate (U5MR) to 25 deaths per 1000 live births by 2030. However, these SDGs seem very unlikely to be reached by a large number of African countries. Huge differences are seen in neonatal, infant, child and under-five mortality between African countries. The neonatal mortality rate was nearly 6 times higher in Angola (48.7 deaths per 1000 live births) compared with Mauritius (8.4 deaths per 1000 live births) while under-five mortality rate ranged from 13.5 and 156.9 deaths per 1000 live births in these two countries respectively, yielding a ratio of nearly 12. As illustrated by Fig. 2.6, a large dispersion is seen in under-five mortality rate between the 47 countries of the WHO African region.

#### 2.2.3.3 Differences Within Countries of the WHO African Region

Although at different levels, economic status, education and residence (rural-urban) are social determinants clearly affecting U5MR in countries of the WHO region (Table 2.5).

In the 23 countries for which disaggregated data is available, children living in the poorest households ($Q_1$) are much exposed to death before their fifth birthday than their counterparts living in the richest households ($Q_5$). The ratio $Q_1/Q_5$ is greater than 2 in 9 countries and ranges from 1.15 in Chad to 2.7 in Togo. Figure 2.7 illustrates clearly the gradient in the three countries independently of the level of under-five mortality rate average.

As shown in Fig. 2.8, the gradient induced by education seems sharper in WHO region countries. In Ethiopia and Uganda, children born from mothers without education are more than three times likely to die before their fifth birthday than their counterparts born from mothers with secondary or higher level of education. This comparison shows how action on a social determinant of health like education can reduce the early childhood mortality.

Although with less variation than economic status and education level, living in rural or urban areas also affects the under-five mortality rate in African countries. Figure 2.9 shows that while only two countries have U5MR in urban zones greater

**Table 2.5** Under-five mortality rate by country, economic status, education level and residence

| Country | Economic status | | | | | Education level | | | Residence | | National |
|---|---|---|---|---|---|---|---|---|---|---|---|
| | Q1 | Q2 | Q3 | Q4 | Q5 | None | Primary | Secondary or higher | Rural | Urban | Average |
| Benin DHS 2017–2018 | 108 | 124 | 106 | 103 | 60 | 109 | 94 | 77 | 106 | 81 | 96 |
| Cameroon DHS 2011 | 184 | 143 | 120 | 87 | 72 | 175 | 126 | 76 | 153 | 93 | 128 |
| Chad DHS 2014 | 159 | 123 | 142 | 133 | 138 | 139 | 179 | 131 | 149 | 141 | 148 |
| Ethiopia DHS 2011 | 136 | 120 | 97 | 99 | 84 | 119 | 87 | 36 | 114 | 82 | 82 |
| Gambia DHS 2013 | 69 | 67 | 70 | 59 | 34 | 68 | 66 | 37 | 68 | 53 | 62 |
| Ghana DHS 2014 | 91 | 73 | 61 | 55 | 64 | 92 | 73 | 54 | 74 | 64 | 70 |
| Guinea DHS 2012 | 166 | 146 | 139 | 116 | 67 | 138 | 127 | 67 | 147 | 88 | 123 |
| Kenya DHS 2014 | 56 | 63 | 52 | 57 | 47 | 51 | 59 | 50 | 55 | 56 | 56 |
| Liberia DHS 2013 | 129 | 110 | 101 | 111 | 99 | 120 | 108 | 96 | 118 | 104 | 113 |
| Mali DHS 2012 | 112 | 117 | 129 | 90 | 61 | 106 | 120 | 60 | 113 | 64 | 104 |
| Mozambique DHS 2011 | 130 | 105 | 113 | 95 | 90 | 108 | 113 | 77 | 111 | 100 | 108 |
| Namibia DHS 2013 | 67 | 68 | 65 | 56 | 30 | 78 | 89 | 54 | 64 | 54 | 59 |
| Niger DHS 2012 | 143 | 167 | 167 | 162 | 112 | 157 | 121 | 90 | 162 | 82 | 153 |
| Nigeria DHS 2013 | 187 | 187 | 126 | 100 | 72 | 178 | 127 | 85 | 166 | 39 | 144 |
| Rwanda DHS 2014 | 82 | 76 | 66 | 56 | 38 | 87 | 63 | 37 | 68 | 50 | 67 |
| Senegal DHS 2017–18 | 76 | 65 | 67 | 49 | 30 | 71 | 38 | 34 | 63 | 43 | 60 |
| Sierra Leone DHS 2013 | 185 | 177 | 188 | 168 | 143 | 180 | 169 | 146 | 181 | 157 | 175 |
| South Africa DHS 2016 | 37 | 43 | 21 | 17 | 17 | 27 | 62 | 28 | 29 | 28 | 29 |
| Togo DHS 2013 | 119 | 108 | 97 | 78 | 44 | 107 | 89 | 62 | 105 | 68 | 94 |
| Uganda DHS 2016 | 88 | 79 | 73 | 69 | 53 | 105 | 76 | 29 | 68 | 52 | 64 |
| Tanzania DHS 2015 | 77 | 86 | 73 | 77 | 73 | 82 | 78 | 60 | 74 | 86 | 78 |
| Zambia DHS 2013 | 99 | 83 | 78 | 72 | 58 | 108 | 81 | 64 | 84 | 72 | 81 |
| Zimbabwe DHS 2015 | 102 | 90 | 96 | 68 | 52 | 108 | 106 | 69 | 92 | 60 | 82 |

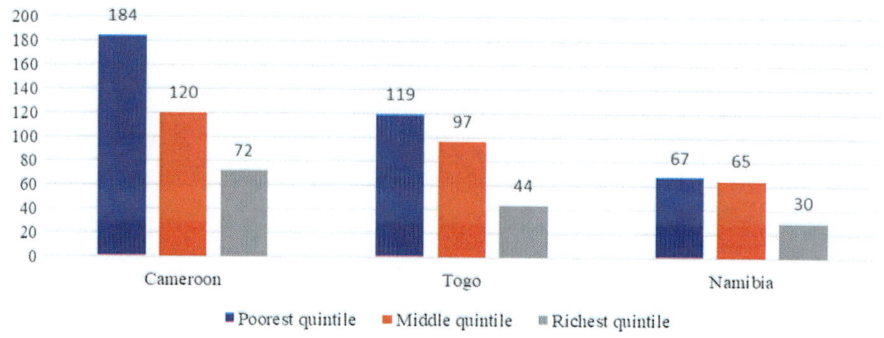


**Fig. 2.7** Gradient induced by economic status on under-five mortality rate, 2015

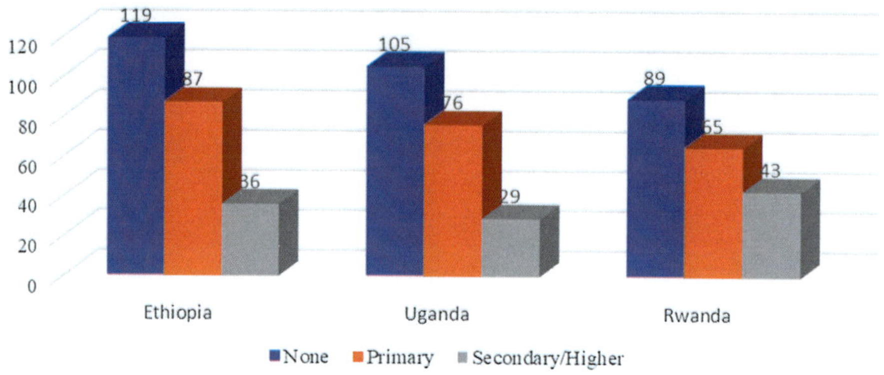


**Fig. 2.8** Gradient induced by education on under-five mortality rate, 2015

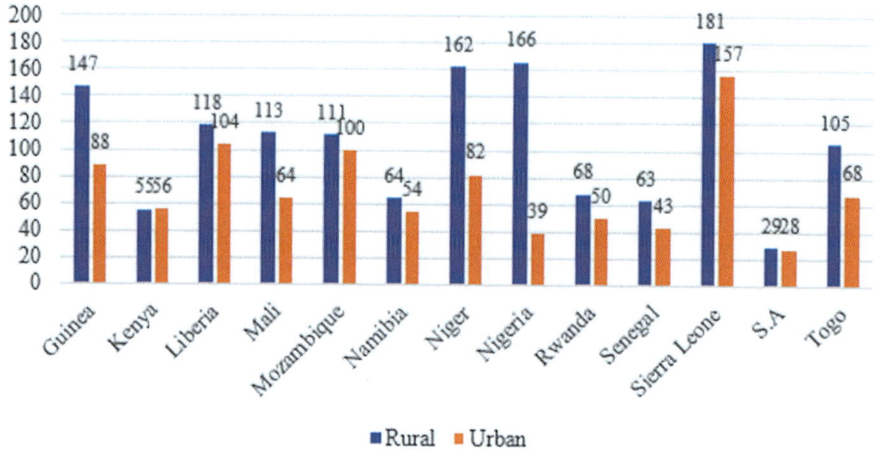


**Fig. 2.9** U5MR by residence in different countries of the WHO African region

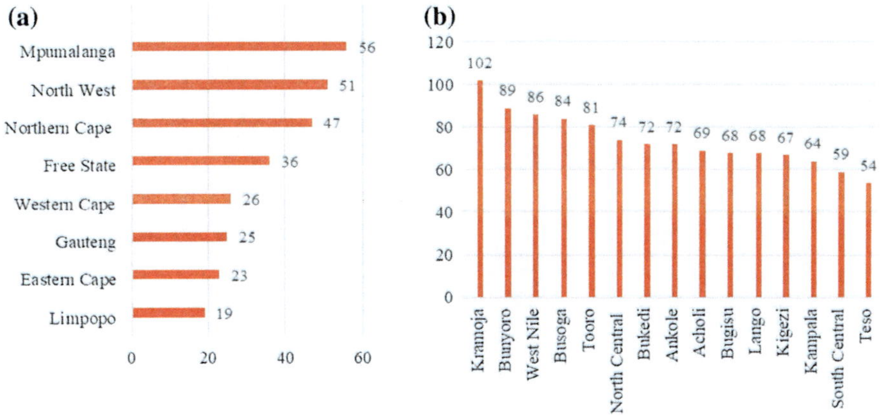


**Fig. 2.10** **a** U5MR by province in South Africa, **b** U5MR by region in Uganda

**Table 2.6** Under-five mortality rate by regions in WHO African countries

| Country | Geographic disparity | | | | | Gap | |
|---|---|---|---|---|---|---|---|
| | Region1 | Region2 | Region3 | Region4 | Region5 | Difference | Ratio |
| Benin DHS 2017–2018 | 64 | 87 | 98 | 104 | 129 | 65 | 2 |
| Cameroon DHS 2011 | 68 | 100 | 121 | 168 | 191 | 128 | 2.8 |
| Chad DHS 2014 | 67 | 99 | 145 | 203 | 230 | 163 | 3.4 |
| Ethiopia DHS 2011 | 39 | 59 | 88 | 94 | 125 | 86 | 3.2 |
| Gambia DHS 2013 | 38 | 52 | 63 | 70 | 92 | 54 | 2.4 |
| Ghana DHS 2014 | 47 | 61 | 80 | 92 | 111 | 64 | 2.4 |
| Guinea DHS 2012 | 70 | 104 | 129 | 163 | 194 | 124 | 2.8 |
| Kenya DHS 2014 | 42 | 57 | 64 | 72 | 82 | 40 | 2 |
| Lesotho DHS 2014 | 59 | 76 | 95 | 101 | 111 | 52 | 1.9 |
| Mali DHS 2012 | 59 | 96 | 111 | 116 | 121 | 62 | 2 |
| Namibia DHS 2013 | 38 | 45 | 68 | 79 | 97 | 59 | 2.5 |
| Niger DHS 2012 | 51 | 80 | 140 | 160 | 210 | 159 | 4.1 |
| Nigeria DHS 2013 | 90 | 100 | 131 | 160 | 185 | 95 | 2 |
| Rwanda DHS 2014 | 42 | 60 | 62 | 66 | 86 | 44 | 2 |
| Senegal DHS 2017–18 | 34 | 55 | 74 | 80 | 89 | 55 | 2.6 |
| South Africa DHS 2016 | 17 | 25 | 36 | 47 | 56 | 39 | 3.3 |
| Togo DHS 2013 | 63 | 79 | 96 | 113 | 130 | 67 | 2.1 |
| Uganda DHS 2016 | 59 | 72 | 84 | 89 | 102 | 43 | 1.7 |
| Tanzania DHS 2015 | 56 | 65 | 79 | 88 | 95 | 39 | 1.7 |
| Zambia DHS 2013 | 63 | 73 | 88 | 98 | 115 | 52 | 1.8 |
| Zimbabwe DHS 2015 | 50 | 67 | 80 | 101 | 112 | 62 | 2.2 |

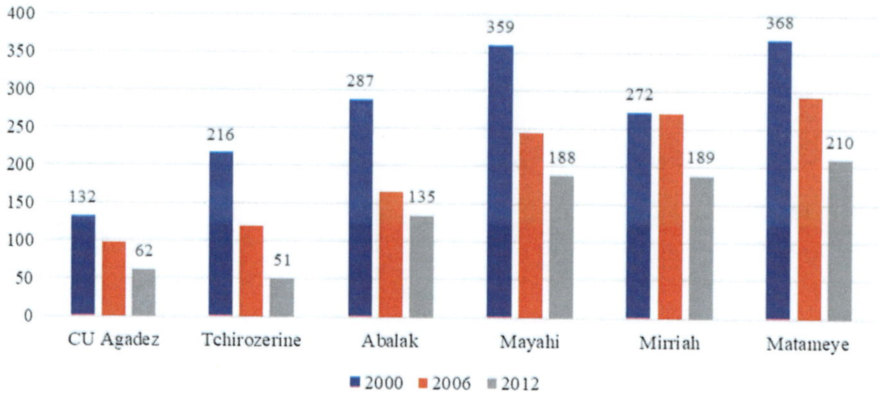


**Fig. 2.11** Evolution with time of U5MR by department in Niger

than in urban areas, two-thirds of ratios (rural/urban) fall between 1 and 1.5 with Nigeria having a ratio of 4.25 meaning that children in rural areas are 4.25 times more exposed to death before age 5 than children living in urban areas.

Like in other WHO regions [2, 3, 6], geographic situation in terms of regions, governorates, departments or cities of WHO African countries exhibits large disparities, showing that in Ethiopia, Chad, South Africa and Niger, children living in the region with the highest U5MR are 3.2, 3.3, 3.4 and 4.1 respectively, more likely to die before age 5 than their counterparts living in the region with the lowest level of U5MR (Fig. 2.10). More generally, Table 2.6 shows that all ratios are greater than 1.7.

Despite a noticeable decrease in the average under-five mortality rate during the last decades in all African countries, inequalities between regions, department, provinces or cities of the same country persist. In average, the under-five mortality decreased in Niger between 2000 and 2012. However, the ratio of U5MR between the departments of Matameye and Tchirozerine increased from 1.7 (368/216) to 4.1 (210/51) during the same period (Fig. 2.11).

## 2.3 Conclusion

The 47 countries of the WHO African region are struggling to reduce mortality and improve well-being of their populations. Most of them are afflicted by the burden of communicable disease like HIV/AIDS, tuberculosis, malaria, neglected diseases and others. Although at a lower level, compared with the other WHO regions, many African countries are now also suffering from non communicable diseases like cardiovascular diseases, cancer and diabetes. Beside undernutrition, many African countries are exposed to risk factors like high blood pressure, overweight/obesity, smoking and alcohol. Maternal mortality and infant mortality remain very high in the WHO African region compared to other WHO regions. Moreover, most of health indicators are showing huge gaps between different categories of the population and large territorial disparities. In this chapter, we showed that avoidable health inequalities can and must be reduced by efficiently acting on social determinants of health like economic status, education level, residence (urban-rural) and territorial disparities between regions, provinces, departments or cities. Health decision makers in African countries are called to act urgently to improve health conditions of the whole population by leaving no one behind as stipulated by the sustainable development goals.

## References

1. Baschieri A (2014) Health inequities in the eastern mediterranean region selected country case studies. In: EMRO technical publications series 40. World Health Organization, p 68
2. Boutayeb A, Boutayeb W, Lamlili ENM (2018) A mini review of health inequity, territorial disparities and socio-economic inequalities in morocco. Int J Manag Appl Sci 4(7):23–29
3. Boutayeb A, Lamlili ENM, Boutayeb W (2018) Health inequity and territorial disparity in under-five mortality between and within who-emr countries. Int J Manag Appl Sci 4(8):71–79
4. Braveman P (2006) Health disparities and health equity: concepts and measurement. Annu Rev Public Health 27:167–194
5. Hosseinpoor AR, Bergen N, Schlotheuber A, Victora C, Boerma T, Barros AJ (2016) Data resource profile: who health equity monitor (hem). Int J Epidemiol 45(5):1404–1405e
6. Omer AS, Bezruchka S, Longhi D, Kelly Z, Brown M, Hagopian A (2014) The effects of household assets inequality and conflict on population health in sudan. Afr Popul Stud 28(3):1216–1232
7. Pan American Health Organisation (2019) Socioeconomic inequalities in health. https://www.paho.org/salud-en-las-americas-2017/?tag=health-equity. Accessed 18 Feb 2019
8. The World Bank Group (2019) The world bank available from. https://data.worldbank.org/indicator/SP.DYN.LE00.IN?locations=ZG. Accessed 15 Feb 2019
9. UNDP (2017) Inequality-adjusted human development index (IHDI). http://hdr.undp.org/en/content/inequality-adjusted-human-development-index-ihdi. Accessed 18 Mar 2018
10. UNDP (2018) Human development indices and indicators 2018 statistical update. http://hdr.undp.org/sites/default/files/2018_human_development_statistical_update.pdf. Accessed 13 Apr 2019
11. UNDP (2019) Human development report 2019 focusing on inequality. http://hdr.undp.org/en/towards-hdr-2019. Accessed 18 March 2018
12. UNICEF (2019) Multiple indicator cluster surveys (mics). http://mics.unicef.org/. Accessed 18 Feb 2019
13. United Nations (2015) Transforming our world: the 2030 agenda for sustainable development. Resolution adopted by the General Assembly
14. United Nations Statistics Division (2006) Millennium development goal indicators database. http://millenniumindicators.un.org/unsd/mi/mi_goals.asp. Accessed 18 March 2018
15. USAID (2019) Demographic health surveys (dhs). https://dhsprogram.com/. Accessed 18 Feb 2019
16. WHO Commission on Social Determinants of Health and World Health Organization (2008) Closing the gap in a generation: health equity through action on the social determinants of health: Commission on Social Determinants of Health final report. World Health Organization
17. Working Group for Monitoring Action on the Social Determinants of Health (2018) Towards a global monitoring system for implementing the rio political declaration on social determinants

of health: developing a core set of indicators for government action on the social determinants of health to improve health equity. Int J Equity Health 17:1–27
18. World Health Organization and others (2011) Rio political declaration on social determinants of health. In: World conference on social determinants of health. Rio de Janeiro, pp 19–21
19. World Health Organization and others (2018) Atlas of african health statistics 2018: Universal health coverage and the sustainable development goals in the who african region

# Chapter 3
# Under-Five Mortality Rate in Sudan: Statistical Analysis of Social Determinants of Health and Health Equity

**Mohammed Abdu, Mohamed E. N. Lamlili, Nabil Azouagh and Ahmed Ouazza**

**Abstract** The focus on health equity has grown in importance, leading to a widespread recognition that action on Social Determinants of Health is crucial for reducing inequalities in health. Sudan was among the first countries which adopted a roadmap for Health in All Policies. However, efficient actions to reduce health inequalities need to be enhanced. This paper illustrates the need to act on Social Determinants of Health to reduce health inequalities in Sudan. Descriptive statistics was used to get summarised information. Statistical significance of differences was tested by Pearson's chi-squared. For the interaction between the 13 variables at the same time, Principal Components Analysis was carried out. As an attempt to explain Under-Five Mortality Rate (U5MR) by the remaining variables Multiple Regression was applied. Huge gaps were found between the 18 states. Contraception varied from 26.5% in Khartoum to 2.9% in Central Darfur; home delivery increased from 27.1% in Northern to 91.4% in West Kordofan and early childbearing was higher in Blue Nile (23.4%) than in Northern (8.6%). Under-five mortality rate is nearly four times higher in East Darfur (112) than in Northern (30). A ratio greater than two was indicated for mother education and income. A lower gap was seen for milieu and gender. The difference was statistically significant for education (p-value $<0.005$), income (p-value $<0.001$) and states (p-value $<0.0001$). The U5MR in Sudan is influenced

M. Abdu
Department of Health Information & Research Evidence, Federal Ministry of Health, Khartoum, Sudan
e-mail: moh85150@gmail.com

M. E. N. Lamlili (✉) · N. Azouagh · A. Ouazza
Laboratory of Stochastic and Deterministic Modelling (LaSDM), Faculty of Sciences, University Mohamed Ier, Oujda, Morocco
e-mail: mohamed.lamlili@gmail.com

N. Azouagh
e-mail: azouaghnabil@gmail.com

A. Ouazza
e-mail: ouazzaahmed@gmail.com



A. Boutayeb (ed.), *Disease Prevention and Health Promotion in Developing Countries*,
https://doi.org/10.1007/978-3-030-34702-4_3

by social determinants of health like milieu, gender, education, income and territoriality. A large gap was found between states in term of U5MR. Serious efforts must be devoted to reducing heath inequalities by acting on social determinants of health in Sudan. Furthermore, in order to control the U5MR in Sudan we need to act simultaneously on Contraception, use of improved water, Literacy young women and stunted.

## 3.1 Background

During the last two decades, the focus on health equity has grown in importance, leading to a widespread recognition that action on social determinants of health (SDH) is crucial for reducing and reversing the growing unfair and remediable inequalities in health [2]. In 2008, the World Health Organisation Commission on SDH released its report "Closing the gap in a generation: health equity through action on the social determinants of health", stressing that "reducing health inequities is an ethical imperative and that social injustice is killing people on grand scale" [5]. In 2011, the Rio Political Declaration on Social Determinants of Health indicated five key points to reduce health inequalities: (1) better governance, (2) participation, (3) reorienting the health sector, (4) global governance and (5) progress monitoring [7]. In 2016, the technical meeting on measuring and monitoring action on the social determinants of health proposed a framework and a basket of core indicators [6]. Worldwide and independently of the economic level, all governments are called to act on SDH to reduce avoidable inequalities in health and to use the framework for country action to promote Health in All Policies (HiAP) [8]. Sudan is one of the first countries which adopted a roadmap for Health in All Policies [1]. However, real and efficient actions to reduce health inequalities remain insufficient and need to be enhanced.

In 2014, Omer et al. studied the effect of household assets inequality and conflict on population health in Sudan. They considered life expectancy, infant mortality, stunting, adequacy of food consumption, teenage birth rates and vaccination coverage for young children and found that outcomes were significantly worse in the states with more unequal asset distribution and worse outcomes was also predicted by conflict status [3].

The main objective of this paper is to show how under-five mortality in Sudan is related to social determinants of health like territorial context (between states), income, education and milieu (rural-urban). Given the importance of monitoring, it is useful to analyse data provided by the Multiple Indicator Cluster Survey (MICS5) carried out by UNICEF in 2014 [4] and to make a starting point for comparison with MICS6 planned for 2019 especially in terms of implementing HiAP to reduce health inequalities between and within the 18 states of Sudan.

## 3.2 Methods

First of all, descriptive statistics are used to get summarised information on 13 variables observed on 18 states as given by the Multiple Indicator Cluster Survey (MICS5) carried out by UNICEF in 2014. Secondly, Pearson's chi-squared was used to test statistical significance of differences according to milieu (rural-urban), education, income and territoriality (between states). Thirdly, in order to get a summary of information on the interaction between all variables (indicators) at the same time, Principal Components Analysis (PCA) was used to select the first and second factors (F1 and F2). The corresponding eigenvalues give the percentages of information summarised by these factors respectively (F1: 69% and F2: 8%). Variables are then projected on the circle of correlation and countries on the first plan (F1 $\times$ F2). The more the variables are near the circle, the better will be the interpretation. In the meantime, a projection of states on the first plan should lead to a classification according to the scores of each state with regard to the variables under consideration. Additional information may be obtained by the third and fourth axis, but the interpretation is then conditional to what was given by the precedent factors. Fourth, we used a linear multiple regression to see how U5MR may be explained by the other 12 variables. Due to the fact that all variables are correlated to each other we selected the most correlated one which is the variable of contraception use. As a result 64.9% of the variability of the U5MR is explained by the variability of the contraception use. We also tried a multiple regression on the principal components of the 12 variables without improving the quality of adjustment. Finally, we turned to a an exponential model, where we consider many regression of the logarithm of U5MR ($ln(U5MR)$) on crossed variables resulting from the 12 remaining ones, taking in consideration the principle of parsimony, this technique has improved the quality of adjustment where we succeed to explain almost 80% of U5MR by using a crossed variable: Contraception use * use of improved water * literacy young women * stunted.

## 3.3 Results and Discussion

In Sudan, inequalities in health are seen directly in access to health services and health care like vaccination, healthy nutrition, contraception, antenatal visits, delivery assistance and postnatal care. Consequently, gaps are found in impacts like life expectancy and mortality. However, health inequalities are also linked to variables like education, early childbearing, access to drinking water and sanitation.

Territorial disparity is one of the main problems challenging health authorities in Sudan. Indeed, huge gaps and inacceptable health inequalities are found between the 18 states. For instance, contraceptive use (any method) is relatively low in all states but it varies from 26.5% in Khartoum to 2.9% in Central Darfur; home delivery increases from 27.1% in Northern to 91.4% in West Kordofan and early childbearing

(a) (b)

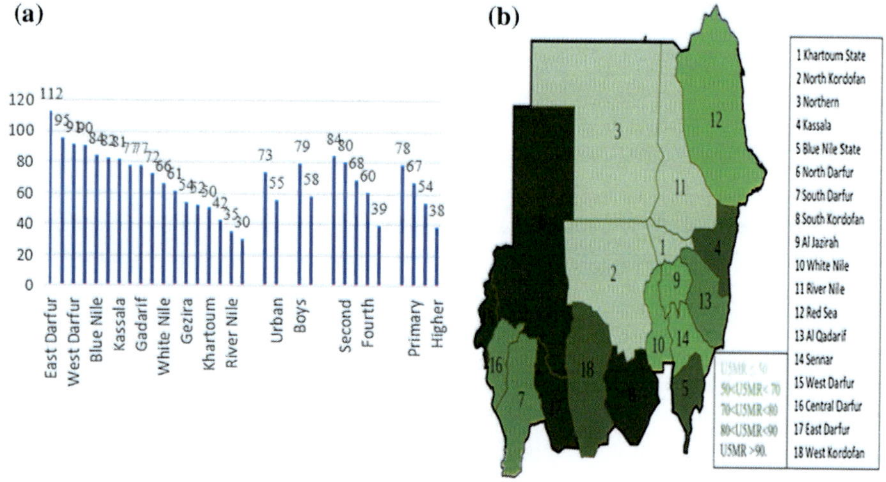


**Fig. 3.1** **a** U5MR by SDH (rounded data worked out from MICS 2014 Sudan with kind permission of UNICEF), **b** U5MR illustrated by a gradient colour covering the 18 states of Sudan

(girls between 15 and 18 years of age) is nearly three times higher in Blue Nile (23.4%) than in Northern (8.6%).

As illustrated by Fig. 3.1a, under-five mortality rate shows a noticeable difference by milieu (rural-urban); gender (boys-girls); education level; income (approximated by household assets) and territorially by states. Indeed, children are nearly four times more likely to die before their fifth birthday in East Darfur (112 deaths per 1000 live births) than in Northern (30 deaths per 1000 live births). A ratio greater than two is also indicated when comparing U5MR according to the level of mother education (no education: 78 vs higher: 38) and income (poorest quintile: 84 vs richest quintile: 39). Finally, a relatively lower gap is seen between rural children (73) and their urban counterparts (55) and between boys (79) and girls (58). More importantly, the Pearson's chi-squared test shows that the difference is statistically significant for education (p-value $<0.005$), income (p-value $<0.001$) and states (p-value $<0.0001$). Figure 3.1b shows the map of Sudan with a gradient colour classifying the 18 states in five groups according to the level of U5MR in each state. A first group including four states having an U5MR less or equal than 50; a second group comprising four states with U5MR greater than 50 and less than 70; a third group of three states having U5MR between 70 and 80; a fourth group of three states with U5MR greater than 80 and less than 90 and finally a fifth group of four states with U5MR greater or equal than 90.

In order to illustrate the gaps between the whole set of the 18 states, we carried out Principal Component Analysis (PCA) as a multivariate data analysis using the 18 states for individuals and 13 variables (U5MR, stunting, under-weight, vaccination, contraceptive use, early child bearing, antenatal access, home delivery, postnatal access, early education, literacy of young women, use of improved drinking water, use of improved sanitation). Table 3.2 shows values of the 13 variables as collected by UNICEF through the Multiple Indicator Cluster Survey (MICS) carried out in 2014 in the 18 states of Sudan [3].

The PCA allows to deal with all the 13 variables simultaneously. It starts giving the correlation between all the variables as indicated in Table 3.1. In particular, under-five mortality rate is seen to have a correlation greater than 0.5 or less than −0.5 with 10 out of 12 variables and it is especially negatively highly correlated ($r < -0.7$) with four variables (contraception use, postnatal new born, young women literacy and sanitation) and positively highly correlated with home delivery ($r = 0.769$). Table 3.1 also shows the correlation of each variable with the other 12 variables.

Then projecting variables on the circle of correlation (Fig. 3.2a) and states on the first plan (axis F1 × axis F2) (Fig. 3.2b) allows interesting illustration (1) explicitly between variables, (2) explicitly between states and (3) implicitly between variables and states. The quality of representation depends on the percentage of information explained by each axis and is mathematically given by eigenvalues. In our case, the first plan summarises nearly 77% of information (first axis F1: 68.55% and second axis F2: 8.21%). Figure 3.2 shows a net opposition between a set of five variables well represented on the left-hand side and another set of eight variables also well represented on the right-hand side. Combining the graphic illustration with data in Table 3.1, we can see, for example that U5MR is positively correlated with stunting, under-weight, home delivery and early childbearing and negatively correlated with the remaining eight variables. This classification indicates obviously, that a strategy to reduce U5MR should aim to decrease stunting, under-weight, home delivery and early childbearing and/or to enhance access to vaccination, antenatal visits, postnatal care, contraception, early education, literacy of young women, improved drinking water and sanitation. Now, coming to the sketch of states on the first (horizontal) axis provided by PCA, we see again a display of the 18 states, with three states (Northern, Khartoum and River Nile) isolated on the right-hand side opposed to a set of nine states on the left-hand side while the six remaining states are projected between the two previous sets. Again, combining the graphic illustration with data in Table 3.2, we can see that U5MR has a value less than 50 in Khartoum (49.8), River Nile (35.1) and Northern (30) whereas its value is greater than 77 in Central Darfur (77.4), West Kordofan (82), North Darfur (90.3) and East Darfur (111.7) (the fourth states completely on the left-hand side of axis 1). Similar comparisons can be made for stunting, under-weight, home delivery and early childbearing as well as for the 13 remaining variables. (Data extracted with kind permission of UNICEF from MICS 2014 Sudan, Final Report). U5MR is expressed in deaths per 1000 live births while all the other variables are expressed as %.

Additional information can be obtained by the second axis F2 but the interpretation is then conditional to the information provided by the first factor F1. For instance, we see that Khartoum and Northern have nearly the same projection on the horizontal axis F1 but they appear opposed on the vertical axis F2 mainly due to the opposition of the two variables: use of improved water (Khartoum 86.9% vs Northern 93.8%) and antenatal visits (at least 4 visits) (Khartoum 81.9% vs Northern 66.5%). A similar opposition is seen on the left-hand side between East Darfur (antenatal visits 46.8%

**Table 3.1** Correlation between the 13 variables considered in PCA

| | U5MR | Stunted | Underweight | Vaccination measles | Contraception use | Early childbearing | Antenatal visits | Home delivery | Postnatal new born | Early education | Literacy young women | Use of improved water | Improved sanitation |
|---|---|---|---|---|---|---|---|---|---|---|---|---|---|
| U5MR | 1 | 0.635 | 0.615 | −0.521 | −0.804 | 0.398 | −0.433 | 0.769 | −0.746 | −0.624 | −0.753 | −0.517 | −0.741 |
| Stunted | | 1 | 0.874 | −0.444 | −0.771 | 0.641 | −0.615 | 0.715 | −0.799 | −0.768 | −0.747 | −0.542 | −0.723 |
| Underweight | | | 1 | −0.472 | −0.703 | 0.407 | −0.661 | 0.69 | −0.753 | −0.709 | −0.707 | −0.397 | −0.747 |
| Vaccination measles | | | | 1 | 0.643 | −0.342 | 0.406 | −0.596 | 0.555 | 0.478 | 0.475 | 0.506 | 0.57 |
| Contraception use | | | | | 1 | −0469 | 0.689 | −0.889 | 0.914 | 0.831 | 0.848 | 0.486 | 0.833 |
| Early childbearing | | | | | | 1 | −0.299 | 0.514 | −0.453 | −0.609 | −0.545 | −0.408 | −0.441 |
| Antenatal visits | | | | | | | 1 | −0.708 | 0.787 | 0.728 | 0.644 | 0.284 | 0.699 |
| Home delivery | | | | | | | | 1 | −0.94 | −0.908 | −0.921 | −0.392 | −0.938 |
| Postnatal new born | | | | | | | | | 1 | 0.869 | 0.909 | 0.401 | 0.875 |
| Early education | | | | | | | | | | 1 | 0.874 | 0.298 | 0.884 |
| Literacy young women | | | | | | | | | | | 1 | 0.345 | 0.851 |
| Use of improved water | | | | | | | | | | | | 1 | 0.474 |
| Inproved sanitation | | | | | | | | | | | | | 1 |

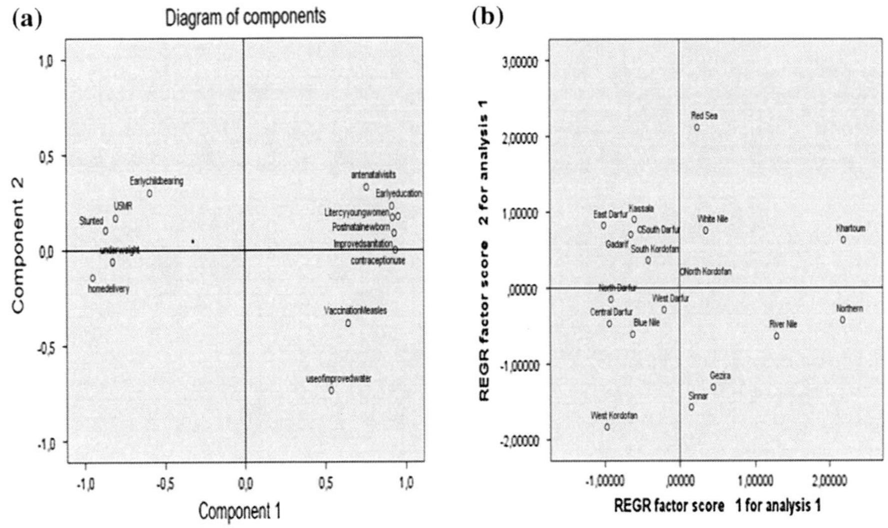


**Fig. 3.2** **a** Projection of variables on the circle of correlations, **b** Projection of states on the first plan ($F1 \times F2$)

and improved water 45.1%) and West Kordofan (antenatal visits 28.1% and improved water 86%).

More importantly, the PCA offers also the opportunity for a critical analysis. For instance, Table 3.2 indicates that North Kordofan (41.9) has the third smallest U5MR which is less than U5MR in Khartoum (49.8) while this state is projected near zero on the first axis, far away from the group of Northern, Khartoum and River Nile. In fact, the four variables positively correlated with U5MR (stunting, underweight, home delivery and early childbearing) all have values in North Kordofan (40.8, 32.4, 74.5 and 14.7) greater than in Khartoum (29.5, 23.2, 35.7 and 9.4) and on the other side, the remaining 13 variables negatively correlated with U5MR all have values in North Kordofan (74.5, 14.7, 57.7, 31.3, 9.4, 58.8, 69.8 and 30) smaller than in Khartoum (89.7, 26.5, 81.9, 57.4, 56.2, 82.6, 86.9 and 85.4). Consequently, we can conclude that the U5MR given for North Kordofan may be under estimated. The multiple regression technique provide a model which helps one understand how the typical value of the dependent variable (U5MR) changes when any one of the 12 independent variables is varied, while the others are fixed. The first attempt is a linear regression model which was carried out by step wise regression using SPSS software. Since all variables are correlated, this method chooses contraception use variable which is the most correlated one with U5MR. We have succeeded to explain 63.9% of the variability of U5MR, see details in Fig. 3.3. We intended to use the multiple regression of U5MR on the principle components of the 12 remaining variables, but we renounced to use it because it did not improve the explanation of U5MR (it barely reached the vicinity of 59%). That's why we proposed to consider a regression between $ln(U5MR)$ and a variety set of crossed variables from the 12

**Table 3.2** Values of 13 variables observed in the 18 states of Sudan

| | U5MR | Stunted | Underweight | Vaccination measles | Contraception use | Early childbearing | Antenatal visits | Home delivery | Postnatal new born | Early education | Literacy young women | Use of improved water | Inproved sanitation |
|---|---|---|---|---|---|---|---|---|---|---|---|---|---|
| Northern | 30 | 22.6 | 21.9 | 97.1 | 22.9 | 8.6 | 66.5 | 27.1 | 48.2 | 47.3 | 91.5 | 93.8 | 95 |
| River Nile | 35.1 | 29.5 | 32.2 | 95.5 | 21.3 | 15.1 | 52.9 | 43.6 | 45.7 | 36.1 | 79.8 | 88.3 | 61.9 |
| Red Sea | 61.3 | 45.4 | 33.6 | 67.3 | 9.6 | 15.5 | 53.4 | 51.5 | 32.4 | 37.6 | 71.9 | 33.2 | 56 |
| Kassala | 80.5 | 48.8 | 42 | 73 | 7.9 | 22.6 | 54 | 71.5 | 27.2 | 12.2 | 48.4 | 57.2 | 34.1 |
| Gadarif | 76.7 | 46 | 37.7 | 86.4 | 9.5 | 18.8 | 44.8 | 79.5 | 20.8 | 16.2 | 42.8 | 27.7 | 12.6 |
| Khartoum | 49.8 | 21.9 | 23.2 | 89.7 | 26.5 | 9.4 | 81.9 | 35.7 | 57.4 | 56.2 | 82.6 | 86.9 | 85.4 |
| Gezira | 53.5 | 41.6 | 32.4 | 96.7 | 12.2 | 13.5 | 50.5 | 62.5 | 28.5 | 21 | 66.4 | 88.9 | 49.9 |
| White Nile | 65.8 | 36.6 | 29.8 | 89.1 | 15.6 | 14.5 | 45.5 | 63.4 | 32.7 | 26.2 | 67.5 | 32.7 | 38.8 |
| Sinnar | 51.6 | 38.1 | 36.4 | 87.4 | 13.5 | 13.1 | 43.5 | 73.7 | 24.5 | 24.8 | 54 | 88.7 | 28.9 |
| Blue Nile | 83.9 | 46.7 | 35.3 | 90.6 | 7.1 | 23.4 | 42.7 | 86.1 | 15.8 | 13.3 | 36.1 | 71.3 | 42.8 |
| North Kordofan | 41.9 | 40.8 | 32.4 | 74.5 | 14.7 | 20.9 | 57.7 | 76.1 | 31.3 | 9.4 | 58.8 | 69.8 | 30 |
| South Kordofan | 95.4 | 40.6 | 34.8 | 75.2 | 9 | 15.9 | 59.3 | 85 | 16.2 | 21.9 | 49.2 | 60.1 | 20.9 |
| West Kordofan | 82.1 | 42.5 | 38.7 | 67.5 | 6.1 | 14 | 28.1 | 91.4 | 12.4 | 4.3 | 32.9 | 86 | 11.6 |
| North Darfur | 90.3 | 45.9 | 44.9 | 67.5 | 3.7 | 11.8 | 36.9 | 88.9 | 15.8 | 13.7 | 56 | 50.6 | 13.8 |
| East Darfur | 111.7 | 46.6 | 40.2 | 72.1 | 6.2 | 19.8 | 46.8 | 84.2 | 17.6 | 11.8 | 40 | 45.1 | 17 |
| Central Darfur | 77.4 | 47.2 | 41 | 77.8 | 2.9 | 14.4 | 47.1 | 88.1 | 12.2 | 9.1 | 27.4 | 50.6 | 19.1 |
| West Darfur | 91.4 | 35.2 | 29.4 | 83.4 | 4.1 | 14.6 | 56.1 | 82.5 | 27.1 | 13.5 | 50.1 | 67.5 | 18.3 |
| South Darfur | 71.9 | 34.2 | 29.4 | 58.9 | 5.4 | 19.1 | 40.9 | 88.6 | 19 | 17.3 | 49.3 | 46.6 | 29 |

**Model Summary[b]**

| Model | R | R Square | Adjusted R Square | Std. Error of the Estimate | Change Statistics | | | | | Durbin-Watson |
|---|---|---|---|---|---|---|---|---|---|---|
| | | | | | R Square Change | F Change | df1 | df2 | Sig. F Change | |
| 1 | ,800[a] | ,639 | ,617 | 13,858 | ,639 | 28,374 | 1 | 16 | ,000 | 2,711 |

a. Predictors: (Constant), contraception use
b. Dependent Variable: U5MR

**Coefficients[a]**

| Model | | Unstandardized Coefficients | | Standardized Coefficients | t | Sig. | 95,0% Confidence Interval for B | |
|---|---|---|---|---|---|---|---|---|
| | | B | Std. Error | Beta | | | Lower Bound | Upper Bound |
| 1 | (Constant) | 98,048 | 6,283 | | 15,606 | ,000 | 84,730 | 111,367 |
| | contraception use | -2,596 | ,487 | -,800 | -5,327 | ,000 | -3,629 | -1,563 |

a. Dependent Variable: U5MR

**Fig. 3.3** Output of linear multiple regression model

```
            Estimate     Std. Error   t value   Pr(>|t|)
(Intercept)  4.546e+00   6.149e-02    73.928  < 2e-16 ***
X1          -2.198e-07   2.825e-08    -7.782 7.93e-07 ***
---
Signif. codes:  0 '***' 0.001 '**' 0.01 '*' 0.05 '.' 0.1 ' ' 1

Residual standard error: 0.1708 on 16 degrees of freedom
Multiple R-squared:  0.791,   Adjusted R-squared:  0.7779
F-statistic: 60.55 on 1 and 16 DF,  p-value: 7.927e-07
```

**Fig. 3.4** Output of the regression of ln(U5MR) on $X_1$: Contraception* use of improved water *Literacy young women * stunted

remaining ones. After a large numbers of attempts we succeed to reach the vicinity of 80% of explanation by regressing $ln(U5MR)$ on $X_1$ which is the crossed variable resulting from the product of Contraception use, use of improved water, Literacy young women and Stunted, see Fig. 3.4. Thus, the final resulting model is giving as follows:

$$U5MR = \exp(4.546) * \exp(-2.198 * 10^{-7} X_1) + \varepsilon \tag{3.1}$$

Thus, by acting simultaneously on these four variables contained in $X_1$ (Contraception use, use of improved water, Literacy young women and Stunted), we can influence and control the infant mortality rate with a high percentage of 80%. Indeed, the augmentation value of $X_1$ entail a reduction in U5MR.

## 3.4 Conclusion

Using descriptive statistics, statistics for decision (Pearson's chi-squared test) and multivariate analysis (Principal Component Analysis), we have graphically illustrated and pragmatically proved that U5MR in Sudan is influenced by social determinants of health like milieu (rural-urban), gender (boys-girls), education level, income (as approximated by household assets) and territorial disparity between states. In particular, our study has shown that a large gap is found between states according to the 13 variables in general and especially in term of under-five mortality. As we indicated in the introduction section, if Sudan is to be really considered as a pioneer in terms of Health in All Policies, serious efforts must be devoted to reducing inacceptable heath inequalities by acting on social determinants of health. Furthermore, by acting simultaneously on Contraception use, use of improved water, Literacy young women and Stunted, we may reduce and control the under-five mortality rate. The next Multiple Indicator Cluster Survey planned for 2019 (Sudan MICS19) could be a first test.

## References

1. Abdalla S, Mutaz M (2014) Road map for implementing health in all policies in Sudan
2. Braveman P (2006) Health disparities and health equity: concepts and measurement. Annu Rev Public Health 27:167–194
3. Omer AS, Bezruchka S, Longhi D, Kelly Z, Brown M, Hagopian A (2014) The effects of household assets inequality and conflict on population health in Sudan. Afr Popul Stud 28(3):1216–1232
4. UNICEF (2014) Multiple Indicator Cluster Survey (MICS) final report Sudan
5. WHO Commission on Social Determinants of Health and World Health Organization (2008) Closing the gap in a generation: health equity through action on the social determinants of health: commission on social determinants of health final report. World Health Organization
6. Working Group for Monitoring Action on the Social Determinants of Health (2018) Towards a global monitoring system for implementing the rio political declaration on social determinants of health: developing a core set of indicators for government action on the social determinants of health to improve health equity. Int J Equity Health 17:1–27
7. World Health Organization (2011) World conference on social determinants of health: meeting report, Rio de Janeiro, Brazil
8. World Health Organization (2014) Health in all policies: framework for country action

# Chapter 4
# The Environmental Health Role in Reducing Non Communicable Diseases Through a Healthy Lifestyle

**Abdellatif Maamri and Souad Ben El Mostafa**

**Abstract** The fight against noncommunicable diseases (NCDs) and their risk factors is one of the major challenges of sustainable development in the twenty-first century. These diseases are emerging more and more in low- and middle-income countries, including Morocco. This study examines the role of environmental health in reducing noncommunicable diseases through a literature review of epidemiological profiles of certain diseases such as type 2 diabetes and hypertension; and identifying environmental risks. The results show that 80% of premature deaths due to noncommunicable diseases could have been largely prevented by effective interventions aimed at reducing the level of exposure of individuals and populations to risk factors, namely smoking, malnutrition, inactivity and the harmful consumption of alcohol. In addition, strengthening health systems so that they can provide more effective and equitable care to people affected by noncommunicable diseases will reduce morbidity, disability and mortality by contributing to better health outcomes. The 2018–2030 Montevideo NCD Roadmap, as a priority for sustainable development, is the cornerstone of achieving Goal 3 of the SDGs on NCDs at the level of the Sustainable Development Goals. Morocco, through its national multisectoral strategy for the prevention and control of noncommunicable diseases, is participating to this global effort to combat noncommunicable diseases, the results of which will be predictable in the coming years.

A. Maamri (✉)
Department of Biology, Faculty of Sciences, University Mohamed Ier, Oujda, Morocco
e-mail: abdellatifm@hotmail.com

S. Ben El Mostafa
Higher Institute of Health Nursing and Technical Professions (ISPITS), Ministry of Health, Nador, Morocco
e-mail: souadbenelmostafa@hotmail.fr



A. Boutayeb (ed.), *Disease Prevention and Health Promotion in Developing Countries*,
https://doi.org/10.1007/978-3-030-34702-4_4

## 4.1 Introduction

Health is a major concern for sustainable development, as emphasized in Principle I of the Rio Declaration on Environment and Development in 1992. "Human beings are at the center of sustainable development concerns and entitled to a healthy life and productive in harmony with nature".

Despite the undeniable progress achieved in terms of public health in the last decade, it is clear that the environment is becoming an increasingly strong determinant of health and wellbeing. Environmental factors are responsible for a quarter of human morbidity and mortality [48]. The interdependence between global development, environmental degradation and health is a key issue confronting sustainable development.

According to the World Health Organization (WHO) [52], NCDs are responsible for 41 million of the 57 million deaths worldwide (71%). 15 million of these deaths were premature (aged 30–70 years) in 2016.

In low- and middle-income countries, the burden remains heavy: 78% of deaths are due to noncommunicable diseases and 85% of premature deaths.

There are environmental risk factors that contribute to NCDs. Thus, NCDs caused by environmental risk factors are considered to be one of the major obstacles to sustainable development. The fight against these risk factors is therefore one of the major challenges facing the international community for a secure development in the twenty-first century. Indeed, health can be at the origin of economic slowdown (endemic malaria in African countries is predicted to cause a slowdown in economic growth of up to 1.3% per year) [47]. The pollution of water, air and soil due to nitrogen use is estimated to cost between 150 and 740 euros per person per year in Europe. The degradation of water quality linked to excess nitrogen fertilizers and pesticides used in agriculture costs more than one billion euros to French households, or 215 € per person [1].

The implementation of prevention strategies can also be financially demanding for governments, but also provide economic benefit through improving health to foster economic development. Using air quality as an example in the European Union (EU), the EU's air quality strategy will reduce the number of premature deaths per year caused by fine particles and ozone from 370,000 in 2000 to 230,000 in 2020 [44] [This will result in annual benefits of around 42 billion euros which is more than 5 times the cost of implementing the strategy estimated at 7.1 billion euros per year and 0.05% of EU 25 GDP in 2010]. According to the WHO, Diabetes and heart disease will cost China's national income 558 billion US $ and India, 237 billion. Between 2000 and 2030, the number of people living with diabetes will increase from 171 million to 366 million, including 298 million in low- and middle-income countries [33].

Today, there are 40 million annual deaths caused by noncommunicable diseases, more than any other cause of death. Of these deaths, 15 million occur prematurely in people aged 30 to 70, and 7 million occur in low- and middle-income countries.

Diabetes is recognized as an important cause of premature death and disability. It is one of four priority no communicable diseases (NCDs) targeted by world leaders in the 2011 Political Declaration on the Prevention and Control of NCDs [51]. The declaration recognizes that the impact of diabetes on health and wellbeing, as with many other NCDs, can be largely prevented. This requires an approach that incorporates evidence-based, affordable, cost-effective, and population-wide and multisectoral interventions.

In Morocco, the situation is alarming; NCDs are the main cause of mortality, accounting for 80% of deaths [47]. Morocco's rate of mortality due to NCDs is among the highest in the EMRO region. The probability of dying between 30 and 70 years is 23%.

Morocco has experienced an epidemiological and demographic transition leading to an increase in the burden of NCDs, in particular cancers (11% of deaths), diabetes (12%), cardiovascular diseases (34%), communicable diseases, maternal, perinatal and nutritional diseases (18%), chronic respiratory diseases (4%), trauma (7%), and other noncommunicable diseases 14% [50].

The cost of managing these diseases is very high. According to the Comprehensive Report on Compulsory Health Insurance (AMO) in 2012, 3% of NCD patients consumed 50% of AMO expenses [50].

Among the Sustainable Development Goals (SDGs) [45] to be achieved in 2030, three objectives (3.a, 4 and 5) are directly related to NCDs:

- Target 3.a: Strengthen in all countries, where appropriate, the application of Framework Convention on Tobacco Control (FCTC).
- Target 4: Reduce by one-third, through prevention and treatment, the premature death rate due to the absence of communicable diseases by 2030 and promote mental health and well-being.
- Target 5: Strengthen the prevention and treatment of psychoactive drugs, including narcotics and alcohol, for the treatment of drug addiction.

Additionally, the Montevideo 2018–2030 No communicable Disease Roadmap [36] launched in 2017 is a commitment following agreement between world leaders to reduce by one third premature deaths from non-communicable diseases by 2030 under the United Nations Sustainable Development Program.

## 4.2 Non Communicable Diseases in the Word

The definition of noncommunicable diseases (NCDs), also known as chronic diseases, are diseases that are not transmitted from one person to another. They are of long duration, generally evolve slowly and refer to incomparable affections. Chronic diseases impact patients' lifestyles and living conditions, but also the individual's psychosocial and emotional state.

The four main types of noncommunicable diseases are cardiovascular diseases (heart disease and stroke), cancers, chronic respiratory diseases (such as chronic

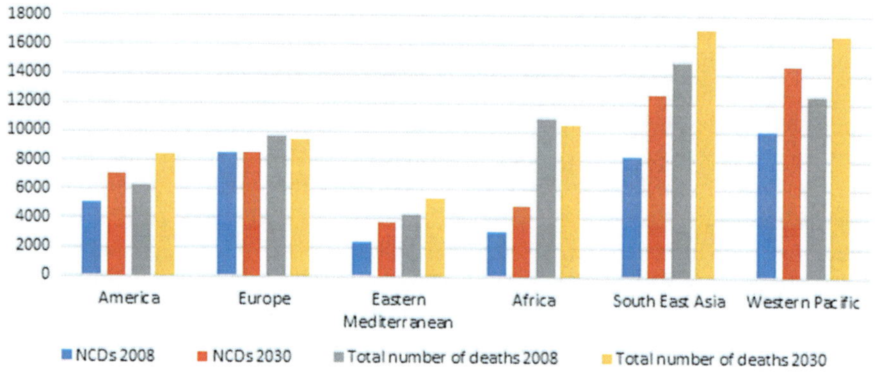


**Fig. 4.1** Distribution of noncommunicable diseases and number of deaths due to non-natural causes (communicable diseases, NCDs and accidents) and their projections in 2030 [47]

obstructive pulmonary disease or asthma) and diabetes. Most are caused by environmental factors including social determinants of health (Fig. 4.1).

Non Communicable Diseases will make more and more deaths in the years to come as confirmed by WHO [47]. These noncommunicable diseases will have their frequencies exploded by 2030 in the different regions of the world as shown in the projection above. In order to estimate the reported prevalence of chronic diseases in Morocco, the 2017–2018 survey showed that 21.0% of the Moroccan population suffers from at least one chronic disease with women more affected than men (24.9% versus 17.1%). The Prevalence is higher in people aged 60 and older with 64.4% [28].

In Morocco mortality from NCDs is the main cause of mortality. It is estimated at 80% according to WHO and premature mortality is estimated at 12%. This exceeds the global average of 70% of deaths and places Morocco among the first countries with high mortality from NCDs in the region of eastern Mediterranean, as illustrated by the graph above (Fig. 4.2). Cardiovascular disease is the leading cause of death (Fig. 4.3).

Berrahou [8] found a significant positive association between hypertension and the following factors: higher age, higher BMI, duration of diabetes and illiteracy. In Morocco, despite the fact that the prevalence of hypertension has slightly decreased between 2000 (33.6%) and 2017 (29.3%) (Fig. 4.4), hypertension continues to cause enormous damage to health. Morocco has set a goal of reducing the prevalence of high blood pressure by 10% by 2029 [29].

Diabetes continues its alarming increase worldwide. In Morocco, the prevalence measured in the survey (2017–2018) was 10.6% (Figs. 4.4 and 4.5), which has increased significantly compared to 2000 (6.6%). Diabetes is one of four priority NCDs in the 2011 NCD Prevention and Control Policy Statement. The global goal for noncommunicable diseases is to bring down the rise of diabetes by the end of 2025 at its level of 2010. In Morocco, the 15% reduction of this increase is the goal to be achieved by 2029 [29].

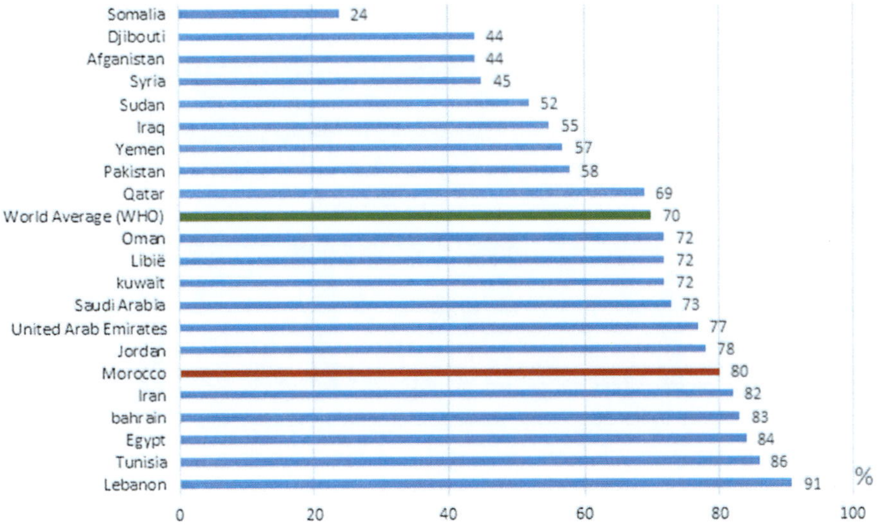


**Fig. 4.2** Deaths from NCDs 2018, (data from [28])

**Fig. 4.3** Causes of death in Morocco due to noncommunicable diseases

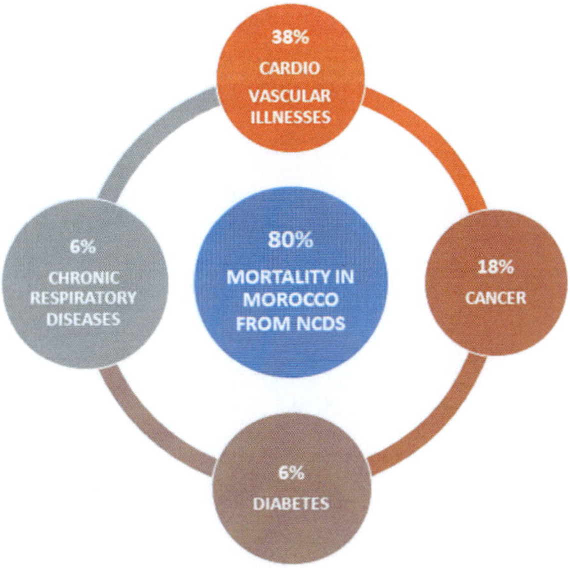


Despite a slight decrease in the prevalence of hypertension between 2000 and 2017, efforts still need to be made to combat this scourge. On the contrary, the prevalence of diabetes has increased exceptionally since 2000, doubling in 2017. High prevalence is noted in women for both diabetes and hypertension (Fig. 4.6).

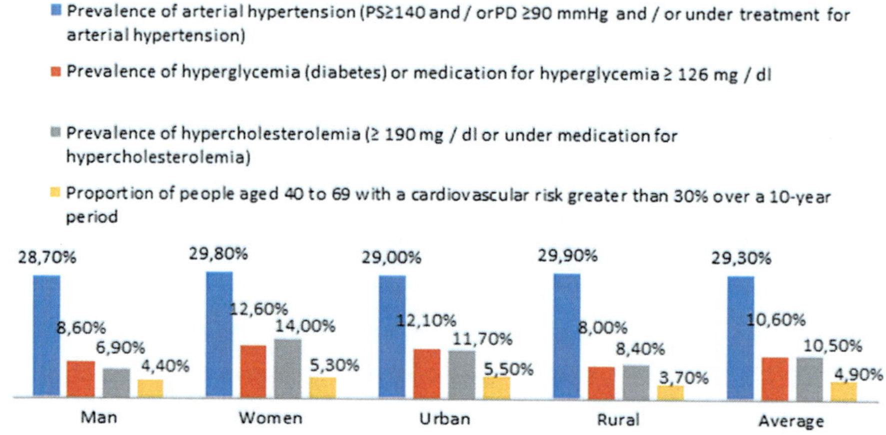


**Fig. 4.4** HTA, diabetes prevalence, hypercholesterolemia and cardiovascular risk in Morocco (data from [29])

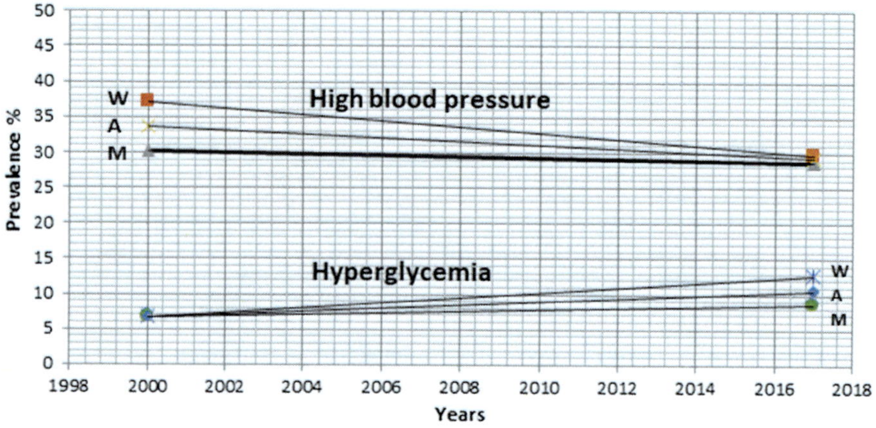


**Fig. 4.5** Evolution of HTA and diabetes prevalence in Morocco between 2000 and 2017 (W: Women, A: Average, M: Men)

## 4.3 Environmental Health

According to the WHO definition—Helsinki Conference—1994 "Environmental health includes aspects of human health, including the quality of life, which are determined by physical, chemical, biological, social, psychosocial and aesthetic of our environment" [46].

It also concerns policies and practices for managing, controlling, and preventing environmental factors that may affect the health of current and future generations, whether local or global. For example, the air quality considers indoor air to planetary

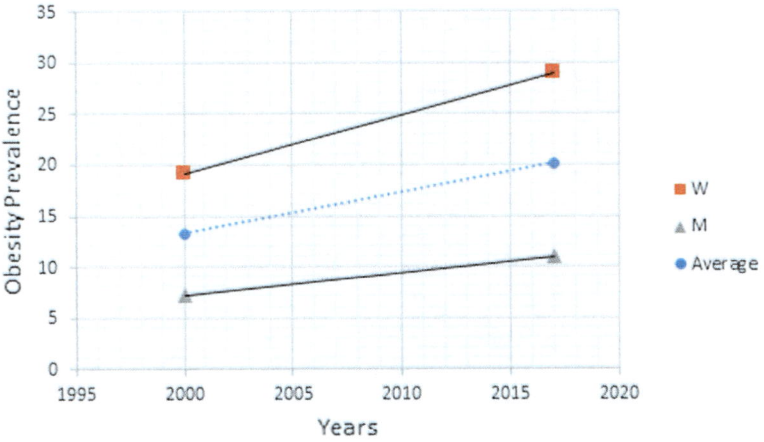


**Fig. 4.6** Evolution of obesity prevalence in Morocco between 2000 and 2017 (W: Women, A: Average, M: Men)

atmosphere—including the consequences of global warming. Hence, it is closely associated with the notion of "public health".

The notion of "environmental health" is a proactive and organized approach, inscribed in the experience. The articulation of health with the environment underlines the continuity that link all living organisms together and the relationship between them (Fig. 4.7).

Worldwide, the mortality rate due to environmental factors is 23%. This represents 12.6 million deaths per year. All areas of the globe are affected by this phenomenon. Southeast Asia and the Western Pacific region remain the WHO regions most exposed to these environmental impacts [35]. In a study of 1,000 people [35], a quarter of respondents reported having a chronic illness. The link between health and the environment is established for 97% of respondents. It is a consistent result for executives, workers and employees, but also for urban and rural populations. There is evidence for an environmental link in 80% of people with chronic illness. For nearly 75%, the primary cause is changing lifestyles (eating habits, sedentary lifestyle, lack of sleep …). The second cause highlighted is the degradation of the quality of the environment. The aging of the population and social fragilities linked to people's economic situation are also contributing factors.

## 4.4 Healthy Lifestyle and Risk Factor

At the general population level, healthy living refers to the practices of various groups within a population to support, improve, maintain or improve health status. At the individual level, a healthy lifestyle is the individual practice of promoting better

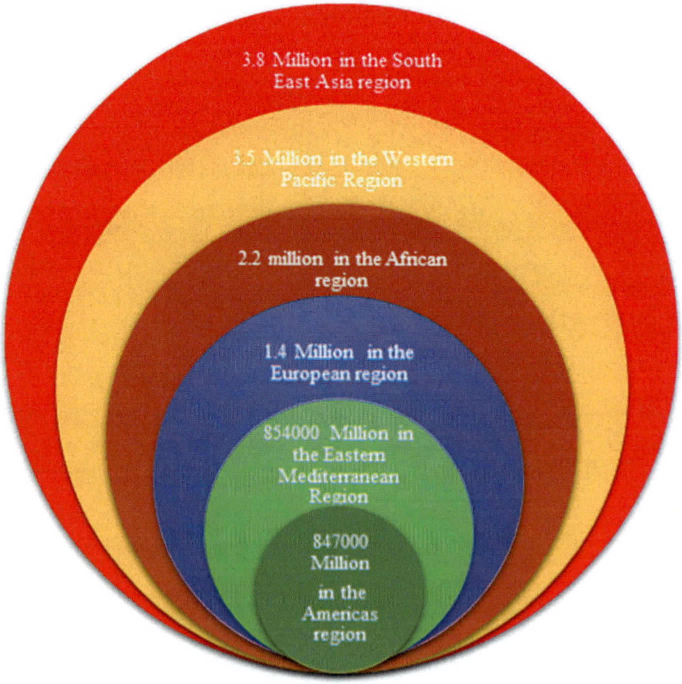


**Fig. 4.7** Worldwide mortality related to environment factors (data from [35])

health, more simply, adopting a healthy lifestyle. For this, a person must have the physical, mental and spiritual capacity to make healthy choices. The Integrated Pan-Canadian Healthy Living Strategy focuses on healthy eating, physical activity, and the effects of these factors on achieving a healthy weight [43].

WHO's "First Global Ministerial Conference on Healthy Lifestyles" and "Non communicable Disease Control" emphasized the role of multisectoral, national, international and behavioral actions to reduce the level of exposure of individuals and populations to modifiable common risk factors like tobacco, unhealthy diet, physical inactivity and alcohol consumption.

A risk factor is any attribute, characteristic or exposure of a subject that increases the probability of developing a disease or suffering a trauma. The most important risk factors for NCDs are, for example, underweight, high blood pressure, tobacco or alcohol consumption, unsafe water, inadequate hygiene or sanitation.

Risk factors for NCDs often begin at the beginning of life and continue into adulthood. However, there is evidence that prevention and treatment interventions are needed to reverse the trend of the no communicable disease epidemic. The Global Plan of Action for Noncommunicable Disease Control provides a roadmap of policy options to be implemented between 2018 and 2023, focusing on modifiable and

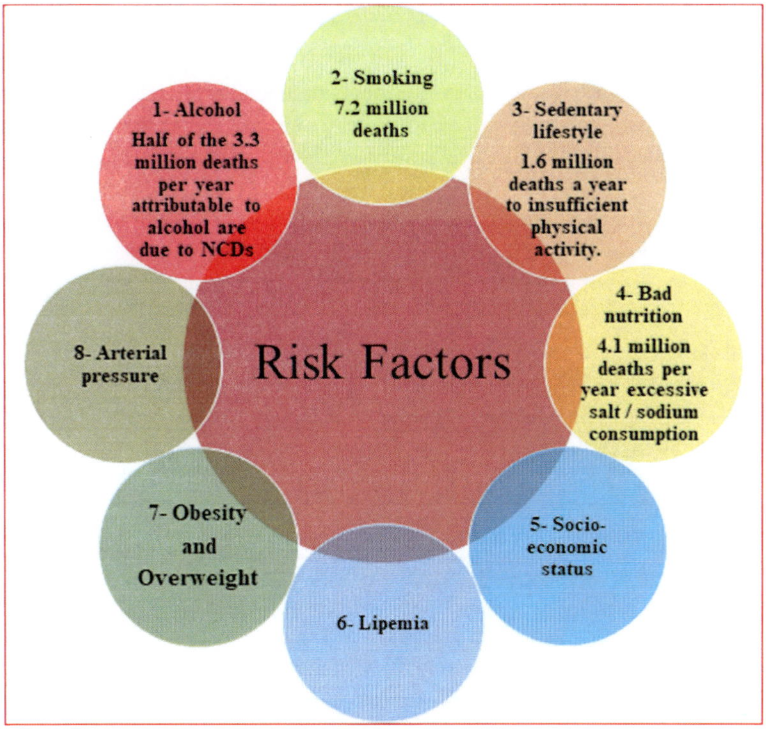


**Fig. 4.8** Risks factors for NCDs 1–4: influence factors related to lifestyle; 5-socio economic factors; 6–8: physiological health factors

common behavioral risk factors for NCDs that are related to the four avoidable noncommunicable diseases [49] (Fig. 4.8).

Studies have shown that four factors have a strong influence on the probability of suffering from a NCD: physical activity, diet, tobacco and alcohol. By acting on these four factors, we promote the health of the population and fight against NCDs. A study published in Switzerland showed that the probability of survival of a person in the next ten years was closely related to the interaction of four factors: physical activity, diet, tobacco and alcohol. The combination of these four factors is comparable to a 10-year age difference: thus, a 65-year-old who has an unbalanced lifestyle has the same chance of survival for the next ten years (67%) as a 75-year-old with a healthy lifestyle (67%) [14].

Other factors include socio-economic factors (awareness, education and access to services which are linked to income, social status and education level). This theme is addressed in the chapter "Social and territorial inequalities in health".

Environmental architectures that promote healthy lifestyle choices can decrease risk factors associated with NCDs and thus decrease their prevalence.

### 4.4.1 Fruit and Vegetable Consumption

Fruits and vegetables are important components of a healthy diet. Reduced consumption of fruits and vegetables is linked to poor health and increased risk of noncommunicable diseases. An estimated 3.9 million deaths worldwide in 2017 were due to insufficient consumption of fruits and vegetables, of which 14% worldwide are associated with gastrointestinal cancer each year, 11% with cardiovascular diseases and 9% with cerebrovascular accidents [31].

As a result, in the context of a healthy diet low in fat, sugar and sodium, the WHO suggests consuming more than 400 g of fruits and vegetables a day to improve overall health and reduce the risk of some noncommunicable diseases.

In Morocco, the STEPS survey on NCD risk factors 2017–2018 showed that the study population consumes fruits 4 times a week while the consumption of vegetables was 6 days per week (Fig. 4.9).

Dietary habits compared to average consumption of other foods were also considered by the study.

Red or white meat is eaten on average 4.2 days a week. Eggs are consumed on average 2.8 days a week and fish has been reported consumed 1.6 days a week on average. Finally, non-alcoholic beverages and commercial fruit juices are consumed on average one day per week (Fig. 4.10).

In rehabilitating the quantities of vegetables and fruits consumed by Moroccans, the survey showed that more than 76% of the population is below the WHO recommendations (Fig. 4.11).

In Europe, according to a recent study, 34.4% of Europeans over 15 years of age do not consume any daily portion of fruit and vegetables and 85.7% of Europeans do not meet the recommendations of 5 fruits and vegetables per day [31].

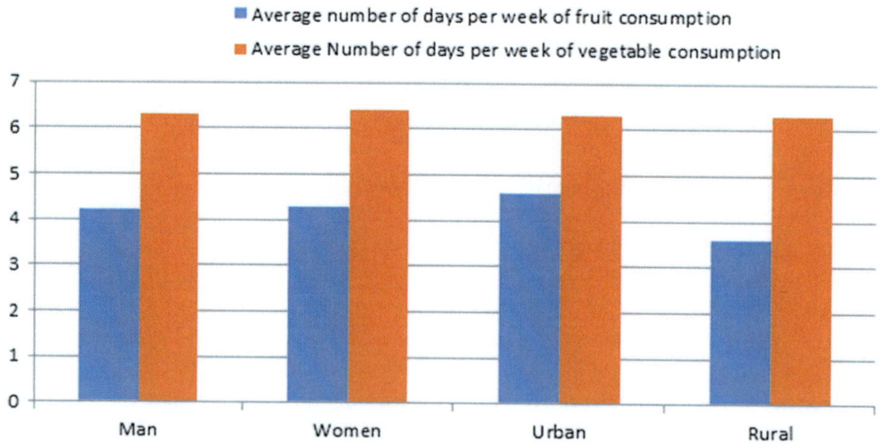


**Fig. 4.9** Consumption of fruits, vegetables and other foods in Morocco (data from [29])

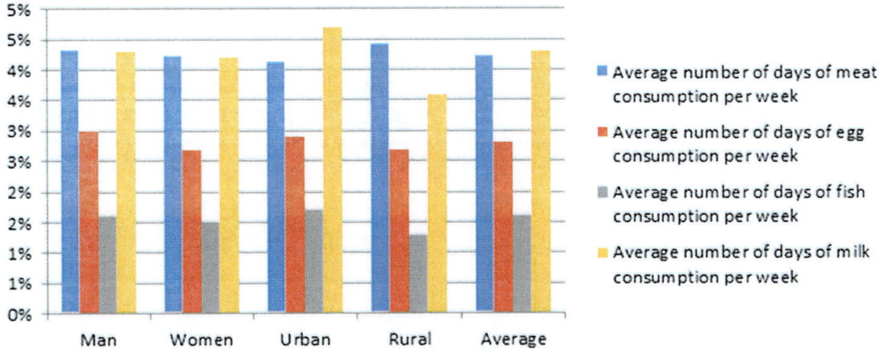


**Fig. 4.10** Consumption of other foods in Morocco (data from [29])

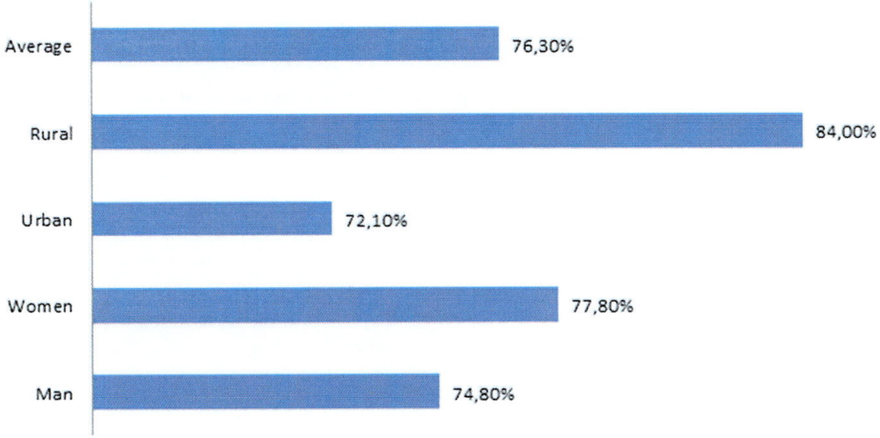


**Fig. 4.11** Percentage of people who consume less than 5 servings of fruits and / or vegetables per day in Morocco (data from [29])

## *4.4.2 Overweight and Obesity*

The World Health Organization defines obesity as "an abnormal or excessive accumulation of body fat that poses a risk to health". The simplest calculation tool is Body Mass Index (BMI in $kg/m^2$).

Obesity and overweight are largely responsible for chronic diseases, especially among women with a very high prevalence of obesity [9, 16]. Women have a significantly higher BMI than their male counterparts [9, 26, 41].

In the United States, the results of the 2015–2016 National Health and Nutrition Survey indicate that 39.8% of adults aged 20 years or older reported being obese, 31.8% being overweight and 7.6% being severely obese [20].

The problem of obesity is not a special issue of high-income countries; it also exists in low- and middle-income countries, where 115 million people are affected by this phenomenon. In Morocco, according to the survey of NCDs [47], 53% of Moroccans are overweight and 20% are obese. Similarly, Atek [4] in his study conducted in Algeria on 4746 subjects found that 66.5% of respondents are overweight and 30.1% are obese. The same author found among 5343 screened subjects, 71.1% overweight and 37% suffering from obesity in Tunisia.

Overweight and obesity are associated with multiple unhealthy health long life health consequences.

Obesity is linked to an increased risk of hypertension, many NCDs (such as diabetes, coronary heart disease, stroke and cancer).

Obesity is the most powerful factor predisposing to diabetes, especially in the case of abdominal distribution. Obesity is able to induce or aggravate insulin resistance, forcing the pancreas to hyper secrete permanently. Berraho [8], in a study of 525 people with type 2 diabetes in Morocco, found that around 74% of their target population was either overweight (43%) or obese (31%). Oudghiri [37], working on blood pressure in 151 women in Morocco, found a strong association between hypertension and BMI/obesity in 81% of cases.

### *4.4.3 Physical Activity and Sedentarity*

Physical activity is an important and variable component of total energy expenditure. In contrast, physical inactivity refers to the lack of physical activity and is considered the leading death factor in the world (6%).

According to the Epidemiological survey of prevalence of risk factors for non-communicable diseases [29], the analysis of the percentage of the target population does not reach the recommended amount of physical activity (150 min of moderate physical activity per week or equivalent) concluded that 21.1% did not respond to this recommendation. Women (26%) are more likely to have sedentary behaviors compared to men (16.1%). The older the age, the more the tendency to sedentarity. This percentage rose to 31.5% among those aged 60–69 and 49.3% among those aged 70 and over (Fig. 4.12).

Urbanization, the mechanization of work as well as that of transport and the nature of leisure activities lead to a growing sedentary lifestyle. Urbanization is causing a change in lifestyles with a sharp increase in the inactivity. In 2009, Africa surpassed the billion inhabitants, of which 395 million (40%) lived in urban areas. In 2050, the total population of African cities will rise to more than 1.23 billion inhabitants or more than 60% of the population (Fig. 4.13).

For Type 2 Diabetes (T2D), the reduction in physical activity is responsible for a decrease in glucose uptake by the muscles and a strengthening of the phenomenon of insulin resistance. Associated with the disappearance of the defenses of thermoregulation [24], this situation creates an environment far away from that of the countrymen

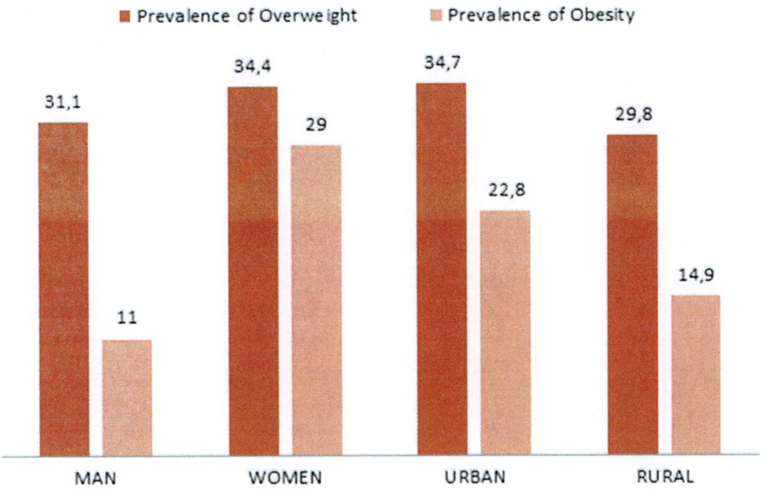


**Fig. 4.12** Overweight and obesity prevalence in Morocco (data from [29])

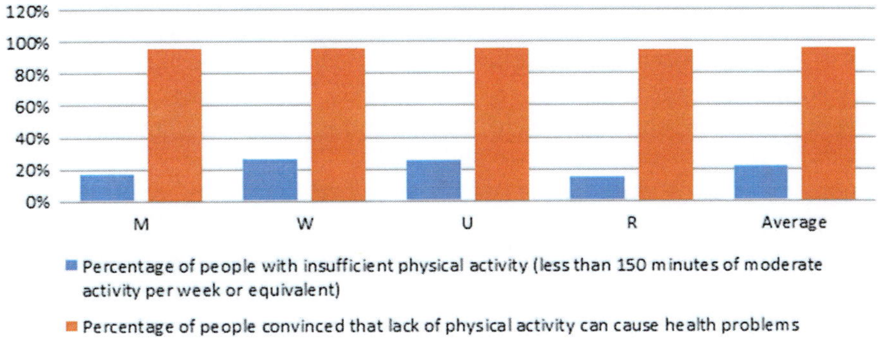


**Fig. 4.13** Physical activity for Moroccans peoples (data from [29])

whose the way of life rests on the physical effort. As a result, the prevalence of T2D is higher among urban dwellers than in rural areas [2, 34, 39].

The hypothesis of a close link between physical activity and the appearance of some chronic diseases such as diabetes is based on epidemiological studies which report, among other arguments, that populations who have abandoned the rural way of life in favor of living in the city have seen an increase in the incidence of diabetes [13]. Regular exercise associated with a balanced diet has long been considered the cornerstone of prevention and treatment of type 2 diabetes [32].

Recognizing the potential role of physical activity promotion in the fight against overweight, obesity and diabetes, the World Health Assembly in May 2004 adopted the WHO Global Strategy for Food, physical activity and health [6]. In 2013, WHO adopted Resolution WHA66.10, Global Action Plan for Non Communicable Diseases 2013–2020, which includes a set of goals to be achieved, including the promotion of physical activity [2].

In type 2 diabetics, physical activity can improve their cardiovascular fitness, increase their physical stamina, improve their glycemic control [11, 38], reduce their insulin resistance, improve their lipid profile, lower their blood pressure and maintain a healthy lifestyle and better weight control [5]. It can also reduce the cost of treatment [40], improve quality of life and perceived well-being [7, 30] and reduce the need for insulin in insulin-treated patients [3, 22].

Performed regularly and appropriately, passively [12, 19] or intense or moderate cardiorespiratory [27], it is associated with a very significant reduction in cardiovascular mortality and overall mortality, evaluated between minus 39% and minus 70%. In high-risk groups, physical activity appears to reduce the risk of developing T2D from 47 to 58%. This reduction in incidence seems to persist 10 years after the initial intervention [17].

Aerobic exercise (walking, biking, jogging, etc.) and resistance exercise (with weight machines or counterbalanced) are recommended for most people with diabetes. Walking is the most popular and easiest type of aerobic exercise for middle-aged diabetics who are overweight or elderly. Resistance exercises strengthen lean muscle mass [30] and bone mineral density [7], improving functional abilities and preventing sarcopenia and osteoporosis [23].

Supervised exercise programs improve blood glucose control without a diet being part of the program. These results are usually only obtained after a nutritional intervention if the exercises are not supervised [15, 23].

The follow-up study of the European EPIC cohort shows for the first time that promoting the fight against total physical inactivity regardless of BMI and waist circumference can affect mortality [42]. It must be recalled, however, that the fight against a sedentary lifestyle cannot replace moderate endurance exercises [18, 25].

A previously sedentary diabetic with limited exercise tolerance may be required to progressively increase his/her level of physical activity by taking several short exercise sessions (approximately 10 min) during a day [10, 23].

Adherence to different levels of physical activity is positively correlated with the importance of social and psychological factors. The most important criteria are young age, cultural level, lack of motivation barrier, perception of health performance [7, 30] and the desire to combat drug obesity [21].

### *4.4.4 Tobacco and Alcohol*

Smoking, including smoked and non-smoking tobacco products, is currently one of the major risks of some noncommunicable diseases, such as cancer. This burden due to direct consumption as well as to indirect (secondary smoking). In addition, two-thirds of noncommunicable diseases are linked to unhealthy behaviors: more than 7.2 million deaths are attributable to tobacco each year (including exposure to second-hand smoke). In addition, tobacco is the leading preventable cause of cancer.

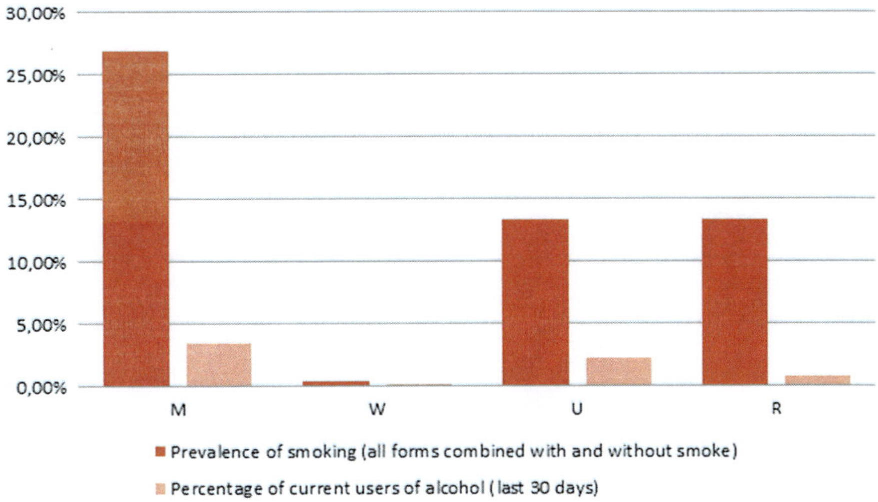


**Fig. 4.14** Smoking prevalence and current user's alcohol % in Morocco (data from [29]) (M: Men; W: Women, U: Urban, R: Rural)

Smokers who die prematurely deprive their families of income, deteriorate their health and slow their economic development.

In Morocco the survey of 2018, showed that 13.4% of the population 18 years and older are currently tobacco users (24.6% of men and 0.6% of women). Compared to the global prevalence of smoking in 2016 at people aged 15 and over, by the numbers are 34% for men and 6% for women (Fig. 4.14).

Alcohol consumption has a significant impact on health. In Switzerland, one in eleven deaths is linked to alcohol. This mortality is mainly due to diseases (cirrhosis of the liver, pancreatitis, cancers, cardiovascular diseases …) as well as trauma (accidents, suicides …) related to alcohol consumption.

## 4.5 Direct Cost of NCDs

The economic burden of NCDs in Morocco is very important. Indeed, 3% of the population AMO who uses Long Term Affective Care (ALD) consumes 47.7% of total expenditure. Moreover, 73% of the expenditures of the ALDs are consumed by the four following conditions:

- Chronic Final Renal Failure: 26.40%;
- Malignant neoplasms: 24%;
- Severe hypertension: 11.70%;
- Diabetes type 1 and 2: 11%.

**Table 4.1** Household expenditures for the 4 NCDs (%) compared to total household expenditures in Morocco [29]

| | |
|---|---|
| Total Expenditure of the 4 NCDs | 777 millions US$ |
| Total household expenditures for the 4 NCDs | 364 millions $US |
| Expenditures for the 4 NCDs as (%) of total health expenditure | 13.9% |
| Household spending for the 4 NCDs (%) relative to total household expenditures | 12.2% |
| Household expenditures for the 4 NCDs (%) compared to total NCD expenditures | 46.9% |

The costs of care for noncommunicable diseases quickly deplete household resources. The exorbitant costs of these diseases, often with long and onerous treatment and the loss of family support, drive millions of people into poverty every year and stifle development.

In Morocco, household expenditures for the 4 NCDs (%) compared to total NCD expenditures are almost 50% (Table 4.1).

There is a strong link between poverty and noncommunicable diseases. The rapid growth of noncommunicable diseases is expected to be an obstacle to poverty reduction initiatives in low-income countries, in particular because of rising household-related health expenditures.

As a result, vulnerable and socially disadvantaged people get sick and die faster than those at a higher social level, particularly because they are at greater risk of exposure to harmful products, such as tobacco, poor eating habits and because they have limited access to health services.

## 4.6 Prevention and Control of Noncommunicable Diseases in Morocco

In 2013, a global plan of action for the prevention and control of NCDs 2013–2020 has been developed with 9 global targets and 25 indicators [49]. A framework for action for the implementation of the United Nations Political Declaration on NCDs has been put in place and which defines the commitments as well as the strategic interventions of countries. The targets set by Morocco's NCD country by 2029, compared to WHO's voluntary targets are as follows (Fig. 4.15).

To control these diseases, it is urgent to promote healthy living and address the main common risk factors and their underlying determinants. Critically: smoking, poor diet, sedentary lifestyle and the harmful use of alcohol.

Addressing modifiable risk factors is not the only way to combat noncommunicable diseases. Acting on the social determinants of health in Morocco is also essential

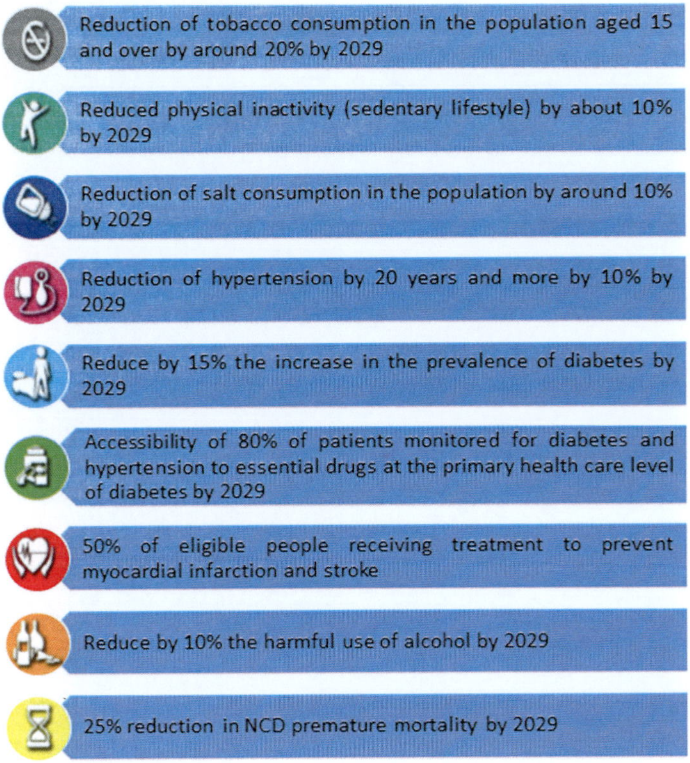


**Fig. 4.15** Global plan of action for the prevention and control of noncommunicable diseases 2019–2029 in Morocco (data from [29])

to achieve the objectives of the Global Action Plan for the Prevention and Control of Non Communicable Diseases 2019–2029 in Morocco (Fig. 4.16).

For example, air pollution is to blame. It accounts for between one-quarter and one-third of stroke-related morbidity, cardiovascular events, heart attacks, chronic lung cancer and chronic obstructive pulmonary disease (COPD), and more pneumonia. deaths in children. Thus, air pollution is also one of the main risk factors leading to premature morbidity and mortality. In regions such as Asia, it is even the most important risk factor. Interventions to improve air quality should target the entire population.

There is a strong link between poverty and noncommunicable diseases. The rapid growth of noncommunicable diseases is expected to be an impediment to poverty reduction initiatives in low-income countries, in part because of increased household spending on health. When financial resources are limited, the costs of care for non-communicable diseases quickly deplete household resources. The exorbitant costs of noncommunicable diseases, often associated with long and onerous treatment

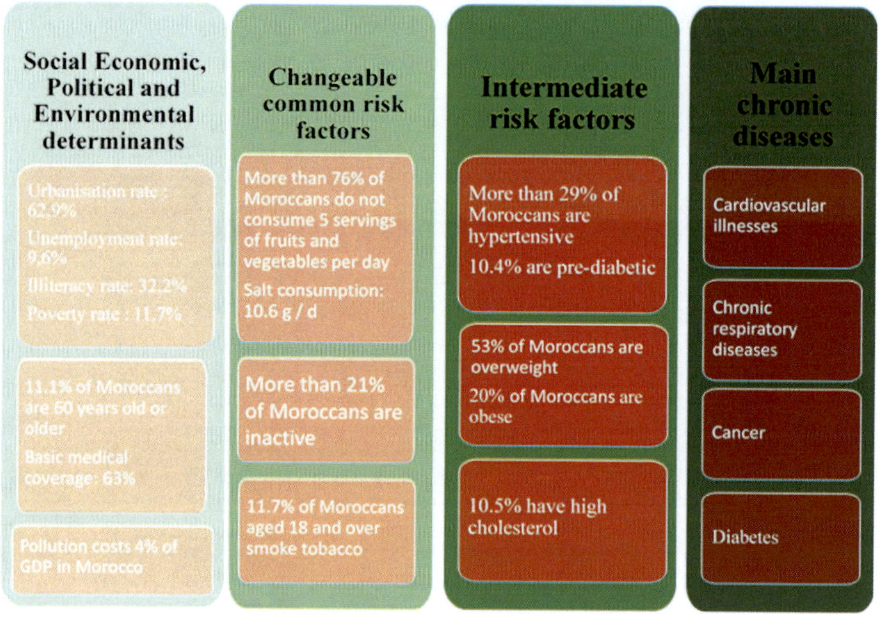


**Fig. 4.16** Chronic diseases and risk factors related to the environment in Morocco

and the loss of family support, drive millions of people into poverty every year and impede development [52].

In addition, vulnerable and socially disadvantaged people get sick and die faster than those of higher social status, especially because they are at greater risk of being exposed to harmful products such as tobacco, poor eating habits and their limited access to health services.

## 4.7 Conclusion

In Morocco, the results of the national survey on NCD risk factors 5 transcribe the growing burden of NCDs and their Risk factors indeed:

- 29.3% are hypertensive;
- 10.6% are diabetic and 10.4% are pre-diabetic;
- 11.7% of Moroccans aged 18 and over smoke tobacco;
- 92.9% never used alcohol for life and 1.7% use alcohol currently;
- 21.1% have a low level of physical activity;
- 76.3% do not meet international consumption recommendations five servings of vegetables and fruits a day;
- 53% are overweight and 20% are obese;
- 10.5% have high blood cholesterol.

The negative impact of noncommunicable diseases on individuals and society is certain. To mitigate this, it is necessary to set up a global and integrated sectoral approach involving different departments (health, finance, transport, education, agriculture, planning, solidarity …), to reduce the risks associated with these diseases and to promoting interventions to avoid and combat them.

To do this, it is important to invest in better management of noncommunicable diseases, based on detection, detection and treatment.

The implementation of the Global Action Plan for Non Communicable Disease Control 2013–2020, with its nine targets for the prevention and care of Non Communicable Diseases, remains one of the safe and effective ways to combat against this scourge of public health and reach the target of sustainable development goals of a decrease of one third by 2030.

## References

1. AEE (2014) La pollution atmosphérique industrielle a un coût économique élevé. Technical report
2. Agence Nationale d'Accréditation et d'évaluation en Santé (2000) Stratégie de prise en charge du patient diabétique de type 2 à l'exclusion de la prise en charge des complications. ANAES, Paris
3. Associazione Medici Diabetologi/Società Italiana di Diabetologia (2018) Standard italiani per la cura del diabete mellito. Italia, Rome
4. Atek M, Traissac P, El Ati J, Laid Y, Aounallah-Skhiri H, Eymard-Duvernay S, Mézimèche N, Bougatef S, Béji C, Boutekdjiret L et al (2013) Obesity and association with area of residence, gender and socio-economic factors in Algerian and Tunisian adults. PloS one 8(10):e75640
5. Balducci S, Iacobellis G, Parisi L, Di Biase N, Calandriello E, Leonetti F, Fallucca F (2006) Exercise training can modify the natural history of diabetic peripheral neuropathy. J Diabetes Its Complicat 20(4):216–223
6. Balducci S, Zanuso S, Nicolucci A, De Feo P, Cavallo S, Cardelli P, Fallucca S, Alessi E, Fallucca F, Pugliese G (2010) Effect of an intensive exercise intervention strategy on modifiable cardiovascular risk factors in subjects with type 2 diabetes mellitus: a randomized controlled trial: the Italian Diabetes and Exercise Study (IDES). Arch Intern Med 170(20):1794–1803
7. Balducci S, Zanuso S, Cardelli P, Salerno G, Fallucca S, Nicolucci A, Pugliese G, Investigators IDESI et al (2012) Supervised exercise training counterbalances the adverse effects of insulin therapy in overweight/obese subjects with type 2 diabetes. Diabetes Care 35(1):39–41
8. Berraho M, El Achhab Y, Benslimane A, Rhazi KE, Chikri M, Nejjari C (2012) Hypertension and type 2 diabetes: a cross-sectional study in morocco (epidiam study). Pan Afr Med J 11(1)
9. Bouguerra R, Alberti H, Salem LB, Rayana CB, Atti J, Gaigi S, Slama CB, Zouari B, Alberti K (2007) The global diabetes pandemic: the Tunisian experience. Eur J Clin Nutr 61(2):160
10. Canadian Agency for Drugs and Technologies in Health (2014) Obesity interventions delivered in primary care for patients with diabetes: a review of clinical effectiveness. Rapid response report
11. Chudyk A, Petrella RJ (2011) Effects of exercise on cardiovascular risk factors in type 2 diabetes: a meta-analysis. Diabetes Care 34(5):1228–1237
12. Church TS, LaMonte MJ, Barlow CE, Blair SN (2005) Cardiorespiratory fitness and body mass index as predictors of cardiovascular disease mortality among men with diabetes. Arch Intern Med 165(18):2114–2120
13. Duclos M, Gautier J (2009) Activité physique et diabète de type 2. Médecine des maladies métaboliques 3(1):31–38

14. EHIS (2019) European health interview survey (EHIS). Reference metadata in Euro SDMX metadata structure (ESMS). Compiling agency: Eurostat, the statistical office of the European Union. Techincal report
15. Ekelund U, Ward HA, Norat T, Luan J, May AM, Weiderpass E, Sharp SJ, Overvad K, Østergaard JN, Tjønneland A et al (2015) Physical activity and all-cause mortality across levels of overall and abdominal adiposity in European men and women: the European Prospective Investigation into Cancer and Nutrition Study (EPIC). Am J Clin Nutr 101(3):613–621
16. El Rhazi K, Nejjari C, Romaguera D, Feart C, Obtel M, Zidouh A, Bekkali R, Gateau PB (2012) Adherence to a Mediterranean diet in Morocco and its correlates: cross-sectional analysis of a sample of the adult Moroccan population. BMC Public Health 12(1):345
17. Engelke K, Kemmler W, Lauber D, Beeskow C, Pintag R, Kalender W (2006) Exercise maintains bone density at spine and hip EFOPS: a 3-year longitudinal study in early postmenopausal women. Osteoporos Int 17(1):133–142
18. Eriksen L, Dahl-Petersen I, Haugaard SB, Dela F (2007) Comparison of the effect of multiple short-duration with single long-duration exercise sessions on glucose homeostasis in type 2 diabetes mellitus. Diabetologia 50(11):2245–2253
19. Gregg EW, Gerzoff RB, Caspersen CJ, Williamson DF, Narayan KV (2003) Relationship of walking to mortality among US adults with diabetes. Arch Intern Med 163(12):1440–1447
20. Hales C, Carroll M, Fryar C, Ogden C (2017) Prevalence of obesity among adults and youth: United States, 2015–2016. NCHS data brief, pp 1–8
21. Haut Commissariat au Plan (2018) Les indicateurs sociaux au maroc. 311p
22. Hu G, Jousilahti P, Barengo NC, Qiao Q, Lakka TA, Tuomilehto J (2005) Physical activity, cardiovascular risk factors, and mortality among finnish adults with diabetes. Diabetes Care 28(4):799–805
23. King H, Kriska AM (1992) Prevention of type II diabetes by physical training: epidemiological considerations and study methods. Diabetes Care 15(11):1794–1799
24. Knowler WC, Barrett-Connor E, Fowler SE, Hamman RF, Lachin JM, Walker EA, Nathan DM (2002) Reduction in the incidence of type 2 diabetes with lifestyle intervention or metformin. N Engl J Med 346(6):393–403
25. Kulinski JP, Khera A, Ayers CR, Das SR, De Lemos JA, Blair SN, Berry JD (2014) Association between cardiorespiratory fitness and accelerometer-derived physical activity and sedentary time in the general population. Mayo Clin Proc 89:1063–1071
26. Lahmam A, Baali A, Hilali MK, Cherkaoui M, Chapuis-Lucciani N, Boëtsch G (2008) Obesity, overweight and body-weight perception in a High Atlas Moroccan population. Obes Rev 9(2):93–99
27. Lumb A (2014) Diabetes and exercise. Clin Med 14(6):673–676
28. Ministère de la santé du Maroc (2018a) Rapport de l'enquête nationale sur les facteurs de risque communs des maladie non transmissibles, steps, 2017–2018. 120p
29. Ministère de la santé du Maroc (2018b) Stratégie nationale multisectorielle de prévention et de contrôle des maladies non transmissibles 2019–2029. 44p
30. Nelson ME, Fiatarone MA, Morganti CM, Trice I, Greenberg RA, Evans WJ (1994) Effects of high-intensity strength training on multiple risk factors for osteoporotic fractures: a randomized controlled trial. Jama 272(24):1909–1914
31. OFS (2018) Rapport annuel 2017 : office fédéral de la statistique, Neuchâtel 2018, 48 pages. Numéro OFS 1237-1700-05. Technical report
32. OMS (2004) Stratégie mondiale pour l'alimentation, l'exercice physique et la santé. Genève, Suisse
33. OMS (2006) Prévenir les maladies chroniques: un investissement vital. Technical report
34. OMS (2014) Activité physique. http://www.who.int/dietphysicalactivity/pa/fr/. Accessed 15 Dec 2018
35. OMS (2016) Prévenir les maladies dans des environnements sains: évaluation globale de la charge de morbidité due aux risques environnementaux. 176p. Technical report, OMS
36. OMS (2017) Feuille de route de montevideo 2018-2030 sur les maladies non transmissibles en tant que priorité du développement durable. Conférence mondiale de l'OMS sur les maladies

non transmissibles Recherche d'une cohérence des politiques pour atteindre la cible 34 de l'ODD 3 sur les MNT, pp 18–20
37. Oudghiri DE, Ruiz-Cabello P, Camiletti-Moirón D, Fernández MDM, Aranda P, Aparicio VA (2016) Influence of weight status on physical and mental health in Moroccan perimenopausal women. Pan Afr Med J 23(1)
38. Quílez Llopis P, Reig García-Galbis M (2015) Control glucémico a través del ejercicio físico en pacientes con diabetes mellitus tipo 2: revisión sistemática. Nutrición Hospitalaria 31(4):1465–1472
39. Raynaud MH (2010) Les origines de l'épidémie de diabète et de maladies cardiovasculaires. Pojet: Double fardeau nutritionne/Pole francophone en Afrique Montréal, Canada: TRANSNUT
40. Ryan AS, Hurlbut DE, Lott ME, Ivey FM, Fleg J, Hurley BF, Goldberg AP (2001) Insulin action after resistive training in insulin resistant older men and women. J Am Geriatr Soc 49(3):247–253
41. Sebbani M, Dali MS, Amine M, Aouar A (2014) Prevalence of type 2 diabetes and factors associated in depression. L'Encephale 40(1):9–14
42. Shuval K, Finley CE, Barlow CE, Gabriel KP, Leonard D, Kohl HW III (2014) Sedentary behavior, cardiorespiratory fitness, physical activity, and cardiometabolic risk in men: the cooper center longitudinal study. Mayo Clin Proc 89:1052–1062
43. The Secretariat for the Intersectoral Healthy Living Network in partnership with the F/P/T Healthy Living Task Group and the F/P/T Advisory Committee on Population Health and Health Security (ACPHHS) (2005) The integrated pan-canadian healthy living strategy
44. UE (2013) Communication from the commission to the european parliament, the council, the european economic and social committee and the committee of the regions. A Clean Air Programme for Europe 12p
45. United Nations (2015) Transforming our world: The 2030 agenda for sustainable development. Resolution adopted by the General Assembly
46. WHO (1994) Déclaration d'Helsinki sur l'action pour l'environnement et la santé en Europe: deuxième Conférence européenne sur l'environnement et la santé, Helsinki, Finlande, 20–22 juin 1994. Technical report WHO Regional Office for Europe
47. WHO (2008) Burden: mortality, morbidity and risk factors. Technical report
48. WHO (2011) Global status report on noncommunicable diseases 2010. Technical report
49. WHO (2013) Global action plan for the prevention and control of noncommunicable diseases 2013–2020. Technical report
50. WHO (2014) Selected NCD expenditure within a full distribution of diseases using SHA 2011 framework in Morocco. Technical report
51. WHO (2016) Action plan for the prevention and control of noncommunicable diseases in the WHO European region. 39p. Technical report
52. WHO (2018) Global status report on noncommunicable diseases 2014. 302p. Technical report

# Chapter 5
# The Growing Trend of Noncommunicable Diseases in Arab Countries

**Wiam Boutayeb**

**Abstract** Being the leading cause of death worldwide, noncommunicable diseases are of the main health challenges of the 21st century. Beside the toll of death, these chronic diseases burden individuals, families and the whole society. Following economic, demographic and geographic transitions most of Arab countries are facing an increasing trend in noncommunicable diseases. Mortality caused by these diseases is greater than 70% of all deaths in 12 countries. Moreover, premature death caused by these diseases reaches 20% in 33% of Arab countries. Risk factors like raised blood pressure, unhealthy diet, smoking, obesity and physical inactivity are well known to contribute to the increasing trend of noncommunicable diseases. Action on social determinants of health such as gender, economic status, education level, marital status can reduce simultaneously the burden of noncommunicable diseases and avoidable/unacceptable health inequalities between different categories of Arab populations.

## 5.1 Introduction

One of the biggest challenges currently facing humanity is noncommunicable diseases (NCDs) which are sweeping the entire globe, with an increasing trend in developing countries [5]. Aware of this challenge, the World Health Organisation and the United Nations are trying to convince governments and health decision makers to act on risk factors behind the increasing prevalence of NCDs. In September 2011, at the United Nations General Assembly in New York, a political declaration was made to strengthen global and national responses to prevent and control NCDs [12, 15]. As stressed by the Assistant Director-General of the World Health Organisation (WHO) in her forward to the NCDs country profile 2018, "e human toll of noncommunicable diseases is unacceptable. These diseases are the leading causes of death worldwide and carry a huge cost that extends beyond health to trap people in poverty, deny them a life of dignity, undermine workforce productivity, and threaten economic prosperity"

W. Boutayeb (✉)
School of High Studies in Engineering, Oujda, Morocco
e-mail: wiam.boutayeb@gmail.com



A. Boutayeb (ed.), *Disease Prevention and Health Promotion in Developing Countries*,
https://doi.org/10.1007/978-3-030-34702-4_5

[16]. According to data released by the World Health Organisation, noncommunicable diseases caused 71% of the world' 57 million deaths that occurred in 2016, with 15 million premature deaths (30–70 years). Nearly 80% of deaths and 85% of premature deaths caused by NCDs occurred in Low- and middle- income countries. The costly and prolonged care of NCDs in low-and middle-income countries often divert the scarce family and societal resources to medical care. Consequently, the lower socio-economic groups have greater prevalence of risk factors, higher incidence of disease and higher mortality [4, 8, 16]. Among the targets fixed for NCDs in the 2030 Agenda for Sustainable Development Goals [13], a global target of a 25% relative reduction in overall mortality from the four major noncommunicable diseases (cardiovascular diseases, cancers, diabetes, and chronic respiratory diseases). Other targets are devoted to the reduction of risk factors including both metabolic risk factors (raised blood pressure, raised blood glucose and obesity) and behavioural risk factors (tobacco, alcohol, physical inactivity, salt/sodium intake, unhealthy diet).

## 5.2 Noncommunicable Diseases in Arab Countries

Most of Arab countries have high rates of noncommunicable diseases. Mortality caused by these diseases is greater than 70% of all deaths in 12 out of 17 countries with available data. The 17 countries may be classified into three main groups: a first group (Lebanon, Tunisia, Egypt, Bahrain and Morocco) with mortality caused by NCDs higher than or equal to 80%, a second group (Jordan, UAE, Algeria, Saudi Arabia, Kuwait, Libya and Oman) with mortality caused by NCDs between 70% and 80%, and a third group (Yemen, Iraq, Sudan and Syria) with mortality caused by NCDs between 40 and 60%. People living in Lebanon are more than twice likely to die from noncommunicable diseases than their counterparts living in Syria (Fig. 5.1 and Table 5.1).

Noncommunicable diseases cause also high rates of premature deaths in Arab countries, with more than 33% of countries experiencing a premature death caused by noncommunicable diseases higher than 20%. There are large gaps between countries, showing that a Yemeni person is, in average, nearly three times more exposed to

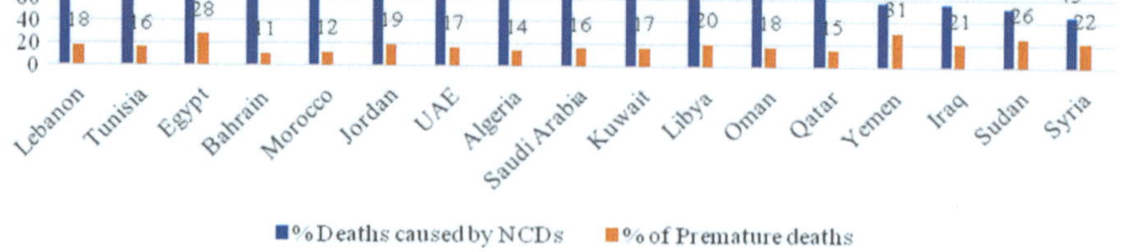


Fig. 5.1 Percent of mortality caused by NCDs and premature deaths in Arab countries

**Table 5.1** Mortality caused by noncommunicable diseases and premature death

| | CVDs % | Cancers % | CRD % | Diabetes % | NCDs % | Risk of premature death from NCDs (30–70 years) % | | |
|---|---|---|---|---|---|---|---|---|
| Algeria | 36 | 13 | 3 | 4 | 76 | M: 15 | F: 13 | Total: 14 |
| Bahrain | 18 | 16 | 3 | 14 | 83 | M: 11 | F: 12 | Total: 11 |
| Egypt | 40 | 13 | 4 | 3 | 84 | M: 32 | F: 24 | Total: 28 |
| Iraq | 27 | 11 | 2 | 4 | 55 | M: 25 | F: 18 | Total: 21 |
| Jordan | 37 | 12 | 3 | 6 | 78 | M: 23 | F: 16 | Total: 19 |
| Kuwait | 41 | 15 | 3 | 3 | 72 | M: 19 | F: 15 | Total: 17 |
| Lebanon | 47 | 16 | 4 | 5 | 91 | M: 20 | F: 15 | Total: 18 |
| Libya | 35 | 12 | 3 | 4 | 72 | M: 24 | F: 16 | Total: 20 |
| Morocco | 38 | 14 | 4 | 6 | 80 | M: 13 | F: 11 | Total: 12 |
| Oman | 36 | 11 | 2 | 8 | 72 | M: 19 | F: 15 | Total: 18 |
| Qatar | 27 | 16 | 1 | 9 | 69 | M: 16 | F: 14 | Total: 15 |
| Saudi Arabia | 37 | 10 | 3 | 3 | 73 | M: 18 | F: 14 | Total: 16 |
| Sudan | 28 | 6 | 3 | 2 | 52 | M: 28 | F: 24 | Total: 26 |
| Syria | 25 | 9 | 2 | 1 | 45 | M: 25 | F: 19 | Total: 22 |
| UAE | 40 | 12 | 5 | 5 | 77 | M: 17 | F: 15 | Total: 17 |
| Tunisia | 44 | 12 | 4 | 5 | 86 | M: 20 | F: 12 | Total: 16 |
| Yemen | 33 | 6 | 4 | 2 | 57 | M: 33 | F: 28 | Total: 31 |

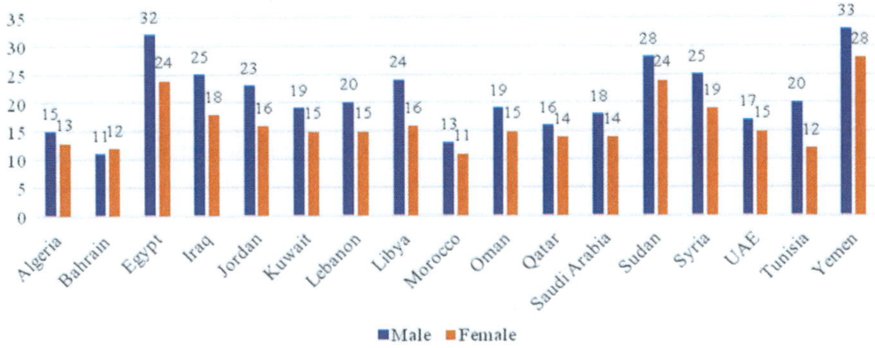


**Fig. 5.2** Premature deaths caused by NCDs in Arab countries by gender

premature death than a Bahraini person (Fig. 5.1 and Table 5.1). Differences may also be seen within each country, but disaggregated data is not available. The average percent of premature deaths is slightly higher in men (21%) than in women (16.5%) (Fig. 5.2 and Table 5.1). The difference between men and women is greater than 5% in 8 countries and reaches 8% in three countries (Egypt, Libya and Tunisia). The Chi square test indicates that gender difference is not statistically different.

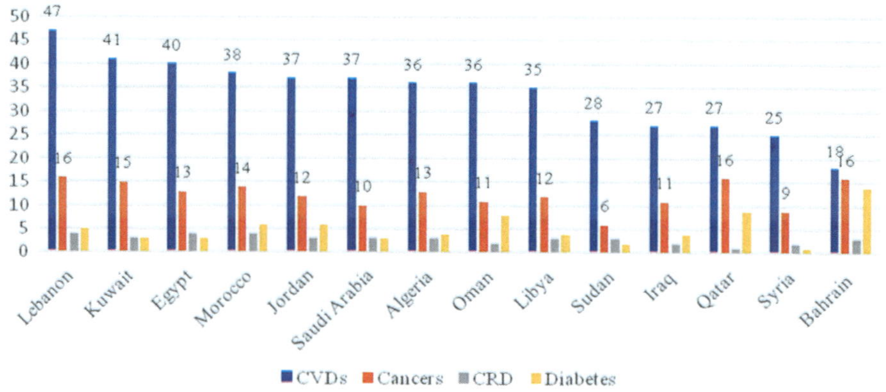


**Fig. 5.3** percent of mortality caused by CVDS, Cancers, Chronic Respiratory Diseases and Diabetes in Arab countries

Cardiovascular diseases are prominent in all Arab countries and mortality caused by these diseases is over 40% in three countries (Lebanon, Kuwait and Egypt). However, the range between the highest level of mortality (47% in Lebanon) and the lowest level of mortality in Bahrain (18%) indicates a ratio of 2.6. Except in three countries (Sudan, Syria and Yemen), cancer is killing between 10 and 20% of people living in Arab countries. Once more, a large gap is seen between the highest level of mortality caused by cancer (16% in Bahrain, Lebanon and Qatar) and the lowest level of mortality caused by cancer (6% in Sudan and Yemen) (Fig. 5.3 and Table 5.1). The trend of diabetes prevalence is increasing in Arab countries. According to the 2017 data released by the International Diabetes Federation (IDF), the number of people with diabetes (20–79 years) in Middle East & North Africa will increase by 110% between 2017 (39 Million) and 2045 (82 Million). Countries of the Gulf are among the countries with the highest diabetes age-adjusted (20–79) comparative prevalence (Saudi Arabia 17.7%, EAU 17.3%, Bahrain 16.5%, Qatar 16.5% and Kuwait 15.8%) [11]. In a previous paper dealing with the rise of diabetes prevalence in the Arab region, it was indicated that human development was highly correlated with diabetes prevalence [6]. As indicated by Fig. 5.3 and Table 5.1, diabetes is killing in average more than 5% of people in the Arab region. The difference is, however, ranging from 1% in Syria to 14% in Bahrain.

Chronic Respiratory Diseases (CRD) are the fourth killer among noncommunicable disease in Arab countries, ranging from 1 to 4% (Fig. 5.3 and Table 5.1).

## 5.3 Risk Factors

The four main noncommunicable diseases discussed in the previous section, namely, CVDs, cancer, diabetes and chronic respiratory diseases have a common denominator which is the risk factors. Indeed, smoking, high blood pressure, obesity and physical

**Table 5.2** Risk factors of noncommunicable diseases in Arab countries

| | Raised blood pressure (%) | | | Raised blood glucose (%) | | | Smoking (%) | | | Obesity adults 18 or + (%) | | | Physical inactivity (%) | | |
|---|---|---|---|---|---|---|---|---|---|---|---|---|---|---|---|
| | M | F | T | M | F | T | M | F | T | M | F | T | M | F | T |
| Algeria | 22 | 21 | 22 | 10 | 11 | 11 | 31 | 1 | 16 | 19 | 34 | 27 | 25 | 39 | 32 |
| Bahrain | 18 | 14 | 16 | 9 | 8 | 9 | 38 | 5 | 27 | 25 | 36 | 29 | | | |
| Egypt | 22 | 23 | 23 | 14 | 18 | 16 | 49 | 0 | 25 | 22 | 40 | 31 | 22 | 38 | 30 |
| Iraq | 20 | 19 | 19 | 13 | 14 | 13 | | | | 21 | 34 | 27 | 37 | 64 | 50 |
| Jordan | 19 | 14 | 16 | 13 | 14 | 13 | | | | 27 | 40 | 33 | 10 | 13 | 10 |
| Kuwait | 20 | 13 | 18 | 15 | 15 | 15 | 40 | 3 | 24 | 33 | 44 | 37 | 60 | 73 | 65 |
| Lebanon | 23 | 17 | 20 | 14 | 11 | 13 | 41 | 26 | 33 | 27 | 35 | 31 | 40 | 33 | 36 |
| Libya | 23 | 19 | 21 | 13 | 14 | 14 | | | | 25 | 39 | 32 | 29 | 40 | 34 |
| Morocco | 24 | 24 | 24 | 13 | 12 | 13 | 48 | 1 | 24 | 19 | 32 | 26 | 20 | 31 | 25 |
| Oman | 17 | 15 | 16 | 7 | 8 | 8 | 16 | 0 | 12 | 20 | 31 | 23 | 27 | 38 | 31 |
| Qatar | 16 | 12 | 15 | 13 | 13 | 13 | 29 | 1 | 22 | 32 | 42 | 34 | 30 | 46 | 34 |
| Saudi Arabia | 21 | 16 | 19 | 15 | 14 | 14 | 26 | 2 | 16 | 31 | 41 | 35 | 44 | 64 | 52 |
| Syria | 21 | 19 | 20 | 11 | 13 | 12 | | | | 19 | 32 | 26 | | | |
| UAE | 15 | 9 | 13 | 8 | 9 | 8 | 38 | 1 | 29 | 27 | 39 | 30 | 36 | 46 | 38 |
| Tunisia | 23 | 22 | 23 | 12 | 13 | 12 | 66 | 1 | 33 | 19 | 35 | 27 | 25 | 33 | 29 |
| Yemen | 23 | 22 | 23 | 8 | 7 | 8 | 28 | 7 | 17 | 10 | 18 | 14 | | | |

inactivity are indicated, at different levels, as risk factors in the four classes of NCDs. Moreover, these risk factors are seen to affect people worldwide with an increasing tendency [5]. In the Arab countries, these risk factors have high and sometimes very high rates (Table 5.2).

### *5.3.1 Blood Pressure*

Hypertension or raised blood pressure constitutes a major risk factor for many non-communicable diseases, including stroke, coronary heart disease and chronic kidney disease. Heart failure, peripheral vascular disease, renal failure, retinal hemorrhage, visual impairment, stroke and dementia (23) can all be caused by complications of uncontrolled hypertension. The World Health Organisation has fixed a global target of 25% relative reduction in the prevalence of raised blood pressure by 2025 [18]. Decision makers in the Arab countries should be really concerned with the reduction target fixed by WHO. Indeed, raised blood pressure affects 20% of the Arab population in average, slightly higher in men (20.5%) than in women (14.5%) and with large gaps between countries ranging from 9% in UAE to 24% in Morocco for women and from 15 to 24% for men in the same countries (Fig. 5.4 and Table 5.2).

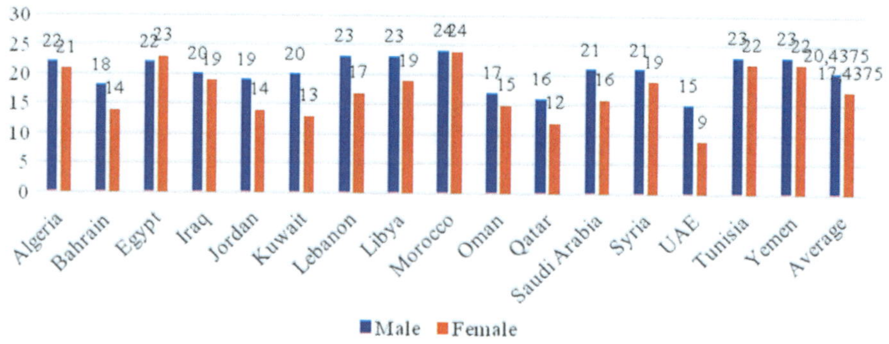


Fig. 5.4 Raised blood pressure by gender in the Arab countries, 2016

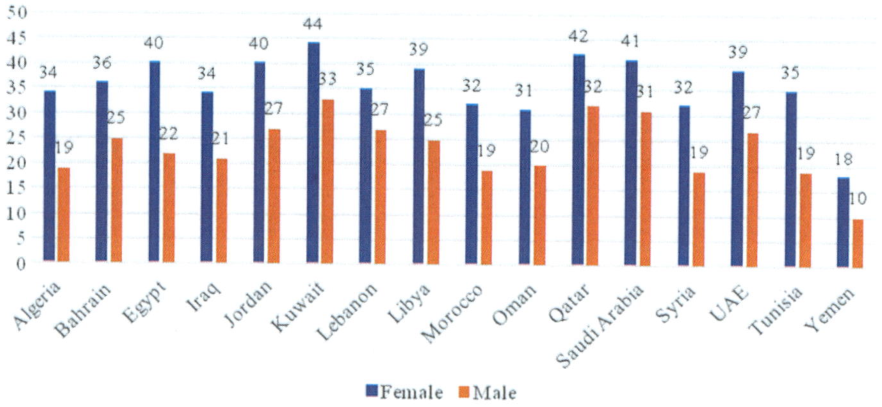


Fig. 5.5 Obesity by gender in the Arab countries, 2016

### 5.3.2 *Obesity*

Nearly 30% of the Arab population is suffering from obesity but large differences are seen between countries and between men and women. As illustrated by Fig. 5.5, women (35.75% in average) are more obese than men (23.5% in average) and the gap between. More precisely, obesity in women ranges from 18% in Yemen to 44% in Kuwait while in men, it varies from 10 to 33% in the same countries.

### 5.3.3 *Smoking*

Smoking in the Arab countries presents a particular feature since, except in Labanon, the percent of smoker women is very low while the percent of men smokers reaches 40% in Kuwait, 41% in Lebanon, 48% in Morocco, 49% in Egypt and jumps to 66% in Tunisia (Fig. 5.6).

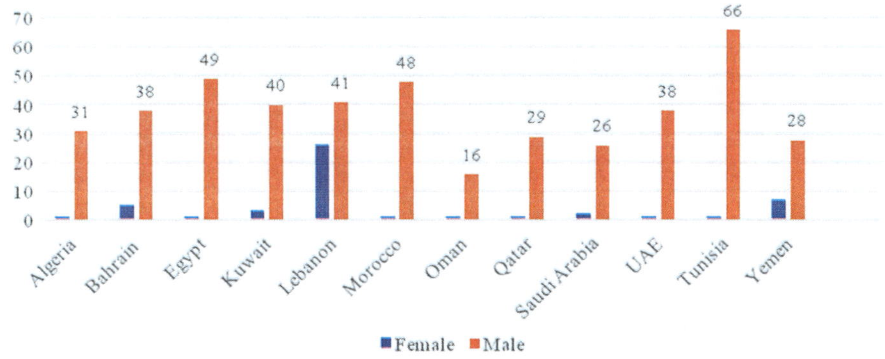


**Fig. 5.6** Smoking by gender in the Arab countries, 2016

### *5.3.4 Physical Inactivity*

Physical activity lowers the risk of stroke, diabetes, hypertension, depression and other diseases. Compared to people who do at least 30 min of moderate-intensity physical activity most days of the week, insufficiently active people have an increased risk of all-cause mortality [18]. Stressing the role of physical activity for well-being and good health in its physical and mental aspects, the Sixty-sixth World Health Assembly in 2013 adopted a global target of a 10% reduction in levels of physical inactivity by 2025 [18]. As in the majority of countries in the world, Arab people are doing less and less physical effort. Iraq and Countries of the Gulf exhibit the higher levels of inactivity while Jordan appears as the country largely the most active. In all countries, women (43% in average) are less active then men (31% in average) but there is a huge gap in physical inactivity between countries, showing a ratio of six or nearly six between men and women living in Kuwait and their counterparts living in Jordan (Fig. 5.7).

## 5.4 Social Determinants of Health and Multimorbidity

During the last two decades, social determinants of health and health equity have known an important development [9]. In 2005, the World Health Organization launched the WHO Commission on Social Determinants of Health which delivered its well-known report in 2008 under the title "Closing the gap in a generation: health equity through action on the social determinants of health". Defined as the conditions in which people are born, grow, live, work and age, including the health system, social determinants of health are seen to be responsible for unfair and avoidable health inequalities within and between countries [10]. In 2011, the Rio Political Declaration on Social Determinants of health adopted by heads of government, ministers and government representatives, stressed that health equity should become part

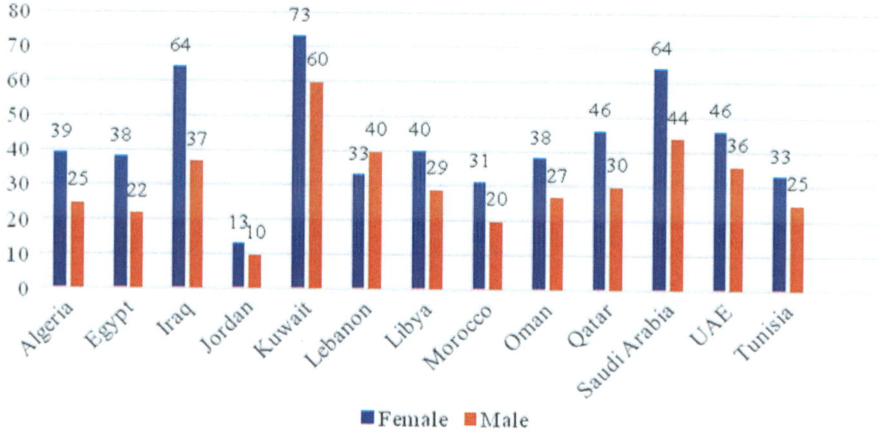


**Fig. 5.7** Physical inactivity by gender in the Arab countries, 2016

**Table 5.3** The 2011 Rio Political Declaration: five Action areas on SDH

| | |
|---|---|
| 1 | Adopt better governance for health and development |
| 2 | Promote participation in policymaking and implementation |
| 3 | Further reorient the health sector towards promoting health and reducing health inequities |
| 4 | Strengthen global governance and collaboration |
| 5 | Monitor progress and increase accountability |

of a government's social and health agenda [17]. For pragmatic strategies in countries, five action areas on social determinants of health were proposed (Table 5.3)

In 2014, a technical report of the WHO Eastern Mediterranean region analysed health iniquities in selected countries of the region. Inequalities were described and analysed between and within selected countries according to many health indicators, including life expectancy, infant and under-five mortality, stunting, coverage of skilled birth attendance, antenatal visits and place of birth. An important finding was that socioeconomic factors together contributed to 60–75% in inequities in skilled birth attendance at delivery [19] (Fig. 5.8).

In order to foster pragmatic action on SDH by national governments, international organizations, and civil society and considering the needs of key indicator users, an interdisciplinary working group (WG) was established by WHO and its Canadian partners, the Public Health Agency of Canada (PHAC), and the Canadian Institutes of Health Research—Institute of Population and Public Health (CIHR–IPPH) in 2016. The working group proposed a core set of the 15–20 selected indicators [14].

Many Arab countries are engaged in the multidimensional transition (economic, demographic, epidemiological and geographical) which is boosting increases in multimorbidity of depression and mental diseases, cardiovascular diseases, diabetes, cancer and respiratory diseases among the whole population but with the highest burden

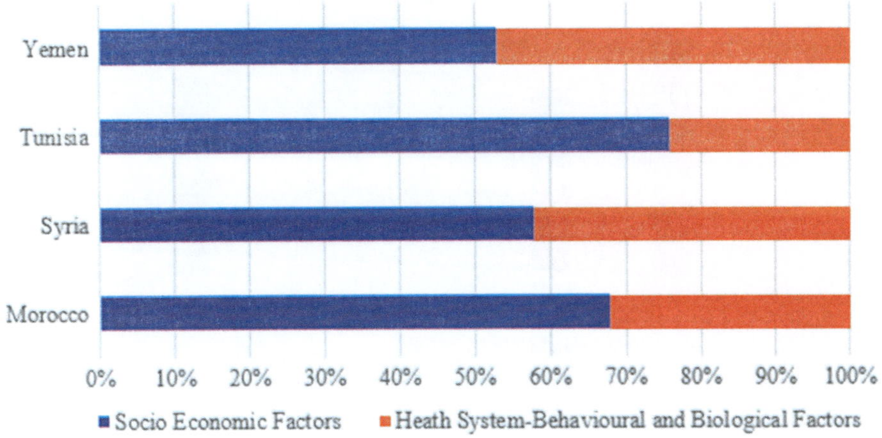


**Fig. 5.8** Contribution of socioeconomic factors in skilled birth attendance *Source* WHO-EMRO [19]

among the least disadvantaged individuals or subpopulation. A previous review on multi-morbidity of noncommunicable diseases and health equity in the WHO Eastern Mediterranean region showed that socio demographic and socioeconomic variables were found to be associated with multimorbidity. Generally, older age, female gender, low education and low income people were seen to be likelier to suffer from multimorbidity [7].

A 6-month registry (Gulf RACE), conducted in six countries of the Arabian gulf in 2007 found that, in the Arab Middle East, patients with acute coronary syndrome (ACS) are about a decade younger compared to their counterparts in developed countries and have a higher prevalence of diabetes, hypertension [20]. Between January 2012 and January 2013, the Gulf COAST registry allowed collecting exhaustive data on patients with confirmed acute coronary syndrome (ACS) from 29 hospitals in four countries: Bahrain, Kuwait, Oman and United Arab Emirates (UAE) [2, 3, 21, 22]. In a previous study using data of the Gulf COAST registry, Al Ali et al. [1] showed how diabetes is affected by social determinants of health like gender, country of residence, education level, marital status and work status. Among the 4061 patients enrolled in the Gulf COAST registry with diagnosed ACS, more than half of them had diabetes (53.26%), with type2 diabetes representing 99%. The mean age was slightly lower in the Gulf registry (60.35 years and 60 years) than in the subpopulation of diabetics (61.97 years and 62 years). The average duration of diabetes was 12.7 years ($\pm$ SD:12.73). Although women represented only 33.59% of patients with ACS, the proportion of women with ACS and diabetes was 40.59%. Consequently, the prevalence of diabetes is higher in women (64.3%) than in men (47.64%) (Fig. 5.9). This difference is statistically significant ($p$-value $< 0.0001$).

The same study [1] found that nearly 80% of diabetes were obese (39.17%) or overweight (38.77%). Again, women (51.56%) were much more affected by obe-

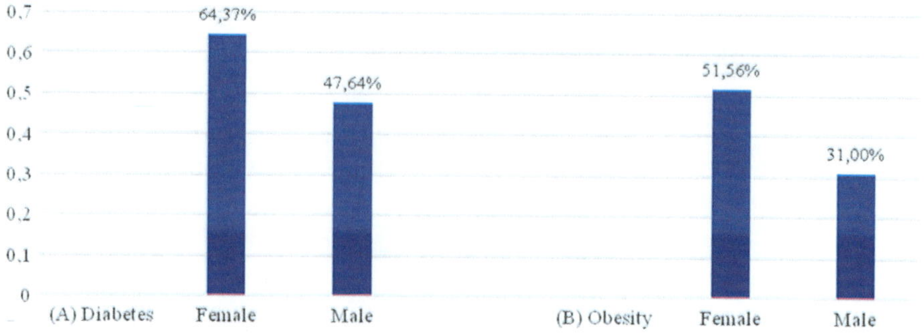


**Fig. 5.9** Prevalence of diabetes and obesity by gender

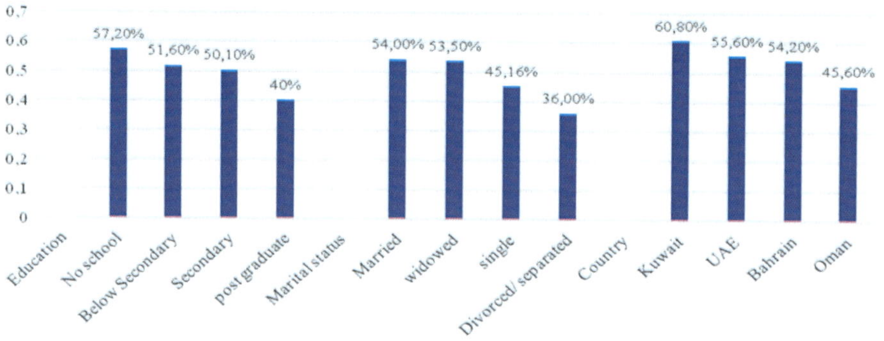


**Fig. 5.10** Prevalence of diabetes by education, marital status and country

sity than men (31%). As indicated by Fig. 5.10, a steepest gradient was seen in the prevalence of diabetes by level of education, marital status and country of residence. Indeed, education level shows a gap between post graduate (40%), secondary (50.1%), below secondary (51.6%) and no school (57.2%). Disaggregation according to marital status follows a similar trend of inequality between divorced/separated (36.11%), single (45.16%), widowed (53.53%) and married (53.96%). Finally, territorial disparity also indicates a clear difference between Oman (45.59%), Bahrain (54.17%), UAE (55.62%) and Kuwait (60.76%). The difference is highly significant ($p$-value $< 0.001$) in the three cases.

Exception is given by work (full or part-time) (52.95%) or no work (53.71%) showing no significant difference in the prevalence of diabetes.

## 5.5 Conclusion

Noncommunicable diseases are one of the biggest challenges currently facing health decision makers in Arab countries. Action on both behavioural risks factors (unhealthy diet, smoking, salt, alcohol, physical inactivity) and metabolic risk factors( raised blood pressure, raised blood sugar, obesity) are needed to halt the increasing trend of noncommunicable diseases and consequently to reduce mortality and especially premature mortality caused by these diseases. Action on social determinants of health like gender, economic status, territory, education level and residence (rural-urban) should contribute to the reduction of noncommunicable diseases as well as the reduction of heath inequalities. Health equity analysis shows that, beside a relatively high prevalence of diabetes in the Gulf countries, there is a disparity according to different social determinants of health. This highlights clearly the crucial need of action on SDH and calls health decision makers in these countries to reorient their action by taking women, no educated and married people, as more exposed to diabetes and hence necessitating more attention. Urgent and efficient actions on social determinants of health are needed to stop (and ideally to reverse) the incredible increasing trend of NCDs in Arab countries. This conclusion agrees pragmatically with a widespread global recognition that "reducing health inequities is an ethical imperative and that social injustice is killing people on grand scale" [10].

## References

1. Al Ali H, Boutayeb W, Boutayeb A (2018) Diabetes and acute coronary syndrome in four countries of the gulf. In: Fourth CVOT Summit in cooperation with D&CVD EASD Study Group, Munich, Germany
2. Al-Roomi F, Khesroh A, Al-Zakwani I, Attur S, Rashed W, Zubaid M (2018) Lifestyle changes among acs survivors in arabian gulf countries (gulf coast registry). Curr Vasc Pharmacol 16(4):363–367
3. Al-Zakwani I, Zubaid M, Alsheikh-Ali AA, Almahmeed W, Rashed W (2018) Effect of evidence-based cardiac drug therapy on mortality in patients with acute coronary syndrome: findings from the gulf coast registry. Cardiovasc Ther 36(6):e12463
4. Boutayeb A (2006) The double burden of communicable and non-communicable diseases in developing countries. Trans R Soc Trop Med Hyg 100(3):191–199
5. Boutayeb A, Boutayeb S (2005) The burden of non communicable diseases in developing countries. Int J Equity Health 4(1):2
6. Boutayeb A, Lamlili ME, Boutayeb W, Maamri A, Ziyyat A, Ramdani N (2012) The rise of diabetes prevalence in the arab region. Open J Epidemiol 2(2):55–60
7. Boutayeb A, Boutayeb S, Boutayeb W (2013) Multi-morbidity of non communicable diseases and equity in who eastern mediterranean countries. Int J Equity Health 12(1):60
8. Boutayeb A, Boutayeb W, Lamlili ME, Boutayeb S (2014) Estimation of the direct cost of diabetes in the arab region. Mediterr J Nutr Metab 7(1):21–32
9. Braveman P (2006) Health disparities and health equity: concepts and measurement. Annu Rev Public Health 27:167–194
10. Commission on Social Determinants of Health and others (2008) Closing the gap in a generation: health equity through action on the social determinants of health: final report of the commission on social determinants of health
11. International Diabetes Foundation (2017) Diabetes atlas 2017. https://www.idf.org/e-library/epidemiology-research/diabetes-atlas/134-idf-diabetes-atlas-8th-edition.html
12. United Nations (2012) Political declaration of the high-level meeting of the general assembly on the prevention and control of non-communicable diseases. https://digitallibrary.un.org/record/720106/files/A_RES_66_2-EN.pdf

13. United Nations (2015) Transforming our world: the 2030 agenda for sustainable development
14. Working Group for Monitoring Action on the Social Determinants of Health (2018) Towards a global monitoring system for implementing the rio political declaration on social determinants of health: developing a core set of indicators for government action on the social determinants of health to improve health equity. Int J Equity Health 17:1–27
15. World Health Organisation (2018) Third united nations high-level meeting on ncds. https://www.who.int/ncds/governance/third-un-meeting/en/
16. World Health Organisation (2019) Noncommunicable diseases country profile. https://www.who.int/nmh/publications/ncd-profiles-2018/en/
17. World Health Organization and others (2011) Rio political declaration on social determinants of health. In: World conference on social determinants of health, Rio de Janeiro, pp 19–21
18. World Health Organization and others (2013) Global action plan for the prevention and control of noncommunicable diseases 2013–2020. http://www.who.int/nmh/events/ncd_action_plan/en/
19. World Health Organization and others (2015) Health inequities in the eastern mediterranean region: selected country case studies
20. Zubaid M, Rashed WA, Almahmeed W, Al-Lawati J, Sulaiman K, Al-Motarreb A, Amin H, Al Suwaidi J, Alhabib K (2009) Management and outcomes of middle eastern patients admitted with acute coronary syndromes in the gulf registry of acute coronary events (gulf race). Acta Cardiol 64(4):439–446
21. Zubaid M, Thani KB, Rashed W, Alsheikh-Ali A, Alrawahi N, Ridha M, Akbar M, Alenezi F, Alhamdan R, Almahmeed W et al (2014) Design and rationale of gulf locals with acute coronary syndrome events (gulf coast) registry. Open Cardiovasc Med J 8:88
22. Zubaid M, Rashed W, Alsheikh-Ali AA, Garadah T, Alrawahi N, Ridha M, Akbar M, Alenezi F, Alhamdan R, Almahmeed W et al (2017) Disparity in st-segment elevation myocardial infarction practices and outcomes in arabian gulf countries (gulf coast registry). Hear Views Off J Gulf Hear Assoc 18(2):41

# Chapter 6
# Magnitude of Overweight, Obesity and Physical Inactivity as Risk Factors of Major Non-communicable Diseases in North African Countries

**Slimane Mehdad, Souad Benaich and Nezha Bouhaddou**

**Abstract** Over the past two decades, overweight, obesity and physical inactivity have been recognized as major risk factors of numerous non-communicable diseases. Their prevalence reached alarming rates among all age-groups, particularly in Low- and Middle Income Countries. In North African countries, available data from official reports released by the WHO, UNICEF and national authorities, as well as research articles (PubMed, Sciencedirect, Scholar Google), published between 2000 and 2018, showed that overweight prevalence in children aged 0–5 years ranged from 1.2 to 14.0%. Among children and adolescents, the prevalence of each of overweight and obesity ranged from 6.3% to 32.5%, and from 2.4% to 9.3%, respectively; while in adults it ranged from 30.0% to 65.4% and from 10.0 % to 35.7%, respectively. Physical inactivity prevalence ranged from 14.6 to 45.8% among adults aged 18 years and older, and from 79.3 to 90.6% among children and adolescents. The prevalence of overweight, obesity and physical inactivity is high in North African populations especially among females. Appropriate interventions are urgently needed to promote physical activity and healthy lifestyle, and to reduce the economic and health burden of overweight and obesity among both children and adults according to a multi-sectoral, multi-disciplinary, and culturally relevant approach.

## 6.1 Introduction

Obesity has become one of the most serious public health issues of the twenty-first century. It has reached epidemic proportions worldwide and its implications regarding both physical and economic health are rising continuously [21]. The global obe-

S. Mehdad (✉) · S. Benaich · N. Bouhaddou
Faculty of Sciences, Laboratory of Animal Physiology, Research Centre of Human Pathologies Genomics, Mohammed V University, Rabat, Morocco
e-mail: slimanemehdad@gmail.com

S. Benaich
e-mail: souad.benaich@gmail.com

N. Bouhaddou
e-mail: bouhaddounezha@gmail.com

 
A. Boutayeb (ed.), *Disease Prevention and Health Promotion in Developing Countries*,
https://doi.org/10.1007/978-3-030-34702-4_6

sity prevalence has nearly tripled over the last four decades. In 2016, overweight and obesity prevalence among adults aged 18 years and over was 39% and 13%, respectively, and more than 18% of children and adolescents aged 5–19 were overweight or obese [56]. The increasing prevalence of overweight and obesity is associated with emergence of many comorbidities including cardiovascular diseases, hypertension, diabetes, dislipidemia, musculoskeletal disorders, asthma, sleep apnea, low self-esteem, psychological problems, and some cancers [31, 44]. Many studies have demonstrated the strong association between overweight and obesity and several major non-communicable diseases (NCDs), and the main pathological events seen in obesity such as chronic low-grade inflammation due to increased leptin levels and oxidative stress are primarily responsible for the development of these diseases [4]. The insufficiency of important organ systems like blood vessels due to increased fat mass in overweight and obese individuals contributes also to the NCDs [7]. Thus, overweight and obesity are among the leading risk factors of morbidity and premature mortality. It is estimated that at least 35.8 million of global disability-adjusted life years are caused by overweight and obesity, and that 2.8 million people die each year as a result of being overweight or obese [56]. Overweight and obesity result from many contributing factors, including individual factors such as genetics and behavior (dietary patterns, physical activity, inactivity, medication use . . .). Other obesogenic factors like food and physical activity environment, education and skills, and food marketing and promotion have resulted in increased prevalence of overweight and obesity [59]. However, the energy imbalance between calories consumed from foods and beverages and calories expended in normal body functions and through physical activity remains the main cause of overweight and obesity [56]. Given their health and socioeconomic negative impacts, overweight and obesity have gained traction for vital prevention and treatment efforts over the last few years all over the world [59]. However, their prevalence is increasing in both developed and developing countries, and the effects of this attention on the disease burden and the associated health care costs remain uncertain [36]. As in many developing countries, the North African countries (Algeria, Egypt, Libya, Mauritania, Morocco, and Tunisia) are experiencing a steady increase in overweight and obesity prevalence due to rapid dietary changes, with increased intake of energy-dense foods, and decline in physical activity among all age groups [5, 17, 21]. Despite their current alarming trends, and recognition of the potential rise in obesity-related diseases, there is little evidence of proper diagnosis, treatment and/or prevention of overweight and obesity in these countries [1]. Accordingly, an analysis of overweight and obesity prevalence and physical inactivity as contributing factors across several countries may provide useful insights into the extent of the problem over time and inform policy and programme interventions to address the challenge in North African countries.

## 6.2 Overweight and Obesity

### *6.2.1 Definitions*

WHO defines overweight and obesity as abnormal or excessive fat accumulation that may impair health [56]. These conditions are classified based on body-mass index (BMI) calculated by mass as measured in kilograms divided by the square of height measured in meters ($kg/m^2$). For adults (individuals above the age of 18 years), overweight is defined as having a BMI between 25 and 30 $kg/m^2$; and obesity is defined as having a BMI greater than or equal to 30 $kg/m^2$. For children and adolescents (individuals under the age of 18 years), classification of overweight and obesity is based on growth references (sex-specific BMI-for-age charts and tables). The main growth references commonly used to assess children weight status are: International Obesity Task Force (IOTF) [8], Centers for Disease Control and Prevention (CDC) [28], and 2007 WHO [35].

### *6.2.2 Prevalence of Overweight and Obesity in North African Countries*

#### 6.2.2.1 Prevalence Among Preschool Children

Overweight and obesity among preschool children in North Africa has increased rapidly in the past three decades. Using the WHO standards, the estimated prevalence and trends of combined overweight and obesity among children aged 0–5 years in this region in 1990, 2000, 2010 and 2020, were 6.1%, 10.3%, 17.0% and 26.6%, respectively [11]. Although there are some surveys on overweight and obesity prevalence among preschool children in this region, the majority of the published papers was not based on nationally representative samples and was more focused on specific areas in their respective country. Available data indicate that overweight prevalence among children aged 0–5 years in Algeria, Egypt, Libya, Mauritania, Morocco and Tunisia ranged from 1.2% in Mauritania to as high as 14.0% in Egypt (Table 6.1). Being obese was least prevalent in Egypt (3.7%) and highest in Tunisia (11.6%).

#### 6.2.2.2 Prevalence Among Children and Adolescents

Currently childhood obesity is one of the major health issues worldwide. There is evidence that childhood obesity leads to adult obesity and predisposes individuals to an increased risk of morbidity and mortality. Its prevalence in children and adolescents has increased substantially worldwide in recent decades [56]. The estimated prevalence of childhood overweight in North African countries ranged from 6.3% in Tunisia to as high as 32.5% in Egypt (Table 6.2). Similarly, the lowest obesity

**Table 6.1** Prevalence of overweight and obesity among preschool children aged 0–5 years in North African countries

| Country | Date of survey | Sample size | Age (year) | Prevalence of overweight | | | Prevalence of obesity | | | References |
|---|---|---|---|---|---|---|---|---|---|---|
| | | | | Total | Males | Females | Total | Males | Females | |
| Algeria | 2012 | | 0–5 | 12.4 | 12.9 | 12.0 | | | | [46] |
| Egypt | 2014 | 3871 | 0–5 | 11.8 | | | 3.7 | | | [41] |
| Libya | 2003 | 7232 | 0–5 | | 13.9 | 12.9 | | | | [15] |
| Mauritania | 2000 | | 0–5 | 3.8 | 3.9 | 3.7 | | | | [47] |
| | 2012 | | 0–5 | 1.2 | | | | | | [54] |
| Morocco | 2004 | 5381 | 0–5 | | 17.8 | 13.2 | 5.1 | | | [15] |
| Tunisia | 2006 | | 0–5 | | 5.6 | 7.2 | | | | [15] |
| | 2011 | 1335 | 4–6 | 9.1 | | | 11.6 | | | [15] |

**Table 6.2** Prevalence of overweight and obesity among children and adolescents in North African countries

| Country | Date of survey | Sample size | Age (year) | Prevalence of overweight | | | Prevalence of obesity | | | References |
|---|---|---|---|---|---|---|---|---|---|---|
| | | | | Total | Males | Females | Total | Males | Females | |
| Algeria | 2011 | 4532 | 13–15 | 13.7 | 10.9 | 16.3 | 3.2 | 3.0 | 3.4 | [50] |
| | 2013 | | <20 | | 21.7 | 30.0 | | 7.7 | 15.3 | [34] |
| | 2015 | | 5–19 | | 31.2 | 30.0 | | 13.9 | 12.4 | [46] |
| Egypt | 2011 | 2568 | 13–15 | 32.5 | 30.7 | 34.1 | 7.0 | 6.8 | 7.1 | [51] |
| | 2014 | 5179 | 11–17 | 31.4 | | | 9.3 | | | [29] |
| | 2013 | | <20 | | 31.5 | 39.5 | | 12.7 | 14.4 | [34] |
| Libya | 2007 | 2242 | 13–15 | 26.0 | 23.4 | 28.7 | 8.2 | 7.6 | 8.7 | [48] |
| | 2013 | | <20 | | 32.5 | 41.7 | | 14.5 | 22.1 | [34] |
| Mauritania | 2010 | 2063 | 13–15 | 22.5 | 17.6 | 28.0 | 3.0 | 1.8 | 4.3 | [34] |
| | 2013 | | <20 | | 5.7 | 14.2 | | 2.8 | 3.8 | [34] |
| | 2014 | 2028 | 11–17 | 24.3 | | | 3.4 | | | [29] |
| | 2018 | | 10–19 | | | | | 2.0 | 5.0 | [55] |
| Morocco | 2016 | 6745 | 13–17 | 13.9 | 10.7 | 17.8 | 3.0 | 2.7 | 3.3 | [53] |
| | 2015 | 1818 | 12–18 | 7.7 | 7.2 | 8.3 | 3.4 | 2.8 | 3.9 | [13] |
| | 2014 | 5756 | 11–17 | 16.6 | | | 3.6 | | | [29] |
| | 2013 | | <20 | | 22.5 | 25.9 | | 7.9 | 9.1 | [34] |
| Tunisia | 2011 | 1335 | 6–12 | 19.7 | | | 5.7 | | | [39] |
| | 2013 | | <20 | | 17.7 | 23.4 | | 4.2 | 4.2 | [34] |
| | 2011 | 1529 | 9–12 | 6.3 | | | 2.4 | | | [29] |
| | 2001 | 1569 | | | 11.6 | 16.1 | | 2.7 | 3.7 | [18] |

prevalence was observed in Tunisia (2.4%) and the highest was observed in Egypt (9.3%). The higher prevalence rates of overweight and obesity in North African children and adolescents, especially Egyptian ones, may be indicative of nutrition transition marked by an over-nutrition [9, 19] as well as an improved socioeconomic status, which have been found previously to be associated with increased sedentary behavior [45], and overweight and obesity [25].

#### 6.2.2.3 Prevalence Among Adults Aged 18 Years and More

There is considerable disparity in overweight and obesity between North African countries. The two countries with the highest adult overweight and obesity prevalence rates are Egypt (63.0 %, and 35.7% respectively), and Libya (65.4 %, and 30.8% respectively) (Table 6.3). Overall, overweight and obesity prevalence is higher among women than men. The gender differences in being overweight and obese have been well documented. Indeed, women generally have a greater proportion of body fat, and are more likely to acquire fat subcutaneously and on their lower extremities because their bodies are more adapted to store fat linked to biological factors involved in reproduction [37]. The childbirth experience increases also the likelihood of obesity [10]. Thus gender is an important social factor contributing to overweight and obesity as well as a biological marker [20]. These higher prevalence rates of overweight and

**Table 6.3** Prevalence of overweight and obesity among adults aged 18 years and more in North African countries

| Country | Date of survey | Sample size | Age (year) | Prevalence of overweight | | | Prevalence of obesity | | | References |
|---|---|---|---|---|---|---|---|---|---|---|
| | | | | Total | Males | Females | Total | Males | Females | |
| Algeria | 2010 | | ≥ 20 | 48.2 | 41.8 | 54.5 | 17.5 | 10.7 | 24.3 | [38] |
| | 2015 | | 25–64 | 46.7 | 36.3 | 53.6 | 16.6 | 8.9 | 21.6 | [61] |
| Egypt | 2013 | | >20 | | 71.2 | 79.4 | | 26.4 | 48.4 | [34] |
| | 2015 | 16671 | 15–59 | | 34.3 | 25.7 | | 26.4 | 50.3 | [30] |
| | 2017 | 6680 | 15–69 | 63.0 | 53.8 | 74.1 | 35.7 | 24.8 | 48.8 | [57] |
| Libya | 2010 | | ≥ 20 | 65.4 | 60.4 | 71.0 | 30.8 | 21.5 | 41.3 | [38] |
| | 2013 | | >20 | | 70.6 | 77.0 | | 30.2 | 57.2 | [34] |
| | 2009 | 3590 | 25–64 | 63.5 | 57.5 | 69.8 | 30.5 | 21.4 | 40.1 | [58] |
| Mauritania | 2013 | | >20 | | 21.4 | 55.7 | | 6.4 | 27.6 | [34] |
| | 2014 | | | 30.0 | 25.0 | 36.0 | 10.0 | 6.0 | 14.0 | [61] |
| | 2015 | | 25–64 | 46.6 | 31.8 | 59.4 | 20.9 | 8.6 | 31.5 | [61] |
| Morocco | 2013 | | >20 | | 54.7 | 52.8 | | 18.1 | 20.9 | [34] |
| | 2013 | | | | 30.8 | 34.7 | | 8.2 | 26.8 | [24] |
| Tunisia | 2005 | 5343 | 35–70 | | 51.7 | 71.1 | | 37.0 | 13.3 | [12] |
| | 2013 | | >20 | | 31.7 | 57.5 | | 15.3 | 12.8 | [34] |
| | 2010 | | ≥ 20 | 55.9 | 47.5 | 64.2 | 23.8 | 13.9 | 33.4 | [38] |

obesity shown in the Table 6.3 indicate that it is time to confront this growing public health problem decisively. North African countries must implement fully the WHO-recommended strategies and interventions to tackle overweight and obesity.

## 6.3 Physical Activity

### *6.3.1 Definitions*

Physical activity is defined as any body movement produced by skeletal muscles action that increases energy expenditure [60]. It comprises all activities, including physical exercise, performed at any intensity and during any time of day or night. The estimates of physical activity level are obtained using questionnaires on frequency, duration and intensity (light, moderate, and vigorous) of all physical activities during a typical week. Based on the compendium of physical activities [2] and the compendium of physical activities for youth [40], physical activities are assigned MET (metabolic equivalent of task) values as follow:

- Moderate-intensity recreational sports are assigned an average MET value equivalent to 4 MET.
- Slow walking, normal-pace walking and brisk walking are assigned MET values of 2.8, 3.5 and 4.5 MET, respectively,
- Vigorous-intensity physical activity and sports (including stair climbing, jogging, running, bicycling, self-defense, weight training and soccer, basketball, handball and singles tennis) are assigned an average value of 8 MET.

The total energy expenditure in MET-min/week is estimated from intensity, duration and frequency of activity. Individuals are subsequently categorized into physically active or inactive based on total physical activity cut-off scores of 1680 MET-min/week (60 min/d $\times$ 7 d/week $\times$ 4 MET), corresponding to 1 h of daily moderate-intensity physical activity [3]. Furthermore, there are two levels of physical inactivity. The first one "inactive" defined as "doing no or very few physical activity at work, at home, for transport or in discretionary time". The second one "insufficiently active" defined as "doing some physical activity but less than 150 min of moderate intensity physical activity or 60 min of vigorous-intensity physical activity a week accumulated across work, home, transport or discretionary domains" [16]. Despite extensive use over 4 decades, physical activity questionnaires have shown limited reliability and validity. The accurate measurement of physical activity has become possible through standardized instruments/devices which record low intensity activities typical of sedentary lifestyle, and provide consistent biological meaning to light, moderate, and vigorous exercise [43].

### 6.3.2 *Health Benefits of Physical Activity*

There is a general consensus that regular and adequate levels of physical activity is likely to protect from excessive fat accumulation and obesity-related diseases including hypertension, coronary heart disease, stroke, diabetes, breast and colon cancer, and depression. Physical activity can also improve mood, sleep quality, and self-esteem, as well as reducing risk of stress, dementia and Alzheimer's disease [60]. Moreover many Authors have suggested that physical activity has a role in increasing resting metabolic rate (which constitutes 60–75% of the daily energy expenditure) and has a positive effect on body composition [27]. In contrast, physical inactivity has been considered as the fourth leading cause of mortality worldwide (6% of deaths). Indeed, people who are physically inactive have a 20–30% increased risk of all-cause mortality compared to those engaged in at least 150 min of moderate-intensity physical activity per week, or equivalent. In addition, approximately 21–25% of breast and colon cancers, 27% of diabetes and approximately 30% of coronary heart disease are attributable to physical inactivity [60].

### 6.3.3 *Prevalence of Physical Inactivity in North African Countries*

#### 6.3.3.1 Prevalence Among Adults Aged 18 Years and More

Latest estimates of the WHO indicate that globally 32% of women and 23% of men aged 18 years and more were insufficiently physically active in 2016. Although health consequences of physical inactivity are well known, the global prevalence of insufficient physical activity did not experience a significant improvement over the past 15 years (28.5% in 2001 vs. 27.5% in 2016) [52]. Data on population-based physical activity in the North African countries are very limited. Table 6.4 presents physical inactivity prevalence among North African adults aged 18 years and more. It summarizes data from World Health reports and Survey data, and information from research articles published in academic journals. Overall, the prevalence of physical inactivity (less than 600 metabolic equivalent (MET) minutes per week, or less than 150 min of moderate activity per week, or less than 60 min of vigorous activity per week) was as low as 14.6% in Tunisia and as high as 45.8% in Libya (Table 6.4). Women were found to be more likely than men to be insufficiently active in all countries. Women's rates of physical inactivity are alarmingly high, particularly in Libya (54.4%), Algeria (49.2%), and Mauritania (47.6%). Overall, the prevalence of physical inactivity among North African adults was higher than the global average (27.5%) reported by the WHO in 2016 [52]. The high levels of physical inactivity among this population are mainly due to a shift away from occupational and domestic activities requiring heavy manual work to the service sector and high technology work

**Table 6.4** Prevalence of physical inactivity among adults aged 18 years and more in North African countries

| Country | Date of survey | Sample size | Age (year) | Prevalence of physical inactivity | | | References |
|---|---|---|---|---|---|---|---|
| | | | | Total | Males | Females | |
| Algeria | 2015 | 4102 | 15–64 | 40.7 | 32.5 | 45.8 | [61] |
| | 2014 | | ≥20 | 40.5 | 31.9 | 49.2 | [38] |
| Egypt | 2012 | 5300 | 15–64 | 32.1 | 23.3 | 42.0 | [26] |
| Libya | 2014 | | ≥20 | 45.8 | 37.3 | 54.4 | [61] |
| | 2009 | 3579 | 25–64 | 43.9 | 36.0 | 51.7 | [26] |
| Mauritania | 2003 | 2726 | | 43.8 | 40.0 | 47.6 | [26] |
| | 2016 | | 18+ | 39.0 | 34.0 | 45.0 | [55] |
| Morocco | 2011 | 2610 | 18+ | 16.5 | 9.4 | 24.2 | [33] |
| | 2011 | 2620 | 18+ | 38.7 | | | [14] |
| Tunisia | 2003 | | ≥20 | 35.9 | 31.5 | 40.3 | [61] |
| | 2008 | 4332 | 18–69 | 14.6 | 11.0 | 18.2 | [22] |

that requires little energy expenditure [32]. Likewise, lack of physical activity during leisure time and increase in using passive transport modes [60].

#### 6.3.3.2 Prevalence Among Children and Adolescents

There are few available data on physical activity at the national level in the North African countries, particularly among children and adolescents. Table 6.5 presents the prevalence of physical inactivity in this Region using data of the Global School-based Student Health Surveys (GSHS). The proportions of physically inactive youth ranged from 79.3% in Algerian to 90.6% in Egyptian. Males were less likely to be physically inactive than females as reported previously [6, 60]. Because of the aforementioned limitations of physical activity questionnaires, the GSHS could over-estimate the prevalence of physical inactivity. For instance a study on physical activity prevalence among 669 Moroccan adolescents aged 15–19 years indicated that 21.1% of participants were found to be physical inactive (8.6% of boys and 32.9% of girls) [23]. Another recent study on objectively measured physical activity and sedentary time among Moroccan children and adolescents (mean age = 10.92 ± 1.55 years,) using a triaxial accelerometer (Actigraph) found that 38.8% of participants reached the recommended moderate and vigorous physical activity levels (≥ 60 min/day) and boys were 8 times more likely to meet this recommendation than girls [6]. Thus using various formats of physical activity questionnaire and standardized instruments/devices in studies aiming to estimate physical inactivity prevalence make interpretation and comparison between the countries, and even in the same country, a difficult task. Nevertheless, high proportions of North African children

**Table 6.5** Prevalence of physical inactivity among children and adolescents in North African countries

| Country | Date of survey | Sample size | Age (year) | Prevalence of physical inactivity | | | References |
|---|---|---|---|---|---|---|---|
| | | | | Total | Males | Females | |
| Algeria | 2011 | 4532 | 13–15 | 79.3 | 68.5 | 89.0 | [49] |
| Egypt | 2006 | 5249 | 13–15 | 90.6 | | | [42] |
| | 2011 | 2568 | 13–15 | 83.5 | 77.0 | 89.7 | [49] |
| Libya | 2007 | 2242 | 13–15 | 83.9 | 79.0 | 89.2 | [49] |
| Mauritania | 2010 | 2063 | 13–15 | 83.7 | 78.5 | 89.1 | [49] |
| Morocco | 2010 | 2924 | 13–15 | 82.6 | | | [42] |
| | 2016 | 6745 | 13–17 | 89.0 | 86.5 | 91.8 | [49] |
| Tunisia | 2008 | 2870 | 13–15 | 81.5 | | | [49] |

and adolescents did not meet the recommended levels of moderate and vigorous physical activity (≥60 min/day) required for promoting health and preventing diseases. The high prevalence of inactivity in this age-group represents a major public health concern in the region.

## 6.4 Conclusions and Perspectives

Over the last decades, North Africa region has experienced rapid dietary and lifestyle changes that have lead to growing overweight and obesity prevalence among all age groups, coupled with a resulting increase in the prevalence of non-communicable diseases. Despite a lack of definite evidence to demonstrate a causal relationship, there is enough certainty that physical inactivity is associated with overweight and obesity. Many studies showed significant correlation of overweight and obesity with insufficient physical activity all over the world, including North African countries. In addition, physical inactivity prevalence and levels of sedentariness reached alarming rates, particularly among children and adolescents. This requires immediate action, and efforts should be made to increase levels of physical activity, especially among young people. There were substantial variations across North African countries. The baseline of comparative and updated information on the magnitude of obesity and overweight as well as physical inactivity provided in this chapter may help health policymakers to set up appropriate interventions to tackle risk factors of overweight and obesity and associated chronic diseases. Such interventions should be primarily focused on nutrition education, physical activity and healthy lifestyle among all age-groups. Studies using harmonized methods, rigorous analytic techniques and a deeper examination of context are needed to design appropriate interventions aiming to address overweight, obesity and physical inactivity, as societal challenges, according to a population-based, multi-sectoral, multi-disciplinary, and culturally relevant approach.

## References

1. Adeboye B, Bermano G, Rolland C (2012) Obesity and its health impact in africa: a systematic review. Cardiovasc J Afr 23(9):512
2. Ainsworth BE, Haskell WL, Whitt MC, Irwin ML, Swartz AM, Strath SJ, O Brien WL, Bassett DR, Schmitz KH, Emplaincourt PO et al (2000) Compendium of physical activities: an update of activity codes and met intensities. Med Sci Sport Exerc 32(9; SUPP/1):S498–S504
3. Al-Hazzaa HM, Musaiger AO, Group AR et al (2011) Arab teens lifestyle study (atls): objectives, design, methodology and implications. Diabetes, Metablc Syndr Obes: Targets Ther 4:417
4. Alwan A et al (2011) Global status report on noncommunicable diseases 2010. World Health Organization
5. Aounallah-Skhiri H, Traissac P, El Ati J, Eymard-Duvernay S, Landais E, Achour N, Delpeuch F, Romdhane HB, Maire B (2011) Nutrition transition among adolescents of a south-mediterranean country: dietary patterns, association with socio-economic factors, overweight and blood pressure. A cross-sectional study in Tunisia. Nutr J 10(1):38
6. Baddou I, El Hamdouchi A, El Harchaoui I, Benjeddou K, Saeid N, Elmzibri M El Kari K, Aguenaou H (2018) Objectively measured physical activity sedentary time among children and adolescents in Morocco: a cross-sectional study. BioMed research international 2018
7. Banjare JB, Bhalerao S et al (2016) Obesity associated noncommunicable disease burden. Int J Health Allied Sci 5(2):81
8. Cole TJ, Bellizzi MC, Flegal KM, Dietz WH (2000) Establishing a standard definition for child overweight and obesity worldwide: international survey. Bmj 320(7244):1240
9. Craigie AM, Lake AA, Kelly SA, Adamson AJ, Mathers JC (2011) Tracking of obesity-related behaviours from childhood to adulthood: a systematic review. Maturitas 70(3):266–284
10. Davis EM, Zyzanski SJ, Olson CM, Stange KC, Horwitz RI (2009) Racial, ethnic and socioeconomic differences in the incidence of obesity related to childbirth. Am J Public Health 99(2):294–299
11. De Onis M, Blössner M, Borghi E (2010) Global prevalence and trends of overweight and obesity among preschool children. Am J Clin Nutr 92(5):1257–1264
12. El AJ, Traissac P, Beji C, Aounallah-Skhiri H, Gaigi S, Kolsteren P, Ben RH Delpeuch F, Marie B (2008) Change in nutritional status of adult women in tunisia from 1996 to 2005: effect of living environment and socio-economic factors. In: 16th European Congress on Obesity, vol 32, pp S215–S215
13. El Kabbaoui M, Chda A, Bousfiha A, Aarab L, Bencheikh R, Tazi A (2018) Prevalence of and risk factors for overweight and obesity among adolescents in Morocco. East Mediterranean Health J 24(6):512–521
14. El Rhazi K, Nejjari C, Zidouh A, Bakkali R, Berraho M, Gateau PB (2011) Prevalence of obesity and associated sociodemographic and lifestyle factors in Morocco. Public Health Nutr 14(1):160–167
15. El-Taguri A, Besmar F, Monem A, Betilmal I, Ricour C, Rolland-Cachera M et al (2009) Stunting is a major risk factor for overweight: results from national surveys in 5 Arab countries. East Mediterranean Health J 15(3):549–562
16. Ezzati M, Lopez AD, Rodgers AA, Murray CJ (2004) Comparative quantification of health risks: global and regional burden of disease attributable to selected major risk factors. World Health Organization, Geneva

17. FAO (2011) PROFIL NUTRITIONNEL DE PAYS ROYAUME DU MAROC. Organisation des Nations Unies pour l'Agriculture (FAO)
18. Gaha R, Ghannem H, Harrabi I, Ben AA, Lazreg F, Fredj A (2002) Study of overweight and obesity in a population of urban school children in Sousse Tunisia. Archives de pediatrie: organe officiel de la Societe francaise de pediatrie 9(6):566–571
19. Galal OM (2002) The nutrition transition in Egypt: obesity, undernutrition the food consumption context. Public Health Nutr 5(1a):141–148
20. Garawi F, Devries K, Thorogood N, Uauy R (2014) Global differences between women and men in the prevalence of obesity: is there an association with gender inequality? Eur J Clin Nutr 68(10):1101
21. GBD (2015) Obesity Collaborators (2017) Health effects of overweight obesity in 195 countries over 25 years. New England Journal of Medicine 377(1):13–27
22. Guthold R, Ono T, Strong KL, Chatterji S, Morabia A (2008) Worldwide variability in physical inactivity: a 51-country survey. Am J Prev Med 34(6):486–494
23. Hamrani A, Mehdad S, El Kari K, El Hamdouchi A, El Menchawy I, El Mzibri, M, Belghiti H, Musaiger AO, Al-Hazzaa HM, Hills AP et al (2015) Physical activity and dietary habits among Moroccan adolescents. Public Health Nutr 18(10):1793–1800
24. Haut-commissariat au plan (2013) Enquête Nationale Anthropométrique (2011) Cahiers du Plan. https://www.hcp.ma/Les-Cahiers-du-Plan-N-43-Mars-Avril-2013_a1248.html. Accessed 26 May 2018
25. Jackson RT, Rashed M, Saad-Eldin R (2003) Rural urban differences in weight body image, and dieting behavior among adolescent Egyptian schoolgirls. Int J Food Sci Nutr 54(1):1–11
26. Kahan D (2015) Adult physical inactivity prevalence in the muslim world: analysis of 38 countries. Prev Med Rep 2:71–75
27. Kiess W, Marcus C, Wabitsch M (2004) Obesity in childhood and adolescence, vol 9. Karger Medical and Scientific Publishers, Basel
28. Kuczmarski R, Ogden C, Guo S, Grummer-Strawn L, Flegal K, Mei Z, Wei R, Curtin L, Roche A, Johnson C (2002) 2000 CDC growth charts for the united states: methods and development. Vital and health statistics Series 11. Data Natl Health Surv 11:1–190
29. Manyanga T, El-Sayed H, Doku DT, Randall JR (2014) The prevalence of underweight, overweight, obesity and associated risk factors among school-going adolescents in seven african countries. BMC Public Health 14(1):887
30. Ministry of Health and Population [Egypt] (2015) Egypt Health Issues Survey 2015. Ministry of Health and Population and ICF International Cairo, Egypt and..
31. Mokdad AH, Ford ES, Bowman BA, Dietz WH, Vinicor F, Bales VS, Marks JS (2003) Prevalence of obesity, diabetes, and obesity-related health risk factors 2001. Jama 289(1):76–79
32. Musaiger AO et al (2011) Overweight and obesity in eastern mediterranean region: prevalence and possible causes. J Obes
33. Najdi A, El Achhab Y, Nejjari C, Norat T, Zidouh A, El Rhazi K (2011) Correlates of physical activity in Morocco. Prev Med 52(5):355–357
34. Ng M, Fleming T, Robinson M, Thomson B, Graetz N, Margono C, Biryukov Mullany EC, S, Abbafati C, Abera SF et al (2014) Global, regional, national prevalence of overweight and obesity in children and adults during 1980–2013: a systematic analysis for the global burden of disease study 2013. The lancet 384(9945):766–781
35. Onis Md, Onyango AW, Borghi E, Siyam A, Nishida C, Siekmann J (2007) Development of a who growth reference for school-aged children adolescents. Bull World Health Organ 85:660–667
36. Pineda E, Sanchez-Romero LM, Brown M, Jaccard A, Jewell J, Galea G, Breda J, Webber L (2018) Forecasting future trends in obesity across Europe: the value of improving surveillance. Obes Facts 11(5):360–371
37. Power ML, Schulkin J (2008) Sex differences in fat storage, fat metabolism, the health risks from obesity: possible evolutionary origins. Br J Nutr 99(5):931–940
38. Rahim HFA, Sibai A, Khader Y, Hwalla N, Fadhil I, Alsiyabi H, Mataria A, Mendis S, Mokdad AH, Husseini A (2014) Non-communicable diseases in the Arab world. The Lancet 383(9914):356–367

39. Reynolds K, Gu D, Whelton PK, Wu X, Duan X, Mo J, He J, Group IC (2007) Prevalence and risk factors of overweight and obesity in China. Obesity 15(1):10–18
40. Ridley K, Ainsworth BE, Olds TS (2008) Development of a compendium of energy expenditures for youth. Int J Behav Nutr Phys Act 5(1):45
41. Saleh M, Anwar W, Habil I, Ishac S (2014) Prevalence of overweight and obesity among a sample of under-five rural children in lower Egypt. Egypt J Community Med 301(1922):1–13
42. Sharara E, Akik C, Ghattas H, Obermeyer CM (2018) Physical inactivity, gender and culture in arab countries: a systematic assessment of the literature. BMC Public Health 18(1):639
43. Shephard RJ (2003) Limits to the measurement of habitual physical activity by questionnaires. Br J Sport Med 37(3):197–206
44. Speiser PW, Rudolf MC, Anhalt H, Camacho-Hubner C, Chiarelli F, Freemark M, Eliakim A, Gruters A, Hershkovitz E, Iughetti L et al (2005) Childhood obesity. J Clin Endocrinol Metablsm 90(3):1871–1887
45. Te Velde SJ, Van Nassau F, Uijtdewilligen L, Van Stralen M, De Craemer Cardon G, M, Manios Y, Brug J, Chinapaw M, (2012) Energy balance-related behaviours associated with overweight and obesity in preschool children: a systematic review of prospective studies. Obes Rev 13:56–74
46. UNICEF (2018a) Nutrition country profile (Algeria). Global nutrition report. https://globalnutritionreport.org/nutrition-profiles/africa/northern-africa/algeria/#profile. Accessed 28 May 2019
47. UNICEF (2018b) Nutrition country profile (Mauritania). Global nutrition report. https://globalnutritionreport.org/nutrition-profiles/africa/western-africa/mauritania/#profile. Accessed 28 May 2019
48. WHO (2007) Global School-based Student Health Survey Libya. https://extranet.who.int/ncdsmicrodata/index.php/catalog/43. Accessed 28 May 2019
49. WHO (2008) Global School-based Student Health Survey (GSHS) Tunisia 2008. https://www.who.int/ncds/surveillance/gshs/tunisia/en/. Accessed 26 Nov 2018
50. WHO (2011a) Global School-based Student Health Survey Algeria. https://extranet.who.int/ncdsmicrodata/index.php/catalog/75. Accessed 28 May 2019
51. WHO (2011b) Global School-based Student Health Survey Egypt. https://extranet.who.int/ncdsmicrodata/index.php/catalog/96. Accessed 28 May 2019
52. WHO (2013) Prevalence of insufficient physical activity. https://www.who.int/gho/ncd/risk_factors/physical_activity_text/en/. Accessed 20 May 2019
53. WHO (2016) Global School-based Student Health Survey Morocco. https://www.who.int/ncds/surveillance/gshs/morocco/en/. Accessed 28 May 2019
54. WHO (2018a) Global Health Observatory/Nutrition Landscape Information System (NLiS). NLiS Country Profile: Mauritania. http://apps.who.int/nutrition/landscape/report.aspx?iso=mrt. Accessed 28 May 2019
55. WHO (2018b) Noncommunicable Diseases (NCD) Country Profiles (Mauritania). https://www.who.int/nmh/countries/mrt_en.pdf?ua=1. Accessed 28 May 2019
56. WHO (2018c) Obesity and overweight. https://www.who.int/news-room/fact-sheets/detail/obesity-and-overweight. Accessed 28 Mar 2019
57. WHO (2019a) Non-communicable diseases and their risk factors. STEPS survey Egypt 2017. WHO
58. WHO (2019b) Non-communicable diseases and their risk factors. STEPS survey Libya 2009. WHO
59. Williams EP, Mesidor M, Winters K, Dubbert PM, Wyatt SB (2015) Overweight obesity: prevalence, consequences, and causes of a growing public health problem. Curr Obes Rep 4(3):363–370
60. World Health Organization and others (2004) Global strategy on diet, physical activity and health. World Health Organization, Geneva
61. World Health Organization and others (2016) Report on the status of major health risk factors for noncommunicable diseases: WHO African Region, 2015. WHO, Regional Office for Africa

# Chapter 7
# Herbal Medicine in Chronic Diseases Treatment: Determinants, Benefits and Risks

**Souad Ben El Mostafa and Abdellatif Maamri**

**Abstract** Phytotherapy as a branch of traditional medicine is one of the most popular remedies in developing countries. Many pharmacological studies have shown the effective effects of some plants in curing or preventing some diseases, such as diabetes and high blood pressure. Herbal medicine is appreciated for several reasons related to the region. In Morocco, it is adopted by a large segment of the population, dominated by women, illiterates and rural residents who are geographically isolated and where poverty is more pronounced. In the absence of political commitment, inappropriate use of plants can lead to serious or even fatal adverse reactions. Efforts have to be made to regulate the sale of these products, qualify service providers and raise consumer awareness.

## 7.1 Introduction

Used since ancient times, traditional practices treatment for some diseases are receiving increasing attention in the context of care health provision and health sector reform. Authorities, healthcare professionals and general population are struggling to ensure safety, effectiveness, quality, availability, preservation and future development of this type of health care [34].

According to the World Health Organization (WHO), traditional medicine (MT) is defined as "*the sum of all knowledge, skills and practices based on the theories, beliefs and experiences of different cultures, whether or not they are explicable, and which are used in the preservation of health, as well as in the prevention, diagnosis,*

S. Ben El Mostafa (✉)
Higher Institute of Health Nursing and Technical Professions (ISPITS), Ministry of Health, Nador, Morocco
e-mail: souadbenelmostafa@hotmail.fr

A. Maamri
Department of Biology, Faculty of Sciences, University Mohamed Ier, Oujda, Morocco
e-mail: abdellatifm@hotmail.com



A. Boutayeb (ed.), *Disease Prevention and Health Promotion in Developing Countries*,
https://doi.org/10.1007/978-3-030-34702-4_7

*improvement or treatment of physical or mental illnesses*" [35]. It integrates, as a result, both drug therapies involving the use of herbal medicines, parts of animals and/or minerals and non-drug therapies such as Chinese acupuncture, manual or spiritual therapies [34].

The practice of traditional medicine can vary greatly between countries or regions. It is influenced by factors such as culture, history and attitudes. It is widespread in developing countries and it's called complementary or alternative medicine (MC) in developed countries where the care system is based mainly on allopathy.

Among the different traditional practices and beliefs, WHO recalls that herbal medicine remains the most popular. This is common in many countries, particularly in Africa, Asia and America [5].

In Africa, more than 80% of people use traditional medicines and pharmacopoeias to deal with health problems. It is practiced in order to maintain a good health, to prevent or treat diseases, especially chronic ones [3, 15, 20, 24, 35]. The failure of conventional pharmaceutical treatments, the high incidence of adverse effects associated with them caused by their association, their high cost and sometimes the insufficiently health infrastructures, particularly in developing countries, have an impact on a large part of the population worldwide to use traditional or complementary medicines [1].

Thanks to its rich culture and diverse flora, Morocco is one of the Mediterranean countries with a long medical tradition and know-how based on medicinal plants. It has a large area of wild aromatic and medicinal plants (PAM) which amounts to 311 862 ha [22]. These plants take part in the national economy. The annual average revenue of the PAM sales is 5.3 million dirhams for an annual quantity of 33,000 tons. WFPs also provide alternative income to local communities and generate in average some 500,000 working days/year [23].

## 7.2 Herbal Medicine in the Treatment of Chronic Diseases

Several ethnobotanical studies carried out throughout the kingdom of Morocco stress on the importance of herbal medicine in the Moroccan population. The rate of medicinal plants utilization for the treatment of chronic diseases in general and diabetes in particular (Figs. 7.1 and 7.2) is significant. Similar results are observed in neighboring countries, including Algeria and sub-Saharan Africa [5, 13, 16, 19, 21, 25, 26, 37, 40].

Tafilalt region (south-east of Morocco) seems to be an excellence pol for the practice of phytotherapy. Empirical knowledge has been transmitted verbally over generations and has been enriched by a strategic geographical location between North Africa, the Sahara and the Sahel, as well as historical events and miscegenation of Amazigh, Jewish and Saharan civilizations and Arab-Muslim [7].

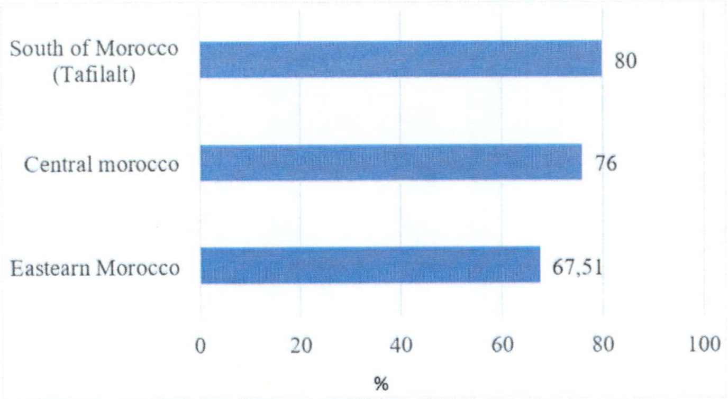


**Fig. 7.1** Use of medicinal plants for chronic diseases

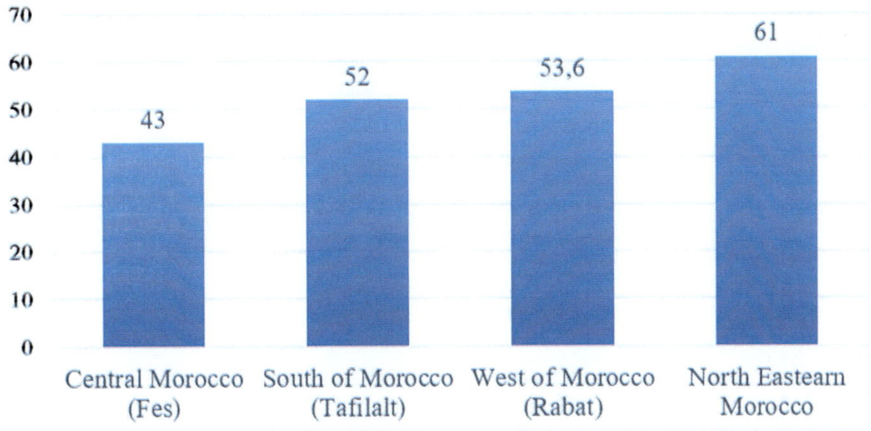


**Fig. 7.2** Use of medicinal plants by diabetics

However, according to the latest national survey on common risks of no communicable diseases [30], the role of traditional medicine in the treatment of chronic diseases is not well demonstrated. The results show that only 3.4% of hypertensive people has already consulted a traditional healer to treat their HTA and 5.3% use traditional medicine without significant difference between the two sexes or between urban and rural areas. Similar values are recorded for diabetics, with values with 5% and 4.9% respectively for those who have ever visited a healer and those who are on traditional therapy. At this level, significant gender and area of residence differences are seen. Women use more traditional remedies and rural citizen are more likely to consult healers (Fig. 7.3).

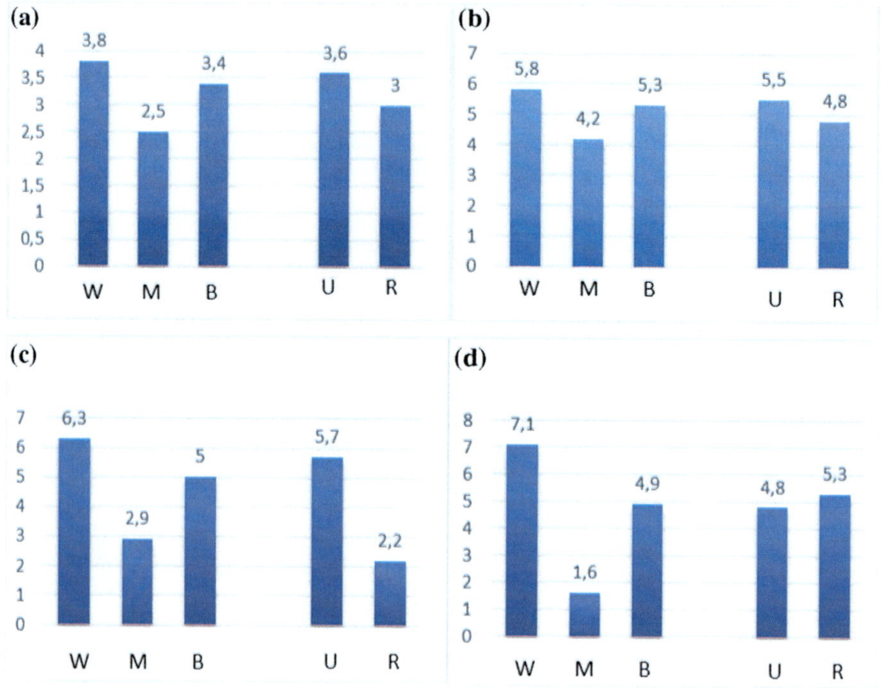


**Fig. 7.3** Hypertensive who have already visited a healer (**a**), hypertensive who use traditional medicine (**b**), diabetics who have already visited a healer (**c**) and diabetics who use traditional medicine (**d**). W: women, M: Mean, B: Both, U: Urban, R: Rural

## 7.3 Demographic and Socio-economic Characteristics of Medicinal Plants Users

Although the data provided by the different surveys are not always ready to be compared and unclear for some parameters, some facts need to be highlighted. Indeed, the majority of ethnobotanical and ethnopharmacological studies undertaken throughout the kingdom show that herbal medicine is adopted by the entire population, regardless of age and level of education, with higher rates of use from adult and illiterate people [9, 13, 18, 26, 27, 37, 40]. According to the same sources, women seem to be more concerned with the use of medicinal plants (Fig. 7.4). This female predisposition, with is also confirmed by the recent Ministry of Health survey [20] can be explained by the fact that women make better use of medicinal properties to relieve the pain of their children and preserve the health of their families trying to avoid heavy material loads, sometimes required by the doctor and the pharmacist [8, 10, 25, 27, 32, 36, 37, 40].

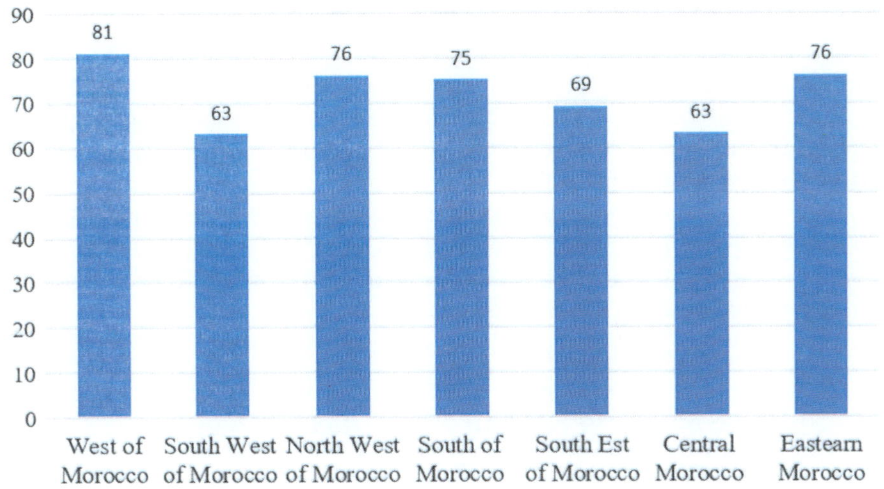


**Fig. 7.4** Women's use of medicinal plants

## 7.4 Reasons Behind Herbal Medicine's Adoption

For several reasons which often associated, herbal medicine is adopted as alternative or complementary medicine to drug treatment. Actually, access to health is open to the entire Moroccan population and even more poorest one, to whom the state provides free primary care. However, geographical isolation areas, limited mean of transport, of healthcare infrastructures and human resources are against the satisfaction of health needs [6]. The case of Tafilalt region (South–East of Morocco) is a good example. Apart from culture and tradition, this region dominated by rural municipalities 109 against 16 urban has the highest poverty rate in the country 21.2% against 8.9% nationally, a negative gap of 12.3 points [31]. The ratios of inhabitants per doctor and per nurse remain relatively high compared to national averages (Table 7.1).

World Health Organization considers that it's unlikely that countries with less than 23 health professionals (doctors, nurses and midwives) per 10,000 population will achieve adequate coverage rates for primary health care interventions [33]. It is therefore obvious that the population of such a region is looking for other care

**Table 7.1** Doctors and Nurses resource in the Draâ-Tafilalt Region [29]

| | Draâ Tafilalt region | National average |
|---|---|---|
| Inhabitants/general doctor | 9951 | 7326 |
| Inhabitants/specialist doctor | 8887 | 3838 |
| Inhabitants/nurse | 1158 | 1091 |

alternatives especially herbal medicine which is easily accessible and widely rooted in its traditions.

In addition, chronic diseases require to follow a set of mandatory requirements to avoid daily discomfort and resulting complications. Oral antidiabetic drugs, for example, are effective in reducing blood glucose, but are often unable to maintain glucose levels around normal values. In such situation, some patients are sensitive to any cure or remission hope and can easily adopt the herbal medicine [17]. It is also pointed out that the seniority of diabetes is a favoring factor to search for other treatment alternatives, especially herbal medicine [36] of which effectiveness has been appreciated by the majority of its users [2, 21, 25, 26].

## 7.5 Pharmacological Properties of Medicinal Plants: Case of Antidiabetic Plants

There are about 500,000 species of plants on earth of which 80,000 have medicinal properties and more than 1,200 are inventoried as antidiabetics and are used for their hypoglycemic and antihyperglycemic properties [4, 28]. Some species are considered as a source of the development of antidiabetic medicines. It is the case of metformin which owes its discovery to *Galega officinalis*. The main popular in Morocco are presented in Table 7.2.

In fact, Plants accumulate secondary metabolites which represent an important source of molecules usable by man in particular in pharmacological field [11]. Most of them are promising, but only a small number has been subject of experimental studies and their actions are highlighted [19].

**Table 7.2** List of some most used antidiabetic plants in Morocco [11]

| Scientific names | Vernacular arabic names |
|---|---|
| *Trigonella foenum-graecum* | Halba |
| *Artemisia herba*-alba | Chih |
| *Citrullus colocynthis* | Hanlel |
| *Olea europaea* | Zitoun |
| *Salvia officinalis* | Salmiya |
| *Coriandrum sativum* | Lkosbr |
| *Nerium oleander* | Defla |
| *Marrubium vulgare* | Merriwa |
| *Allium sativum* | Toum |
| *Prunus amygdalus* | Louz lmar |
| *Ziziphus lotus* | Nbag |
| *Urtica dioica* | Lhariga |

**Table 7.3** List of some plants with multiple activities

| Activity | Plants | References |
|---|---|---|
| Antidiabitic and Hypolipidemiant | *Capparis spinosa* | [14] |
| | *Calamintha officinalis Artemisia herba alba* | |
| | *Rosmarinus officinalis, Ajuga iva* | [12] |
| | *Trigonella foenum-graecum* | |
| Antidiabitic and Hypotensive | *Olea europaea, Salvia officinalis* | |
| | *Lavandula dentata, Origanum compactum* | |
| | *Pistacia lentiscus, Tetraclinis articulata* | |
| | *Nigella sativa, Arbutus unedo* | |
| | *Eugenia caryophyllata, Centaurium Erythraea* | |

Several active ingredients have the ability to generate a hypoglycemic action whose mechanism can be different according to the plants. Among the main constituents there are polysaccharides, peptides, alkaloids, glycopeptides, triterpenoids, amino acids, steroids, flavonoids, phenols, coumarins, inorganic ions and guanidine. Some of them are actually hypoglycemic and may have therapeutic potential, while others produce only hypoglycemia as a side effect of their toxicity, particularly liver toxicity [21]. As the case of conventional oral antidiabetic drugs, these molecules stimulate insulin secretion, increase insulin sensitivity, inhibit intestinal absorption of glucose or reduce its production by the liver. It is also stated that effect of a medicinal plant is never the result of a single substance, but rather an interaction of several molecules [10]. Therefore, an entire plant has properties superior to those of its constituents. The same plant can also be used to treat different diseases. This is the case of some species with antidiabetic, hypolipidemic and/or hypotensive activities (Table 7.3). These results should improve the use of medicinal plants and their total extracts in modern herbal medicine.

## 7.6 Risks Related to the Traditional Use of Plants

Traditional practices of plants that do not respect the rules of use often threatens the consumers quality of live. In Morocco sale of medicinal plants, authorization to exercise this profession and quality control of herbalist are not regulated. Majority of the providers (Herbalists, Aâtars, healers) are aged with a very low education level [3, 13, 16, 25, 26, 40]. In addition, the female trend combined with a high rate of illiteracy may be behind the strong ignorance of toxic potential plants [13, 26].

Interactions between plants and conventional drugs can also produce negative effects such as digestive disorders [21] or a decrease in the effectiveness of treatment that worsens the patient's state of health [39]. Unfortunately, some studies have shown

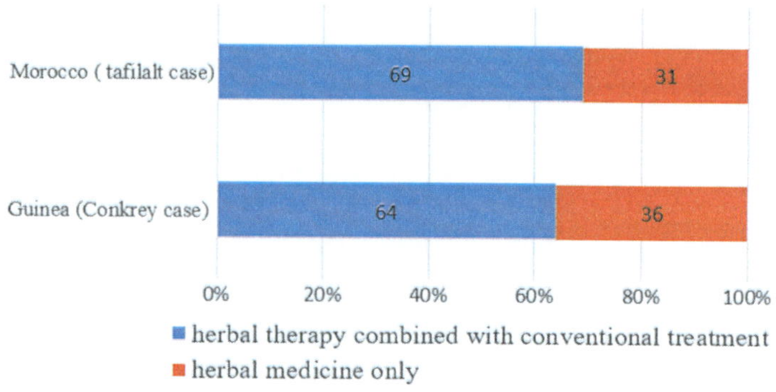


**Fig. 7.5** Modes of use of antidiabetic plants

that a large proportion of patients associate herbal medicine with drug treatment [5, 16] (Fig. 7.5).

The problem is further aggravated by the uncontrolled spread of recipes of medicinal plants through social networks, radio... Botanically different species may have the same vernacular name and misuse of plants can be caused by false identification. In its report of 2017, the Moroccan anti-poison center (CAPM) indicates that deficiency of multisectorial involvement, existence of an informal sector, traditional use of treatments, lack of herbalists training or lack of control throughout the chain from production to sale constitute the causes of any intoxication. If doses are exceeded, use of plants can lead to serious intoxication, a risk of complications and even premature death. 197 cases of plant poisoning were recorded in 2017 [38], this number is undeniably inferior to reality.

## 7.7 Conclusion

Since the 2000s, herbal medicine has known a real expansion throughout the world. Thanks to extensive ethnobotanical and pharmacological research, several species are identified and recognized as having promising effects to cure or prevent certain diseases, including diabetes and hypertension.

In Morocco, the use of medicinal plants is linked to tradition, culture and/or individual needs. This therapy is adopted by a female-dominated population with illiterates and adults tendency. The geographical isolation associated with a high poverty rate also seems to be a determining factor for the practice and adoption of this therapy. In the absence of legislation on medicinal plants, the inappropriate use of plants by such a vulnerable population may lead to serious or even fatal adverse effects. Rigor is required and efforts has to be made to regulate sale of these products, qualify their service providers and raise public awareness of uncontrolled plant use dangers. Accessible and easy to understand information is essential to guide the consumer in his choices.

At the same time, research evaluating the benefit/risk ratio of medicinal plants and clinical studies must be enhanced in order to take advantage of the different virtues of herbal medicine without fear of sometimes dangerous side effects. To this end, WHO encourages the intensification of scientific research and recommends the evaluation of the safety and efficacy of herbal medicines with a view to standardizing their use and integrating them into conventional care systems. It also requires better communication between providers MT/MC, allopath and patients and the provision of scientific information and advice to the general public [34]. In this way, traditional medicines with assured quality, safety and efficiency are proving to be involved in achieving the goal of giving access to care to all people [35].

## References


1. AAmri H (2018) Enquête ethnobotanique à propos des plantes médicinales utilisées dans le traitement traditionnel du vitiligo à marrakech et agadir. PhD thesis, FMP Marrakech, Morocco
2. Alaoui MSB, Satrani B, Boussoula E, Ghanmi M (2018) Etude ethnobotanique des plantes médicinales utilisées dans les provinces du sahara marocain. Int J Innov Appl Stud 24(2):789–801
3. Allali H, Benmehdi H, Dib M, Tabti B, Ghalem S, Benabadji N (2008) Phytotherapy of diabetes in west Algeria. Asian J Chem 20(4):2701
4. Bailey CJ, Day C (1989) Traditional plant medicines as treatments for diabetes. Diabetes Care 12(8):553–564
5. Baldé N, Youla A, Baldé M, Kaké A, Diallo M, Baldé M, Maugendre D (2006) Herbal medicine and treatment of diabetes in Africa: an example from guinea. Diabetes Metab 32(2):171–175
6. Belkhdar H (2014) Phytothérapie au maroc: Entre sciences et charlatanisme, interview
7. Bellakhdar J (1997) La pharmacopée marocaine traditionnelle: Médecine arabe ancienne et savoirs populaires. Ibis press, édition le Fennec et Paris, Casablanca
8. Benkhnigue O, Zidane L, Fadli M, Elyacoubi H, Rochdi A, Douira A (2010) Etude ethnobotanique des plantes médicinales dans la région de mechraâ bel ksiri (région du gharb du maroc). Acta Botanica Barcinonensia 53:191–216
9. Benkhnigue O, Ben Akka F, Salhi S, Fadli M, Douira A, Zidane L (2014) Catalogue des plantes médicinales utilisées dans le traitement du diabète dans la région d'al haouz-rhamna (maroc). J Anim Plant Sci 23:3539–68
10. Bentahar B (2016) Evaluation ethnobotanique des potentialités thérapeutiques de ptychotisverticillata. PhD thesis, FMP Marrakech, Morocco
11. Bnouham M, Mekhfi H, Legssyer A, Ziyyat A (2002) Ethnopharmacology forum medicinal plants used in the treatment of diabetes in Morocco. Int J Diabetes Metab 10:33–50
12. Douira A, Zidane L (2015) Étude ethnobotanique des plantes médicinales utilisées dans le traitement du diabète, et des maladies cardiaques dans la région d'izarène (nord du maroc). J Appl Biosci 86(1):7940–7956
13. Eddouks M, Maghrani M, Lemhadri A, Ouahidi ML, Jouad H (2002) Ethnopharmacological survey of medicinal plants used for the treatment of diabetes mellitus, hypertension and cardiac diseases in the south-east region of Morocco (tafilalet). J Ethnopharmacol 82(2–3):97–103
14. Eddouks M, Hebi M, Ajebli M, El Hidani A, Sulpice T, Burcelin R (2018) Étude de l'activité antidiabétique de capparis spinosa l. et de calamintha officinalis moench chez la souris diabétique. Phytothérapie pp 1–9

15. El-Dahshan NA, Ismail MA, Metwally AS (2015) Use of complementary and alternative medicine among families having patients with chronic diseases: El-mahsama village-ismailia governorate. Therapy 6:139–148
16. El Rhaffari L, Zaid A (2002) Pratique de la phytothérapie dans le sud–est d u maroc (tafilalet). Un savoir empirique pour une pharmacopée rénovée Eu r Cong Ethnopharmacol, pp 293–318
17. Elekofehinti OO (2015) Saponins: anti-diabetic principles from medicinal plants-a review. Pathophysiology 22(2):95–103
18. Ghourri M, Zidane L, Rochdi A, Fadli M, Douira A et al (2012) Etude floristique et ethnobotanique des plantes médicinales de la ville d'el ouatia (maroc saharien). Kastamonu Üniversitesi Orman Fakültesi Dergisi 12(2):218–235
19. Hamza N, Berke B, Cheze C, Le Garrec R, Lassalle R, Agli AN, Robinson P, Gin H, Moore N (2011) Treatment of high fat diet induced type 2 diabetes in C57BL/6J mice by two medicinal plants used in traditional treatment of diabetes in the east of Algeria. J Ethnopharmacol 133(2):931–933
20. Hamza N, Berke B, Umar A, Cheze C, Gin H, Moore N (2019) A review of Algerian medicinal plants used in the treatment of diabetes. J Ethnopharmacol 111841
21. HANAE B (2012) les plantes médicinales et diabète de type 2.(à propos de 199 cas). PhD thesis, Faculté de médecine et de pharmacie, Rabat, Morocco
22. HCEFLCD (2015) Bilan d'activités du Haut-Commissariat aux Eaux et Forêts et à Lutte Contre la Désertification. Contrats programmes 2015. Technical report
23. HCEFLCD (2016) Bilan d'activités du Haut-Commissariat aux Eaux et Forêts et à Lutte Contre la Désertification. Contrats programmes 2016. Technical report
24. Holaly GE, Simplice KD, Charlemagne G, Kodjovi A, Kokou A, Tchadjobo T, Amegnona A, Komlan B, Jacques S (2015) Étude ethnobotanique des plantes utilisées dans le traitement du diabète dans la médecine traditionnelle de la région maritime du togo. Pan Afr Med J 20
25. Jouad H, Haloui M, Rhiouani H, El Hilaly J, Eddouks M (2001) Ethnobotanical survey of medicinal plants used for the treatment of diabetes, cardiac and renal diseases in the north centre region of Morocco (fez-boulemane). J Ethnopharmacol 77(2–3):175–182
26. Laadim M, Ouahidi M, Zidane L, El Hessni A, Ouichou A, Mesfioui A (2017) Ethnopharmacological survey of plants used for the treatment of diabetes in the town of Sidi Slimane (Morocco). J Pharmacogn Phytother 9(6):101–110
27. Lahsissene H, Kahouadji A (2010) Usages thérapeutiques traditionnels des plantes médicinales dans le maroc occidental: cas de la région de zaër. Phytothérapie 8(4):210–217
28. Marles RJ, Farnsworth NR (1995) Antidiabetic plants and their active constituents. Phytomedicine 2(2):137–189
29. Ministère de la Santé, Maroc (2016) Ressources humaines de la santé en chiffre. Technical report
30. Ministère de la santé, Rabat, Maroc (2018) Enquête nationale sur les facteurs de risqué commun des maladies non transmissibles 2017–2018. Technical report
31. Ministère de l'Intérieur, Royaume du Maroc, Direction Générale des Collectivités Locale (2015) La région de drâa-tafilalet, monoraphie générale. Technical report
32. Nabih M (1992) Secrets et vertus thérapeutiques des plantes médicinales utilisées en médecine traditionnelle dans la province de settat. PhD thesis, Faculté de médecine et de pharmacie
33. OMS (2009) Personnel de santé, infrastructures sanitaires et médicaments essentiels. Technical report
34. Organisation Mondiale de la Santé (2002) Stratégie de l'OMS pour la médecine traditionnelle pour 2002–2005. Technical report
35. Organisation Mondiale de la Santé (2013) Stratégie de l'OMS pour la médecine traditionnelle pour 2014–2023. Technical report
36. Selihi Z, Berraho M, El Achhab Y, Nejjari C, Lyoussi B (2015) Phytothérapie et complications dégénératives du diabète de type 2: quelle relation? Médecine des maladies Métaboliques 9(8):792–797
37. Skalli S, Hassikou R, Arahou M (2019) An ethnobotanical survey of medicinal plants used for diabetes treatment in rabat, Morocco. Heliyon 5(3):e01421

38. Soulaymani BR, Soulaymani A (2017) Rapport annuel des analyses toxicologiques capm lab.toxicologie maroc-n 35-4ème trimestre 2017. Technical report
39. Zekkour M (2008) Les risques de la phytothérapie, monographies des plantes toxiques les plus usuelles au maroc. these n 30, doctorat en pharmacie. PhD thesis, Faculté de Médecine et de Pharmacie, Rabat, Morocco
40. Ziyyat A, Legssyer A, Mekhfi H, Dassouli A, Serhrouchni M, Benjelloun W (1997) Phytotherapy of hypertension and diabetes in oriental Morocco. J Ethnopharmacol 58(1):45–54

# Chapter 8
# Artificial Intelligence in Oncology

**Saber Boutayeb and Anass Majbar**

**Abstract** Cancer is a very challenging disease. The medical treatment of cancer has to face the ability of cancer cells to develop a multiple resistance mechanism. Artificial intelligence is the simulation of human intelligence processes by machines in order to perform tasks normally requiring human intelligence, such as decision-making or visual perception. The artificial intelligence in healthcare could improve disease diagnosis, management, and the development of effective therapies. We will focus in this chapter on how artificial intelligence is becoming a reality in oncology daily practice.

## 8.1 A Brief Presentation of Cancer

Cancer is a very smart subversive process. Cancer cells are the results of several conditions:

- Genetic abnormalities that lead to a specific phenotype characterised by an illimited ability of cellular division, an insensitivity to the control signals, the capacity to create its own vascular signal and to develop distant colonies called metastasis,
- The ability to escape from the vigilance of the immune system. This phenomenon is called immunotolerance.

The cancer cells express normal antigens that are present in the normal cells including those related to the Human Leukocyte Antigen (HLA) system that permit to the immune cells to recognise the "non soi" but also many others antigens involved in the capacity acquired by the cancer cells. We know also that the carcinogenesis is a very dynamic process and that the antigen expression on the cancer membrane

S. Boutayeb (✉)
Faculty of Medicine and Pharmacy, Medical Oncology, University Mohamed V, Rabat, Morocco
e-mail: boutayebdr@yahoo.fr

A. Majbar
National Oncology Institute, University Mohammed V,
Rabat, Morocco
e-mail: anass.majbar@um5s.net.ma

 
A. Boutayeb (ed.), *Disease Prevention and Health Promotion in Developing Countries*,
https://doi.org/10.1007/978-3-030-34702-4_8

cell is in perpetual change. This particularity is the fruit of new acquired mutations [11]. In 2000s, fundamental cancer research discovered how the cancer cells interact actively with the immune system in order to inhibit his reaction [6]. In clinical practice, some clinical symptoms are considered as alarming and conduct to clinical work up (radiology, endoscopy and biology). The diagnosis of the solid cancers is based on anatomopathology. The examination by the microscope of tumour samples leads to the diagnosis of cancer. But the exact determination of the cancer subtype is mainly based on the study of the surface antigens by immunochemistry. The major progress made in the biology of cancers was the genome sequencing. Actually, by using modern techniques of genomic, an exact genotyping of each cancer is possible. Major efforts are also done by the scientists in order to correlate these genomic abnormalities to the corresponding proteins expression and by the way to know their exact role. The prognosis and cancer treatment differ basing on the clinical situation. In the localised disease, the goal is to cure. The local therapies such surgery and radiotherapy are the base of treatment. Systemic therapies are used in addition in order to lower the risk of relapse [6, 11]. Whereas the majority of metastatic situations are considered as palliative. Systemic therapies are the principal therapeutic weapons [6]. The specific systemic therapies are divided into:

- Chemotherapies
- Hormonotherapies
- Biotherapies or targeted therapies
- Immunotherapies

The follow up is constituted by physical, radiological and biological examinations. According to their results, doctors discuss the treatment plan adaptations [6].

## 8.2 The Pre ≪ Artificial Intelligence Period ≫

Artificial intelligence (AI) is the simulation of human intelligence processes by machines in order to perform tasks normally requiring human intelligence, such as decision-making or visual perception. The pre "artificial intelligence" period started in the 1990s and was characterised by:

1. The mechanisation and the standardisation of reasoning and process decision [20, 24, 28]: The therapeutic decision in oncology is a multidisciplinary process involving the three major therapeutic specialities (surgery, medical oncology and radiotherapy) supported by the diagnostic specialities such radiology. Each decision should be based on the highest level of evidence-based medicine. The highest level is obtained by phases 3 randomised comparatives trials and meta-analysis comparing two or more interventions (either drugs, surgery or radiotherapy...) The different medical options for diagnosis, treatment and the follow up of each type of cancer are organised under the form of guidelines. The development of each guideline needs an extended systematic review of literature and is the compilation of algorithms. These algorithms are developed by the major scientific societies and updated at least one time a year.

2. The wide use of computers and software in oncology [20, 24, 28].
   The modern medicine has left the written medical observation for the computer medical files. Moreover, oncologists are used to use software to calculate scores and evaluate risks of recurrence.
3. Big data [20, 24, 28].
   Both the fundamental and the clinical have generated a large volume of data. The big jump in technology lead to a better knowledge of cancers with a precise molecular and genetic characterisation. At the same moment, the number of clinical trials has literally exploded.

The challenge was, of course, to use these big data to accelerate the drug development and their efficacy. But moreover, to shift the paradigm by personalising the cancer treatments.

## 8.3 The Current Applications of AI and Futures Trends

### *8.3.1 Precision Medicine*

The principle of precision medicine is that treatments will be tailored to the genetic changes in each person's cancer. Currently the majority of patients are treated depending on the type of cancer, its size, and whether it has spread or not. But an emerging concept of targeted therapies is rapidly growing [24]. The development of molecular characterisation has permitted a novel classification based on the existence of driving mutations which are targeted by specific biologic therapies. Epithelial Growth Factor Receptor (EGFR) mutations and Anaplastic Lymphoma Kinase (ALK)-rearrangements were the first molecular alterations in lung adenocarcinoma -discovered in 2004 and 2007, respectively- that were shown to confer sensitivity to specific targeted therapies, namely tyrosine kinase inhibitors. Nowadays, around 25–30. The use of third generation of EGFR inhibitors or second generation of ALK inhibitors lead to median survival around 4 years versus 1 year with classic chemo [14, 18, 23].

Beyond lung cancers, in the future, each patient at the diagnosis, will have a complete tumoral genome sequencing. His data will be compared at the worldwide level in order to start to most adapted treatment according to the results of clinical trials [24]. The follow up and the evaluation of treatment efficacy will be done by non-invasive technics such as liquid biopsies in order to anticipate the mechanisms of resistance developed by the tumors [24]. In the same way, the drugs toxicities will be managed by comparing the personal data to the huge amount of data collected over the world.

### 8.3.2 Screening in Oncology

Not all cancers can be screened. The screening needs a routine non-invasive test with high sensibility and sensitivity in order to avoid both false positive and false negative results. In daily practice, screening is recommended in few cancers (breast, cervix, colon and prostate). For example, the screening of breast cancer is based on mammography. Screening with mammography is considered effective in reducing breast cancer–related mortality. In many countries, the mammography is read by two radiologists [3, 25]. In context of shortage of health practitioners, automation can relieve some of the burden on radiologists. But more interesting, it seems according the data from clinical trials that the detection accuracy of the algorithm exceeds all of the recommended performance standards for human radiologists [15]. The future of screening will be based also on detection of the lowest levels of circulating tumour DNA, which is commonly found in those with early-stage cancers [1, 8]. Moreover, in a context of routine use of whole genome sequencing in the future, the predictive strategy will allow adapting the screening procedures to the personal risk of cancer [1, 8].

### 8.3.3 Surgery

Within the field of surgical oncology, the adoption of artificial intelligence has been slower compared to other disciplines, probably because of the complex and extreme variability of the interactions with human tissue, and also the lack of awareness or understanding of the potential capabilities of computational approaches in surgical practice [17].

However, there were many advances in the surgical field that will inevitably improve the large adoption of artificial intelligence in the near future. First, surgery has become more dependent on technology in the last three decades. From the adoption of laparoscopy and then robotic surgery, the improvement in medical imaging techniques, image processing with 3D reconstructions, the wide use of electronic health records to capture medical data including per and postoperative monitoring of patients, and the development of very large surgical databases. All these improvements allowed access to a huge quantity of medical data that could be characterized as big data, containing complex patterns that may extend beyond the physician's ability to use traditional data processing techniques such as regression and multivariate analysis for their interpretation [12, 19].

Surgery involves complex decisions including, for example, about the indication for surgery and the surgical technique, the optimal timing for surgery, or the choice between radical versus organ–preserving surgery [17]. Additionally, patients and colleagues expect surgeons to quickly and accurately inform about potential adverse events, the probability for major complications and mortality or risk of cancer recurrence after surgery [17]. These complex assessments are beyond the capabilities of most surgeons [17]. In this context, big data associated with artificial intelligence may help surgeons to overcome these challenges and improve the decision-making process [26]. The most basic application of the big data concept in this context is the creation and exploitation of large clinical databases more than 15 years ago in the USA, followed later on by many other countries in Europe [10, 26]. For example, a recent study used data from the American College of Surgeons National Surgical Quality Improvement Program to explore a novel approach to quantify procedural complexity with the use of a machine learning analysis of the way surgical procedures are described to estimate the inherent risk associated with each procedure. Their hypothesis was that the association between clinical terms and risk can be learned in an entirely data-driven manner without any previous knowledge and extrapolated to inferences about a broad range of surgical procedures. In the exploratory phase, authors used data from 2005 to 2009 to train the model in order to determine the association between Current Procedural Terminology and mortality, morbidity, serious complications, and surgical-site infection and to produce an algorithm capable of generating procedural risk scores. Then, they tested it using the National Surgical Quality Improvement Program data from 2010. They found that the support vector machine approach achieved a greater level of discrimination for determining surgical complications compared with other measures of procedural complexity [27]. More recently, Corey et al. used machine learning models to identify high-risk surgical patients. These authors used automatically curated electronic health record data to train machine learning tools that would predict patients at high risk of postoperative complications. The model created was able to predict postoperative complications better than human experts and the National Surgical Quality Improvement Program calculator, which is a widely used pre-surgical risk prediction model [9]. Similarly, other studies found that machine learning outperformed logistic regression in the prediction of complication for individual patients [2, 13].

Future systems should integrate pre- and intra-operative data, biochemical, radiological and sequencing data to generate algorithms capable to accurately predict patients outcomes from expected duration of stay to personalized complication profile and oncologic outcomes at the touch of a button which would result in improved clinical decision support and better post-surgical care outcomes [21]. Furthermore, a larger scale collaboration between national and international databases would continually improve the accuracy of created algorithms and enhance decision making for cancer patients. In this regard, an artificial intelligence 'colleague' could become in the future a valued member of the surgical multidisciplinary team [17].

Within the operating room, there are many innovations in progress that would enhance surgery precision and increase patients' security. One example would be Intelligent digital assistants. Apple's Siri, Amazon's Alexa, Microsoft's Cortana, Google Now and other virtual assistants have become a firm part of everyday life. They do not only answer user questions via speech but also provide information autonomously and user-oriented. These systems hear and reply in native tongue using a friendly voice and combine the user's available data automatically with contextual knowledge of linked databases [16]. The medical version of intelligent digital assistants would provide an instant verbal interaction to queries, augmented and live overlay of anatomy, resection margins, and vital structures by amalgamating preoperative imaging with the real surgical image [7, 16, 17]. These assistants would control all the operating theatre environment, including lights, insufflation pressures, temperature, table tilt and height, and by using artificial intelligence, automatically change these setting according to the surgical team, procedure, patient and per-operative events [17].

With the development of driverless cars, the idea of autonomous surgical robots might seem like the next step for artificial intelligence and surgery. Autonomous robotic surgery-removing the surgeon's hands-promises enhanced efficacy, safety, and improved access to optimized surgical techniques. Recently, Shademan et al. reported a study comparing the performances of an autonomous surgical robot with expert surgeons in performing a bowel anastomosis. The surgical robot system showed superior efficiency, precision and reproducibility compared with expert surgeons [22]. These developments challenge the current views about the surgical practice and the full potential of interaction between intelligent computers, the surgeon and the patient has yet to be defined [17]. The future patient would probably benefit from close cooperation between surgeons and intelligent computers. This will raise new regulatory, ethical and legal questions that will need to be addressed in the near future [17].

### *8.3.4 Radiotherapy*

The radiotherapy has moved from the 2D techniques to 3D technologies with intensity modulation and the radio-stereotaxy. Artificial Intelligence will provide a qualitative jump by allowing [4, 5]:

- A better and smart automated image segmentation.
- Radiotherapy dose optimization with data driven planning.
- Clinical decision support, powered by treatment and patient outcomes data.

## 8.4 Conclusion

The fields of AI application in oncology are illimited. Artificial Intelligence will not replace doctors. But the next generations of health practitioners should work differently and be completely initiated to the use of new technologies in order to practice a safer and more efficient medicine. But, health community will face emerging challenges such the ethical issues related to artificial intelligence.

## References

1. Aravanis AM, Lee M, Klausner RD (2017) Next-generation sequencing of circulating tumor dna for early cancer detection. Cell 168(4):571–574
2. Arvind V, Kim JS, Oermann EK, Kaji D, Cho SK (2018) Predicting surgical complications in adult patients undergoing anterior cervical discectomy and fusion using machine learning. Neurospine 15(4):329
3. Bergl PA, Wijesekera TP, Nassery N, Cosby KS (2019) Controversies in diagnosis: contemporary debates in the diagnostic safety literature. Diagnosis
4. Bibault JE, Giraud P, Burgun A (2016) Big data and machine learning in radiation oncology: state of the art and future prospects. Cancer Lett 382(1):110–117
5. Brock K (2019) Adaptive radiotherapy: moving into the future. In: Seminars in radiation oncology, vol 29. WB Saunders Ltd, pp 181–184
6. Burotto M, Wilkerson J, Stein W, Bates SE, Fojo T (2019) Adjuvant and neoadjuvant cancer therapies: a historical review and a rational approach to understand outcomes. In: Seminars in oncology. Elsevier
7. Camarillo DB, Krummel TM, Salisbury JK Jr (2004) Robotic technology in surgery: past, present, and future. Am J Surg 188(4):2–15
8. Cohen JD, Li L, Wang Y, Thoburn C, Afsari B, Danilova L, Douville C, Javed AA, Wong F, Mattox A et al (2018) Detection and localization of surgically resectable cancers with a multi-analyte blood test. Science 359(6378):926–930
9. Corey KM, Kashyap S, Lorenzi E, Lagoo-Deenadayalan SA, Heller K, Whalen K, Balu S, Heflin MT, McDonald SR, Swaminathan M et al (2018) Development and validation of machine learning models to identify high-risk surgical patients using automatically curated electronic health record data (pythia): A retrospective, single-site study. PLoS Med 15(11):e1002701
10. Hall BL, Hamilton BH, Richards K, Bilimoria KY, Cohen ME, Ko CY (2009) Does surgical quality improve in the American college of surgeons national surgical quality improvement program: an evaluation of all participating hospitals. Ann Surg 250(3):363–376
11. Hanahan D, Weinberg RA (2011) Hallmarks of cancer: the next generation. Cell 144(5):646–674
12. Kanevsky J, Corban J, Gaster R, Kanevsky A, Lin S, Gilardino M (2016) Big data and machine learning in plastic surgery: a new frontier in surgical innovation. Plastic Reconstr Surg 137(5):890e–897e
13. Kim JS, Arvind V, Oermann EK, Kaji D, Ranson W, Ukogu C, Hussain AK, Caridi J, Cho SK (2018) Predicting surgical complications in patients undergoing elective adult spinal deformity procedures using machine learning. Spine Deform 6(6):762–770
14. Le T, Gerber DE (2019) Newer-generation egfr inhibitors in lung cancer: how are they best used? Cancers 11(3):366
15. Mayo RC, Kent D, Sen LC, Kapoor M, Leung JW, Watanabe AT (2019) Reduction of false-positive markings on mammograms: a retrospective comparison study using an artificial intelligence-based cad. J Digit Imaging 1–7
16. Miehle J, Ostler D, Gerstenlauer N, Minker W (2017) The next step: intelligent digital assistance for clinical operating rooms. Innov Surg Sci 2(3):159–161
17. Mirnezami R, Ahmed A (2018) Surgery 3.0, artificial intelligence and the next-generation surgeon. Br J Surg 105(5):463–465
18. Mok TS, Wu YL, Thongprasert S, Yang CH, Chu DT, Saijo N, Sunpaweravong P, Han B, Margono B, Ichinose Y et al (2009) Gefitinib or carboplatin-paclitaxel in pulmonary adenocarcinoma. N Engl J Med 361(10):947–957
19. Murdoch TB, Detsky AS (2013) The inevitable application of big data to health care. Jama 309(13):1351–1352
20. Nussinov R, Jang H, Tsai CJ, Cheng F (2019) Precision medicine and driver mutations: computational methods, functional assays and conformational principles for interpreting cancer drivers. PLoS Comput Biol 15(3):e1006658

21. Petit C, Bezemer R, Atallah L (2018) A review of recent advances in data analytics for post-operative patient deterioration detection. J Clin Monit Comput 32(3):391–402
22. Shademan A, Decker RS, Opfermann JD, Leonard S, Krieger A, Kim PC (2016) Supervised autonomous robotic soft tissue surgery. Sci Tansl Med 8(337):337ra64–337ra64
23. Shaw AT, Kim DW, Nakagawa K, Seto T, Crinó L, Ahn MJ, De Pas T, Besse B, Solomon BJ, Blackhall F et al (2013) Crizotinib versus chemotherapy in advanced alk-positive lung cancer. N Engl J Med 368(25):2385–2394
24. Sleijfer S, Bogaerts J, Siu LL (2013) Designing transformative clinical trials in the cancer genome era. J Clin Oncol 31(15):1834–1841
25. Strand F, Zackrisson S (2019) Breast cancer imaging-a rapidly evolving discipline. The Breast 46:58–63
26. Targarona E, Balla A, Batista G (2018) Big data and surgery: the digital revolution continues. Cirugia Espanola 96(5):247–249
27. Van Esbroeck A, Rubinfeld I, Hall B, Syed Z (2014) Quantifying surgical complexity with machine learning: looking beyond patient factors to improve surgical models. Surgery 156(5):1097–1105
28. Xu J, Yang P, Xue S, Sharma B, Sanchez-Martin M, Wang F, Beaty KA, Dehan E, Parikh B (2019) Translating cancer genomics into precision medicine with artificial intelligence: applications, challenges and future perspectives. Hum Genetics 138(2):109–124

# Chapter 9
# State of Three Parasitic Diseases in Morocco: Malaria, Schistosomiasis and Leishmaniasis

**Naoual Zitouni**

**Abstract** Malaria, schistosomiasis and leishmaniasis are three parasitic diseases that cause major public health problems worldwide. Morocco has received World Health Organization certification for the elimination of autochthonous malaria, but there is an increase in imported malaria. The autochthonous schistosomiasis has been eliminated; this condition must be maintained and verified by the World Health Organization. Despite this, Morocco is at risk of a re-emergence of these two diseases due to several factors such as: the persistence of vectors, especially *Anopheles labranchiae*, population movements, climate change. Finally, leishmaniasis persists; Morocco is taking several actions to stop the epidemic.

## 9.1 Introduction

Vector-borne diseases are caused by parasites, viruses and bacteria transmitted by vectors such as mosquitoes, sand-flies and molluscs. Each year, more than one billion cases and more than one million deaths worldwide are attributed to vector-borne diseases [29].

According to the latest World Health Organisation (WHO) estimates, major vector-borne diseases are responsible for more than 17% of all infectious diseases. This figure may increase due to the risk of re-emergence as a consequence of climate change. The burden of these diseases is higher in tropical and subtropical areas and disproportionately affects the poorest populations [29].

Malaria, schistosomiasis and leishmaniasis are parasitic diseases linked to poverty and deterioration of living conditions and hygiene. Schistosomiasis and leishmaniasis are classified as neglected tropical diseases by WHO [16, 34]. Thanks to sustained political commitments, considerable efforts have been made to eliminate this group of diseases, particularly in the WHO European Region, which was the first region in the world to have eliminated malaria. However, a significant emergence or re-emergence

N. Zitouni (✉)
Higher Institute of Health Nursing and Technical Professions Oujda (ISPITSO), Oujda, Morocco
e-mail: zitouninaoual@yahoo.fr



A. Boutayeb (ed.), *Disease Prevention and Health Promotion in Developing Countries*,
https://doi.org/10.1007/978-3-030-34702-4_9

of vector-borne diseases has been reported in some areas around the world. Some of these diseases show an increasing tendency to spread to areas where they did not previously exist, to extend their transmission season, to intensify their transmission in areas where they are already present and to reappear in areas from which they were eliminated. This expansion is the result of the intensification and globalization of the exchange and movements of population, man interactions with the environment, and climate change.

As everywhere in the world, Morocco is not protected from this scourge. Indeed, some vector-borne diseases are still a concern. This is the case of autochthonous malaria which, despite its elimination, is likely to be reintroduced due to the existence of favourable conditions, leishmaniasis which is not yet controlled despite the efforts of the public authorities and schistosomiasis for which the stopping of transmission must be maintained.

Morocco has an area of 710.000 $km^2$ and a population of 33.848.242 inhabitants, an annual growth rate of 1.25% and a life expectancy of 74.8 years. The urban population represents 60.3%. Morocco is considered to be a transit country for migrants from sub-Saharan Africa with 77.554 in regular situation and 20.000 in irregular situation [20, 22], which makes it a tropical disease transmission zone.

## 9.2 Malaria

Malaria is the most widespread and deadly infectious disease worldwide [6]. It causes one million deaths/year, 90% of cases are recorded in the tropical areas of Africa and three billion people are at risk of contracting the disease, making it a priority for global health [28].

Malaria is caused by a protozoan parasite of the genus *Plasmodium (P.)*. Five species infect humans: *P. falciparum*, which is the main and most virulent agent, *P. vivax*, *P. ovale*, *P. malariae* and *P. knowlesi*. In Morocco, two species cause autochthonous malaria: *P. falciparum* and *P. vivax*. In addition to these two species, *P. ovale* and *P. malariae* are found in imported malaria cases [12].

Transmission of malaria is done by mosquitoes of the genus *Anopheles (A.)* of the family Culicidae. Some sixty species carry the disease around the world. In Africa, *plasmodium* transmission is mainly via *A. gambiae* [24], in Morocco *A. labranchiae* is the main vector, *A. sergentii* is probably a secondary vector [27].

Anti-malarial action in Morocco began in 1929 after a deadly epidemic. Various vector control measures have led to a drop in the number of cases and the redistribution of disease outbreaks to limited areas [27]. In 1963, Morocco entered a phase of pre-eradication of malaria. The operational phase of the national malaria control programme, established in 1964, reduced autochthonous malaria from 30893 cases in 1963–68 cases in 1998 [32]. This programme led to the elimination of severe falciparum malaria in 1975, while *P. vivax* was not controlled until the late 1990s [14]. In 1998, Morocco adopted the ≪ Global Strategy for the Elimination of autochtonous Malaria ≫ and achieved Certification of Malaria Elimination in 2010; the last case

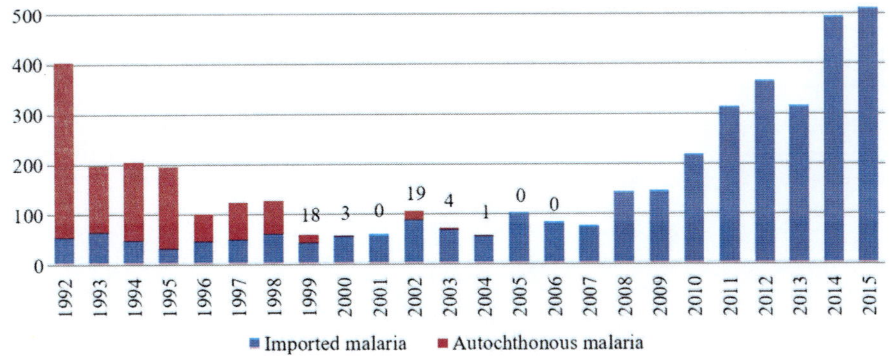


**Fig. 9.1** Cases of malaria in Morocco between 1992 and 2015 *Source* Data provided by the DELM [12]

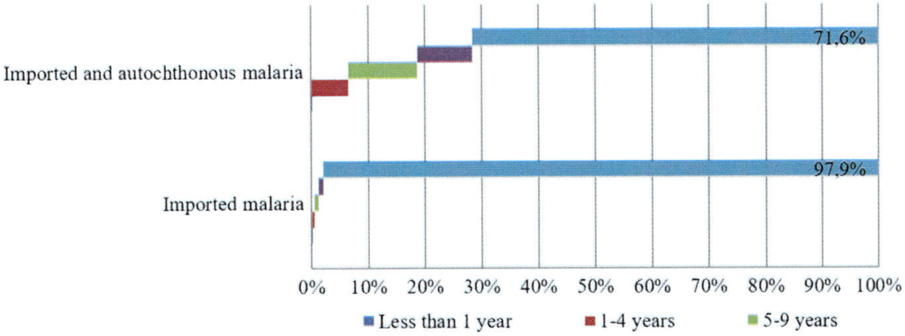


**Fig. 9.2** Malaria cases in Morocco by age of patients *Source* Data provided by the DELM [12]

was recorded in 2004 in Chefchaouen, in the north of the country, in one of the oldest area of malaria in Morocco (Fig. 9.1).

Despite the elimination of autochthonous malaria [36], Morocco is still affected by imported malaria. The first case was registered in 1976 and is becoming more and more frequent. The number of cases increased from 54 in 1992 to 510 in 2015. Thus, imported malaria constituted 16% (720 cases) of total malaria from 1992 to 2004, increasing to 60.8% (2.756 cases) in the period 2005–2015 (Fig. 9.1).

The populations concerned are occasional Moroccan travellers to sub-Saharan Africa, soldiers on humanitarian missions, expatriates and migrants [5]. The proportion of imported malaria is higher among "travellers" than among migrants and refugees [2, 5]. They are generally from urban areas and 98% of them are over 15 years old (Fig. 9.2). Indeed, after the elimination of autochthonous malaria in 2005, 2751 cases of imported malaria were recorded in cities compared to only 5 in rural areas. Before that date, autochtonous malaria was more prevalent in rural areas, where 1051 cases were recorded, compared to 725 urban cases during the period 1992–2004 (Fig. 9.3).

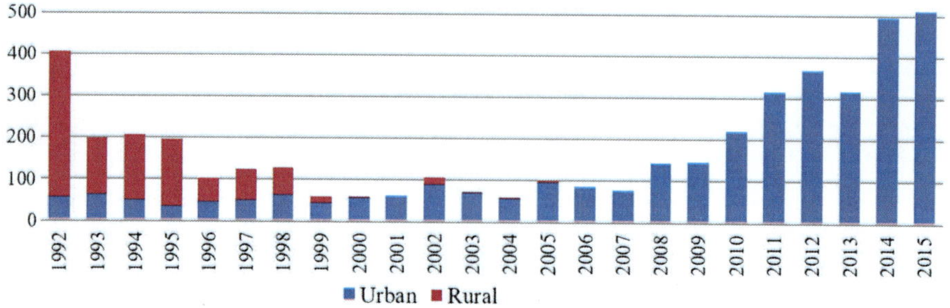


**Fig. 9.3** Cases of malaria in Morocco in urban and rural areas *Source* Data provided by the DELM [12]

## 9.3 Schistosomiasis

Schistosomiasis is the parasitic endemic disease with second highest prevalence in the world, after malaria, with 180 million affected individuals and about 200,000 deaths each year [31]. Africa is the most affected, accounting for 92% of the cases needing preventive treatment, only 28.2% were treated in 2015 [37].

Schistosomiasis is a parasitic disease caused by a flatworm of the *Platyhelminthes* phylum, *Trematoda* class, and genus of *Schistosoma (S.)*. Four species infects humans: *S. mansoni*, *S. japonicum*, *S. intercalatum* and *S. haematobium*. In Morocco, where only *S. haematobium* is present, transmission to humans is necessarily via *Bulinus truncatus* (Phyllum: *Mollusca*. Class: *Gastropoda*).

Schistosomiasis seems to have been present in Morocco since the 16th century [35] according to Carosse [7] it dates back to the 11th century. The first case was detected in 1914 in Marrakech by Job [7]. Since the 1950s, several investigations have shown that the disease is present in the Saharan side of the Atlas mountains [35], in the southern oases and the north-western plains [3, 4].

From 1967 onwards, the disease spread rapidly to other areas of Morocco, due to the development of irrigation systems and population displacements [4]. The situation became serious in 1973 with the registration of 13416 cases [4], which led to the implementation of the preparatory phase of the schistosomiasis control programme in 1976.

The period between 1977 and 1981 was a planning phase and choosing the control strategy to be adopted and the organization responsible for its management. The operational phase lasts from 1982 to 1993 and its objectives were to control infection and transmission along four axes: parasite control (through case detection and treatment) and host control (through physical and chemical actions), education/information and intersectoral collaboration [4, 26].

The process of eliminating schistosomiasis began in 1994 [35], 10 years after its implementation, there was only an average of 352 cases/year, which fell to less than 5 cases/year between 2004 and 2015. The interruption of schistosomiasis transmission was effective from 2004 [1, 26, 35], the last indigenous cases recorded were in

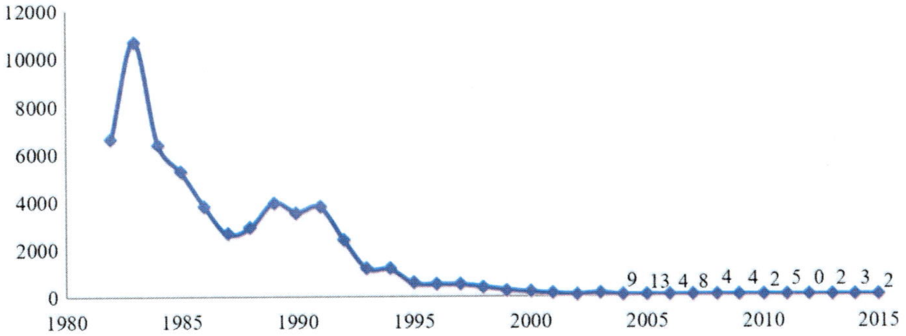


**Fig. 9.4** Cases of schistosomiasis in Morocco between 1982 and 2015 *Source* Data provided by the DELM [12]

2003 [8]. They are children from Tata under the age of 14. The majority of cases between 2003 and 2015 were reported in old schistosomiasis foci, 60% of which were recorded in Tata (Fig. 9.4).

Epidemiological investigations carried out for all cases reported between 2004 and 2007, confirm that they are all either cases imported from foreign countries, or residual cases over 17 years of age. Screening is done by direct urinalysis or biopsy that has revealed a low parasitic content [35]. On the other hand, and according to WHO recommendations [33], molecular tests on *Bulinus*, from the last transmission areas, have shown the absence of *S. heamatobium*, as well as the absence of any serological trace of the parasite DNA in children aged 0–16 years [1]. With the elimination target achieved, Morocco began a phase of consolidation of the elimination of schistosomiasis in 2005.

Currently, Morocco is registered by the World Health Organisation among the countries that must verify if the transmission has actually been interrupted [28]. Until the establishment of a certification process for countries that have not reported schistosomiasis cases for at least 10 years [28], The World Health Organization recommends the creation of an international commission to carry out an appropriate evaluation for each country [31].

## 9.4 Leishmaniasis

As early as the 10th century, leishmaniasis was described and attributed to the "bite of a mosquito" by Arab doctors Al Boukhari and Avicenne, while pathogens were only discovered in the 19th century by Mc Naught and Cunnigham [13]. It is one of the most neglected parasitic diseases in the world [23] and affects between 700,000 and 1 million new cases/year and causes between 20,000 and 30,000 deaths/year [21]. It is linked to poverty, unsanitary housing and malnutrition.

It is caused by a flagellated protozoan parasite of the family *Trypanosomitidae*, genus *Leishmania (L.)* which has more than 20 species. It is transmitted by the bite of the female sandfly (*Diptera, Nematocera*) of the family *Psychodidae*. More than 90 species transmit leishmaniasis and there are 70 animal species, including humans, which can constitute a natural reservoir. The disease comes in three forms: visceral, cutaneous and mucocutaneous leishmaniasis.

In Morocco, cutaneous and visceral leishmaniasis has been rife for a century [13], they are the most frequent, the cutaneous and mucosal form is rare and recent [17]. Cutaneous leishmaniasis is caused by two parasites *L. tropica* and *L. major*. The latter is transmitted by *Phlebotomus papatasi*, the reservoir being a rodent of the family *Gerbilidae*: *Meriones shawi*. The disease is mainly found in palm groves. *L. tropica*, the reservoir of which is Man, is transmitted by *Phlebotomus sergenti* it is mainly found in the semi-arid regions of Morocco it is related to thuya forests [9, 23].

Visceral leishmaniasis is caused by *L. infantum* whose main vector is *Phlebotomus perniciosus* and rarely *Phlebotomus ariasi* and *Phlebotomus longicuspis*, the reservoir of the parasite is the dog [23]. The disease is sporadic in the north of the country, especially in humid and subhumid areas [11]. It is usually found in rural areas. Nevertheless, there is more and more urban cases [19] and in previously unaffected areas [10].

Morocco is ranked third in the world by the high prevalence of leishmaniasis [15]. From 1922 to 2016, 78.498 cases of leishmaniasis were recorded, 93% of them in the last 30 years. Cutaneous leishmaniasis is the most common in Morocco, accounting for 92% of the notifications with 72.047 cases against 6.451 cases of visceral leishmaniasis (Table 9.1).

Both forms are rapidly growing, progressively for visceral leishmaniasis, and according to peaks for the cutaneous form. Between 2008 and 2011, there is an explosion of cases of cutaneous leishmaniasis due to slowdown of epidemiological surveillance and the reduction of indoor residual spraying [30] after the cessation of transmission of autochthonous malaria (Figs. 9.5 and 9.6).

Faced with this epidemic situation, Morocco launched, in 1997, the national program for surveillance and fight against leishmaniasis. It is based on 3 main actions

**Table 9.1** Leishmaniasis cases recorded from 1922 to 2016 in Morocco according to time periods

| Periods | Leishmaniasis cutaneous | Visceral | Total cases | % |
|---|---|---|---|---|
| 1922–1957 | 9 | 21 | 30 | 0.04% |
| 1957–1978 | 952 | 67 | 1019 | 1.30% |
| 1979–1984 | 384 | 3866 | 4250 | 5.41% |
| 1985–2015 | – | 2497 | – | 93.25% |
| 1985–2016 | 70702 | – | 73199 | |
| Total | 72047 | 6451 | 78498 | |

*Source* Data provided by the DELM [12]

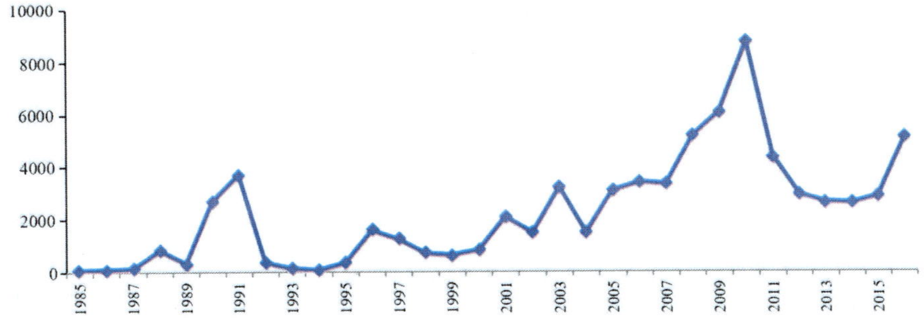


**Fig. 9.5** Cases of visceral leishmaniasis between 1985 and 2015 *Source* Data provided by the DELM [12]

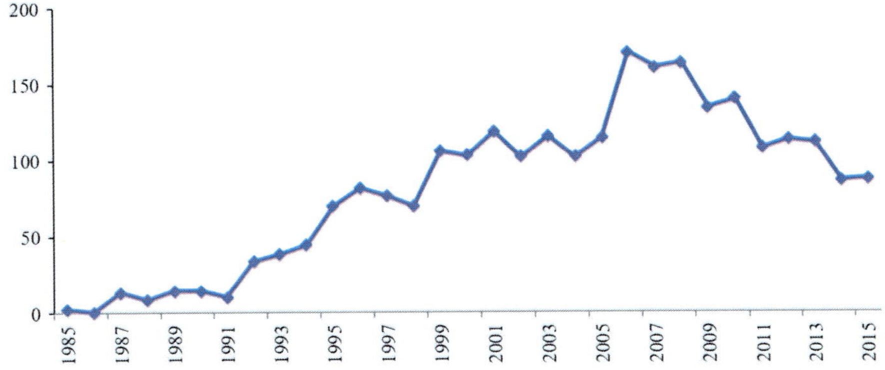


**Fig. 9.6** Cases of cutaneous leishmaniasis in Morocco between 1985 and 2015 *Source* Data provided by the DELM [12]

according to the recommendations of the WHO [23]. Mass screening of exposed foci, early medical care of 100% of detected cases and control of vectors and reservoir hosts animals. These actions are reinforced by information and education of the population concerned and intersectoral collaboration. The objectives of this program are to detect 75% of the estimated cases of cutaneous leishmaniasis and eliminate deaths due to visceral leishmaniasis by 2021 and ultimately to eliminate leishmaniasis by 2030 [11].

## 9.5 Conclusion

After decades of effort, autochthonous malaria has certainly been eradicated, but imported cases are increasing, which presents, in a context of climate, demographic and behavioural change, a risk of re-emergence, especially since its vector is still present.

Transmission of autochthonous schistosomiasis has been interrupted in Morocco. It must be verified by the WHO in order to no longer classify Morocco as an endemic country. In this case too, there is a risk of re-emergence. Indeed, since 2013, there has been a re-emergence and persistence of schistosomiasis in Corsica after 50 years of absence [25] in the WHO European Region, which was considered free of schistosomiasis.

Leishmaniasis is a public health problem; Morocco is in the midst of an epidemic. Cutaneous leishmaniasis is on the rise, visceral leishmaniasis is reaching new areas [10] and we can also see the appearance of the cutaneous-mucous form. In the long term, climate change will also play a role in the increase in leishmaniasis [18] Faced with this epidemic situation, Morocco must strengthen and revitalize its efforts to combat it.

## References

1. Amarir F, El Mansouri B, Fellah H, Sebti F, Mohammed L, Handali S, Wilkins P, El Idrissi AL, Sadak A, Rhajaoui M (2011) National serologic survey of haematobium schistosomiasis in Morocco: evidence for elimination. Am J Trop Med Hyg 84(1):15–19
2. Askling HH, Nilsson J, Tegnell A, Janzon R, Ekdahl K (2005) Malaria risk in travelers. Emerg Infect Dis 11(3):436–441
3. Barkia H, Barkia A, Nhammi H, Belghyti D (2011) La schistosomiase au maroc: de sa découverte à l'après-élimination. East Mediterr Health J 17(3):250–256
4. Barkia H, Barkia A, Yacoubi R, Alemad A, El Kharim K, Belghyti D (2014) Contribution of mobile teams to efforts to eliminate schistosomiasis at schistosoma haematobium in Morocco-narrative review article. Iran J Public health 43(9):1167–1175
5. Benseddik N (2013) Le paludisme d'importation á l'hôpital militaire Moulay Ismail de Meknes. Dissertation, University of Fes
6. Candolfi E (2005) Le paludisme transfusionnel, les mesures de prévention. Transfusion clinique et biologique 12(2):107–113
7. Carrosse J (1930) La bilharziose vésicale dans le sud marocain (schistosoma hæmatobium). Annales de Parasitologie Humaine et Comparée 8(2):161–164
8. Direction d'Epidémiologie et de Lutte contre les Maladies (2003) Données épidémiologiques des maladies sous surveillance, Bilan année 2003. Bulletin d'Epidémiologie et Santé Publique 9
9. Direction d'Epidémiologie et de Lutte contre les Maladies (2010) Lutte contre les leishmanioses: Guide des activités
10. Direction d'Epidémiologie et de Lutte contre les Maladies (2017) Bulletin d'Epidémiologie et Santé Publique 40(74)
11. Direction d'Epidémiologie et de Lutte contre les Maladies (2018) Bulletin d'Epidémiologie et Santé Publique 56(76)
12. Direction d'Epidémiologie et de Lutte contre les Maladies (2019) Publications. https://www.sante.gov.ma/Pages/ADM_Centrale/DELM.aspx
13. El Alami S (2009) Quatre vingt cinq années de Leishmaniose au Maroc. Dissertation, Université Mohammed V of Rabat
14. El Mehdi S, Qacif H, Zyani M (2015) Les circonstances de découverte du paludisme d'importation: expérience du service de médecine interne de l'hôpital militaire avicenne de marrakech. PhD thesis, Thèse de médecine. Faculté de médecine et de pharmacie. Université Cadi-Ayyad

15. Hotez PJ, Savioli L, Fenwick A (2012) Neglected tropical diseases of the middle east and north Africa: review of their prevalence, distribution, and opportunities for control. PLoS Negl Trop Dis 6(2):e1475
16. Hotez PJ, Pecoul B, Rijal S, Boehme C, Aksoy S, Malecela M, Tapia-Conyer R, Reeder JC (2016) Eliminating the neglected tropical diseases: translational science and new technologies. PLoS Negl Trop Dis 10(3):e0003895
17. Iguermia S, Harmouche T, Mikou O, Amarti A, Mernissi F (2011) Mucocutaneous leishmaniasis in Morocco, evidence of the parasite's ecological evolution? Med et Maladies Infect 41(1):47–48
18. Kahime K, Boussaa S, Bounoua L, Fouad O, Messouli M, Boumezzough A (2014) Leishmaniasis in Morocco: diseases and vectors. Asian Pac J Trop Dis 4:S530–S534
19. Kahime K, Boussaa S, Nhammi H, Boumezzough A (2017) Urbanization of human visceral leishmaniasis in Morocco. Parasite Epidemiol Control 2(4):1–6
20. Mghari M (2007) La migration irrégulière au Maroc. Centre d'Etudes et de Recherches Démographiques (CERED), Rabat, Maroc
21. Organisation Mondiale de la Santé (2019) Leishmaniasis. https://www.who.int/news-rooms/fact-sheets/detail/leismaniasis. Accessed 25 May 2019
22. Organisation Mondiale de la Santé (2016) Stratégie de coopération oms-maroc: 2017–2021. Technical report, Organisation mondiale de la Santé. Bureau régional de la Méditerranée orientale
23. Organisation Mondiale de la Santé (2010) La lutte contre les leishmanioses: rapport de la réunion du comité OMS d'experts de la lutte contre les leishmanioses. In: La lutte contre les leishmanioses: rapport de la réunion du comité OMS d'experts de la lutte contre les leishmanioses
24. Pasteur Institut (2013) Le paludisme. http://www.pasteur.fr/fr/centre-medical/fiches-maladies/paludisme. Accessed 20 Oct 2018
25. Ramalli L, Mulero S, Noël H, Chiappini JD, Vincent J, Barré-Cardi H, Malfait P, Normand G, Busato F, Gendrin V et al (2018) Persistence of schistosomal transmission linked to the Cavu river in southern Corsica since 2013. Eurosurveillance 23(4)
26. Rollinson D, Knopp S, Levitz S, Stothard JR, Tchuenté LAT, Garba A, Mohammed KA, Schur N, Person B, Colley DG et al (2013) Time to set the agenda for schistosomiasis elimination. Acta Trop 128(2):423–440
27. Trari B, Carnevale P (2011) De la préélimination à l'élimination du paludisme au maroc. quels risques pour l'avenir? Bulletin de la Societe de pathologie exotique 104(4):291–295
28. World Health Organization (2013) Schistosomiasis: progress report 2001–2011 and strategic plan 2012–2020
29. World Health Organization (2017) Maladie á transmission vectorielle. http://www.who.int/mediacentre/factsheets/fs87/fr. Accessed 20 June 2019
30. World Health Organization (2016) World malaria report 2015. World Health Organization
31. World Health Organization and others (2004) Schistosomiase et géohelminthiases: prévention et lutte: rapport d'un comité d'experts de l'OMS
32. World Health Organization and others (2007) Le paludisme au maroc: une lutte sans relache, une perspective d'elimination. Technical report
33. World Health Organization and others (2009) Elimination of schistosomiasis from low-transmission areas: report of a who informal consultation, salvador, bahia, brazil, 18-19 August 2008. Technical report, World Health Organization, Geneva
34. World Health Organization and others (2010) Working to overcome the global impact of neglected tropical diseases: first who report on neglected tropical diseases. Technical report, World Health Organization, Geneva
35. World Health Organization and others (2012) Elimination de la schistosomiase au maroc: une réalite et un succes apres trois décennies de lutte
36. World Health Organization and others (2013) World malaria report 2012. http://www.who.int/malaria/publications/world_malaria_report_2012/report/en/. Accessed 20 Oct 2018

37. World Health Organization and others (2017) Schistosomiasis and soil-transmitted helminthiases: number of people treated in 2016-schistosomiase et géohelminthiases: nombre de personnes traitées en 2016. Weekly Epidemiological Record Relevé épidémiologique hebdomadaire 92(49):749–760

# Part II
# Mathematical Modelling and Epidemiological Studies

# Chapter 10
# Global Properties of a Diffusive HBV Infection Model with Cell-to-Cell Transmission and Three Distributed Delays

**Khalid Hattaf and Noura Yousfi**

**Abstract** In this chapter, we develop a mathematical model for hepatitis B virus (HBV) infection with two modes of transmission, spatial diffusion for both HBV DNA-containing capsids and viruses, and three distributed delays. The first delay is for the production of productively infected hepatocytes, the second for the production of matured capsids and the third for the production of matured virions with the corresponding probabilities of survival. The global properties of the model are explored. Furthermore, an application of our main results is presented and discussed.

## 10.1 Introduction

Hepatitis B is a viral infection caused by the hepatitis B virus (HBV) which is a member of Hepadnaviridae family of viruses that infects liver cells namely hepatocytes. The HBV infection can eventually become acute or chronic in nature. With dominant immune responses, the acute illness resolves in majority of cases after lasting for several weeks [1]. But the persistent chronic illness potentially lead to range of severe diseases such as liver cirrhosis, hepatocellular carcinoma (HCC), membranous glomerulonephritis and acute necrotizing vasculitis [1]. From the World Health Organization (WHO), an estimated 257 million people are living with HBV infection (defined as hepatitis B surface antigen positive), and 8,87,000 people are dead in 2015 due to HBV complications including cirrhosis and HCC [2].

Mathematical modeling is considered as an effective tool to understand HBV infection dynamics, and gains insights into the mechanisms of HBV infection in vivo. Many mathematical models have been proposed in order to describe the dynamics of HBV infection by using ordinary differential equations (ODEs), delay differential

---

K. Hattaf (✉)
Centre Régional des Métiers de l'Education et de la Formation (CRMEF), Casablanca, Morocco
e-mail: k.hattaf@yahoo.fr

N. Yousfi
Laboratory of Analysis, Modelling and simulation (LAMS), Faculty of Sciences Ben M'sik, Hassan II University of Casablanca, 7955 Sidi Othman, Casablanca, Morocco
e-mail: nourayousfi@gmail.com



A. Boutayeb (ed.), *Disease Prevention and Health Promotion in Developing Countries*,
https://doi.org/10.1007/978-3-030-34702-4_10

equations (DDEs), as well as partial differential equations (PDEs). Nowak et al. [3] designed and investigated a simple HBV infection model comprising a system of three ODEs for uninfected hepatocytes, infected hepatocytes and free virus. Min et al. [4] pointed out that the basic model in [3] might not be suitable for HBV infection since it demonstrated unreasonable relationship between the number of hepatocytes and susceptibility to infection. They amended this basic model by incorporating a standard incidence function instead of mass action term for the infection process. In [5], the authors further extended this model by incorporating time delay for virus production. Li et al. [6] extended the basic model in [3] by replacing the constant source term for uninfected hepatocytes with the logistic hepatocyte growth and proved the existence of Hopf bifurcation. Eikenberry et al. proposed and investigated the dynamics of an HBV infection model with both logistic hepatocyte growth and standard incidence function in [7]. They pointed out the possibility of sustained oscillations which might lead to acute liver failure. Wang et al. [8] improved the model presented in [4] by incorporating the cytokine-mediated cure for infected hepatocytes and carried out the global analysis. Hews et al. [9] identified a Hopf and a homoclinic bifurcation point and showed their dependence on the basic reproduction number and the intrinsic growth rate of hepatocyte for an HBV infection model with logistic hepatocyte growth and standard incidence function. In [10], Yousfi et al. modeled the adaptive immune response in HBV infection and discussed a possible explanation of the immune response failure to the infection. Pang et al. presented and analyzed an HBV infection model with cytotoxic T lymphocyte (CTL) immune responses by taking into account the role of cytolytic and noncytolytic mechanisms and the export of precursor CTL cells from the thymus in [11]. Manna and Chakrabarty [12] investigated the global dynamics of an HBV infection model with HBV DNA-containing capsids. Some other ODE or DDE driven models for HBV infection and their analysis can be found in [13–15]. Furthermore, a recent HBV infection model formulated by fractional differential equations (FDEs) is proposed and analyzed in [16].

The models discussed above do not consider the spatial diffusion of related populations by assuming cells and viruses are well-mixed, but it is evident that such spatial mobility plays a significant role in many biological processes [17, 18]. In recent years, many researchers incorporated spatial mobility in HBV infection models and studied their dynamics. Wang and Wang [19] introduced a diffusive HBV infection model by considering the random mobility of viruses in liver and neglecting the diffusion of susceptible and infected hepatocytes, and they established the existence of traveling waves by using geometric singular perturbation method. Wang et al. [20] considered the delayed version of the model and carried out several numerical simulations to demonstrate the effects of diffusion and delay together on the dynamics. The existence of traveling waves for this delayed model is proved analytically by constructing a pair of upper and lower solutions in [21]. Xu and Ma [22] further extended this model by considering saturation response of the infection process. Chí et al. considered the model with standard incidence function and studied global stability in [23]. Zhang and Xu [24] studied a similar type of model with Beddington-DeAngelis functional response and showed the existence of traveling wave solutions for conditions in term of basic reproduction number. Hattaf and Yousfi [25] proposed a delayed diffusive HBV infection model with general incidence rate and studied stability by using linearization method and by constructing appropriate Lyapunov functionals. Shaoli et al. considered a diffusive HBV infection model with CTL immune response and nonlinear incidence rate and analyzed it in [26]. Manna and Chakrabarty [27] investigated the global properties of a diffusive HBV infection model with capsids and presented an appropriate dynamically consistent non-standard finite difference (NSFD) scheme. The delayed version of this model was analyzed in [28]. Some other diffusion driven viral infection models and their analysis can be found in [29–32]. In 2019, Manna and Hattaf [33] proposed and investigated a reaction-diffusion HBV infection model with capsids, three discrete delays, adaptive immunity and general incidence rate that includes many cases existing in the literature such as the classical bilinear incidence rate, the Beddington-DeAngelis functional response, the Crowley-Martin functional response and the Hattaf–Yousfi functional response.

All the above cited models that are formulated by ODEs, DDEs, FDEs and PDEs considered only the classical virus-to-cell infection. In reality, the virus can spread by two fundamental modes, one by virus-to-cell infection through the extracellular space and the other by cell-to-cell transfer involving direct cell-to-cell contact [34–36]. To better describe the dynamics of HBV infection in within human body, by taking into account both modes of transmission, we propose the following model:

$$\begin{aligned}
\frac{\partial H}{\partial t} &= s - \mu H(x,t) - f\big(H(x,t), I(x,t), V(x,t)\big)V(x,t) - g\big(H(x,t), I(x,t)\big)I(x,t),\\
\frac{\partial I}{\partial t} &= \int_0^\infty f_1(\tau)e^{-\alpha_1\tau}[f\big(H(x,t-\tau), I(x,t-\tau), V(x,t-\tau)\big)V(x,t-\tau)\\
&\quad + g\big(H(x,t-\tau), I(x,t-\tau)\big)I(x,t-\tau)]d\tau - \delta I(x,t),\\
\frac{\partial D}{\partial t} &= d_D\Delta D + a\int_0^\infty f_2(\tau)e^{-\alpha_2\tau}I(x,t-\tau)d\tau - (\beta+\delta)D(x,t),\\
\frac{\partial V}{\partial t} &= d_V\Delta V + \beta\int_0^\infty f_3(\tau)e^{-\alpha_3\tau}D(x,t-\tau)d\tau - cV(x,t),
\end{aligned} \tag{10.1}$$

where $H(x,t)$, $I(x,t)$, $D(x,t)$ and $V(x,t)$ are the densities of the uninfected hepatocytes, infected hepatocytes, HBV DNA-containing capsids, and the virions at position $x$ and time $t$, respectively. Uninfected hepatocytes are produced at rate $s$, die at rate $\mu H$ and become infected by contact with virions at rate $f(H,I,V)V$ and by contact with infected hepatocytes at rate $g(H,I)I$. The parameter $\delta$ is the death rate of infected hepatocytes and capsids. The parameters $a$, $\beta$ and $c$ are, respectively, the production rate of capsids from infected hepatocytes, the rate at which the capsids are transmitted to blood which gets converted to virions, and the clearance rate of virions. In addition, we assume that the virion or hepatocyte cell contacts a susceptible hepatocyte at time $t-\tau$ and the cell becomes infected at time $t$, where $\tau$ is a random variable taken from a probability distribution $f_1(\tau)$. The factor $e^{-\alpha_1\tau}$ accounts for the probability of surviving from time $t-\tau$ to time $t$, where $\alpha_1$ is the death rate for infected but not yet virus-producing cells. Also, we assume that the time spent in the production of matured intracellular HBV DNA-containing capsids is a random variable with a probability distribution $f_2(\tau)$. The probability of survival of immature capsids is given by $e^{-\alpha_2\tau}$ and the average life time of an immature capsid is given by $\frac{1}{\alpha_2}$. In the same, we assume that the time necessary for the newly produced capsids to become virions is a random variable with a probability distribution $f_3(\tau)$. The factor $e^{-\alpha_3\tau}$ accounts for the probability of surviving from time $t-\tau$ to time $t$, where $\frac{1}{\alpha_3}$ is the average life time of an immature virion. The probability distribution functions $f_1(\tau)$, $f_2(\tau)$ and $f_3(\tau)$ are assumed to satisfy $f_i(\tau) \geq 0$ and $\int_0^\infty f_i(\tau)d\tau = 1$ for $i = 1, 2, 3$. Finally, $d_D$ and $d_V$ are the diffusion coefficients of capsids and virions, respectively with $\Delta$ being the Laplacian operator.

As in [37–39], the incidence functions $f(H, I, V)$ and $g(H, I)$ for both modes of infection are continuously differentiable and satisfy the following hypotheses:

$(H_0)$ g(0,I) = 0, for all $I \geq 0$; $\frac{\partial g}{\partial H}(H, I) \geq 0$ (or $g(H, I)$ is a strictly monotone increasing function with respect to $H$ when $f \equiv 0$) and $\frac{\partial g}{\partial I}(H, I) \leq 0$, for all $H \geq 0$ and $I \geq 0$.

$(H_1)$ $f(0, I, V) = 0$, for all $I \geq 0$ and $V \geq 0$,

$(H_2)$ $f(H, I, V)$ is a strictly monotone increasing function with respect to $H$ (or $\frac{\partial f}{\partial H}(H, I, V) \geq 0$ when $g(H, I)$ is a strictly monotone increasing function with respect to $H$), for any fixed $I \geq 0$ and $V \geq 0$,

$(H_3)$ $f(H, I, V)$ is a monotone decreasing function with respect to $I$ and $V$.

Biologically, the four hypotheses hypotheses are reasonable and consistent with the reality. For more details on the biological significance of these four hypotheses, we refer the reader to the works [37, 39–41].

It is very important to note that our model described by system (10.1) includes many special cases. For example, we get the diffused HBV infection model proposed by Manna in [28] when $f_1(\tau) = \delta(\tau - \tau_1)$, $f_2(\tau) = f_3(\tau) = \delta(\tau), \alpha_1 = \alpha_2 = \alpha_3 = 0$, $f(H, I, V) = kH$ and $g(H, I) = 0$, where $\delta(.)$ is the Dirac delta function and $k$ is a positive constant rate describing the infection process. When we neglect the diffusion of capsids, the cell-to-cell transmission mode and consider only the case when $f_i(\tau) = \delta(\tau - \tau_i)$ for $i = 1, 2, 3$, we obtain the PDE model introduced in [31]. When we ignore the HBV DNA-containing capsids and the cell-to-cell transmission mode, we get the diffusive and delayed HBV model [25] which is the generalization of the PDE models presented in [19, 20, 22–24, 30]. Further, the diffusive and delayed viral infection model proposed by Geng et al. [32] is a particular case of our model (10.1).

In this study, we consider system (10.1) with initial conditions

$$\begin{aligned} &H(x,\theta) = \phi_1(x,\theta) \geq 0, \quad I(x,\theta) = \phi_2(x,\theta) \geq 0, \\ &D(x,\theta) = \phi_3(x,\theta) \geq 0, \quad V(x,\theta) = \phi_4(x,\theta) \geq 0, \ (x,\theta) \in \bar{\Omega} \times (-\infty, 0], \end{aligned} \tag{10.2}$$

and Neumann boundary conditions

$$\frac{\partial D}{\partial \nu} = \frac{\partial V}{\partial \nu} = 0, \ on\ \partial\Omega \times (0, +\infty), \tag{10.3}$$

where $\Omega$ is a bounded domain in $\mathbf{R}^n$ with smooth boundary $\partial\Omega$, and $\dfrac{\partial}{\partial\nu}$ denotes the outward normal derivative on $\partial\Omega$. From the biological point of view, the Neumann boundary conditions mean that the capsids and virions do not move across the boundary $\partial\Omega$.

## 10.2 Well-Posedness and Equilibria

In this section, we focus on the existence, uniqueness, positivity and boundedness of solutions of problem (10.1)–(10.3) as they represent the densities of hepatocytes, capsids and virions. Further, we establish the basic reproduction number and equilibria of our model.

Let $\mathbb{X} = C(\bar{\Omega}, \mathbf{R}^4)$ be the Banach space of continuous functions from $\bar{\Omega}$ into $\mathbf{R}^4$, and $\mathcal{C}_\alpha = C_\alpha((-\infty, 0], \mathbb{X})$ be the Banach space of continuous functions $\varphi$ from $(-\infty, 0]$ into $\mathbb{X}$, where $\varphi(\theta)e^{\alpha\theta}$ is uniformly continuous on $(-\infty, 0]$ and $\|\varphi\| = \sup_{\theta\leq 0}\|\varphi(\theta)\|_{\mathbb{X}} e^{\alpha\theta} < \infty$ with $\alpha$ is a positive constant. For convenience, we identify an element $\varphi \in \mathcal{C}_\alpha$ as a function from $\bar{\Omega} \times (-\infty, 0]$ into $\mathbf{R}^4$ defined by $\varphi(x, \theta) = \varphi(\theta)(x)$. For any continuous function $\omega(.) : (-\infty, \sigma) \to \mathbb{X}$ for $\sigma > 0$, we define $\omega_t \in \mathcal{C}_\alpha$ by $\omega_t(\theta) = \omega(t + \theta)$, $\theta \in (-\infty, 0]$. It is easy to show that $t \mapsto \omega_t$ is a continuous function from $[0, \sigma)$ to $\mathcal{C}_\alpha$.

**Theorem** *For any given initial condition $\phi \in \mathcal{C}_\alpha$ satisfying (10.2), there exists a unique solution of the problem (10.1)–(10.3) defined on $[0, +\infty)$ and this solution remains non-negative and bounded for all $t \geq 0$.* □

*Proof* For any $\varphi = (\varphi_1, \varphi_2, \varphi_3, \varphi_4)^T \in \mathcal{C}_\alpha$ and $x \in \bar{\Omega}$, we define $F = (F_1, F_2, F_3, F_4) : \mathcal{C}_\alpha \to \mathbb{X}$ by

$$
\begin{aligned}
F_1(\varphi)(x) &= s - \mu\varphi_1(x, 0) - f\big(\varphi_1(x, 0), \varphi_2(x, 0), \varphi_4(x, 0)\big)\varphi_4(x, 0)\\
&\quad - g\big(\varphi_1(x, 0), \varphi_2(x, 0)\big)\varphi_2(x, 0),\\
F_2(\varphi)(x) &= \int_0^\infty f_1(\tau)e^{-\alpha_1\tau}[f\big(\varphi_1(x, -\tau), \varphi_2(x, -\tau), \varphi_4(x, -\tau)\big)\varphi_4(x, -\tau)\\
&\quad + g\big(\varphi_1(x, -\tau), \varphi_2(x, -\tau)\big)\varphi_2(x, -\tau)]d\tau - \delta\varphi_2(x, 0),\\
F_3(\varphi)(x) &= a\int_0^\infty f_2(\tau)e^{-\alpha_2\tau}\varphi_2(x, -\tau)d\tau - (\beta + \delta)\varphi_3(x, 0),\\
F_4(\varphi)(x) &= \beta\int_0^\infty f_3(\tau)e^{-\alpha_3\tau}\varphi_3(x, -\tau)d\tau - c\varphi_4(x, 0).
\end{aligned}
$$

Then the problem (10.1)–(10.3) can be rewritten as the following abstract functional differential equation:

$$
\begin{aligned}
&\omega'(t) = A\omega + F(\omega_t), \qquad t > 0,\\
&\omega(0) = \phi \in \mathcal{C}_\alpha,
\end{aligned}
\tag{10.4}
$$

where $\omega = (H, I, D, V)^T$, $\phi = (\phi_1, \phi_2, \phi_3, \phi_4)^T$ and $A\omega = (0, 0, d_D\Delta D, d_V\Delta V)^T$. Obviously, we see that $F$ is locally Lipschitz in $\mathcal{C}_\alpha$. It follows from [42–46] that there exists a unique local solution of system (10.4) on $[0, T_{max})$, where $T_{max}$ is the maximal existence time for solution of (10.4).

Clearly, $\mathbf{0} = (0, 0, 0, 0)$ is a lower-solution of the problem (10.1)–(10.3). Hence, $H(x, t) \geq 0$, $I(x, t) \geq 0$, $D(x, t) \geq 0$ and $V(x, t) \geq 0$.

By the first equation of (10.1), we have

$$\frac{\partial H}{\partial t} \leq s - \mu H(x, t), \tag{10.5}$$

which implies that

$$H(x, t) \leq \max\left\{\frac{s}{\mu}, \max_{x\in\bar{\Omega}} \phi_1(x, 0)\right\}, \forall (x, t) \in \bar{\Omega} \times [0, T_{max}).$$

Hence, $T$ is bounded. Let

$$T(x, t) = I(x, t) + \int_0^\infty f_1(\tau)e^{-\alpha_1\tau} H(x, t-\tau)d\tau.$$

The integral in $T(x, t)$ is well-defined and differentiable with respect to $t$, due to $H$ being bounded. Then

$$\begin{aligned}\frac{\partial T}{\partial t} &= s\int_0^\infty f_1(\tau)e^{-\alpha_1\tau}d\tau - \mu\int_0^\infty f_1(\tau)e^{-\alpha_1\tau} H(x, t-\tau)d\tau - \delta I(x, t)\\ &\leq s\eta_1 - \rho_1 T(x, t),\end{aligned}$$

where $\rho_1 = \min\{\mu, \delta\}$ and

$$\eta_i = \int_0^\infty f_i(\tau)e^{-\alpha_i\tau}d\tau, \quad i = 1, 2, 3. \tag{10.6}$$

Thus,

$$T(x, t) \leq \max\left\{\frac{s\eta_1}{\rho_1}, \max_{x\in\bar{\Omega}} T(x, 0)\right\}, \forall (x, t) \in \bar{\Omega} \times [0, T_{max}).$$

This implies that $I$ is bounded.

From the boundedness of $I$ and (10.1)–(10.3), we deduce that $D$ satisfies the following system

$$\begin{cases}\dfrac{\partial D}{\partial t} - d_D\Delta D \leq a\rho_2\eta_2 - (\beta + \delta)D,\\ \dfrac{\partial D}{\partial \nu} = 0,\\ D(x, 0) = \phi_3(x, 0) \geq 0,\end{cases} \tag{10.7}$$

where $\rho_2 = max\left\{\frac{s\eta_1}{\rho_1}, \max_{x\in\bar{\Omega}} T(x, 0)\right\}$.

According to Lemma 1 in [39], we have

$$D(x,t) \le \max\left\{\frac{a\rho_2\eta_2}{\beta+\delta}, \max_{x\in\bar{\Omega}}\phi_3(x,0)\right\}, \forall (x,t) \in \bar{\Omega}\times[0,T_{max}).$$

Similarly to above, we deduce that

$$V(x,t) \le \max\left\{\frac{\beta\rho_3\eta_3}{c}, \max_{x\in\bar{\Omega}}\phi_4(x,0)\right\}, \forall (x,t) \in \bar{\Omega}\times[0,T_{max}),$$

where $\rho_3 = \max\left\{\frac{a\rho_2\eta_2}{\beta+\delta}, \max_{x\in\bar{\Omega}}\phi_3(x,0)\right\}$.

From the above, we have proved that $H(x,t)$, $I(x,t)$, $D(x,t)$ and $V(x,t)$ are bounded on $\bar{\Omega}\times[0,T_{max})$. By the standard theory for semilinear parabolic systems [47], we deduce that $T_{max} = +\infty$. This completes the proof. ■

Obviously, system (10.1) has always one infection-free equilibrium $E_f(H_0,0,0,0)$, where $H_0 = \frac{s}{\mu}$, which represents the healthy state. So, we define the basic reproduction number of (10.1) as follows

$$\mathcal{R}_0 = \frac{a\beta\eta_1\eta_2\eta_3 f(\frac{s}{\mu},0,0) + c(\beta+\delta)\eta_1 g(\frac{s}{\mu},0)}{\delta c(\beta+\delta)}. \tag{10.8}$$

The other equilibrium of (10.1) satisfies:

$$\begin{aligned}
&s-\mu H - f(H,I,V)V - g(H,I)I &&= 0,\\
&\eta_1\big(f(H,I,V)V + g(H,I)I\big) - \delta I &&= 0,\\
&a\eta_2 I - (\beta+\delta)D &&= 0,\\
&\beta\eta_3 D - cV &&= 0,
\end{aligned}$$

which leads to

$$a\beta\eta_1\eta_2\eta_3 f\big(H, \frac{\eta_1(s-\mu H)}{\delta}, \frac{a\eta_1\eta_2\eta_3\beta(s-\mu H)}{c\delta(\beta+\delta)}\big) + c(\beta+\delta)\eta_1 g(H, \frac{\eta_1(s-\mu H)}{\delta}) = c\delta(\beta+\delta). \tag{10.9}$$

We have $I = \frac{\eta_1(s-\mu H)}{\delta} \ge 0$, which implies that $H \le \frac{s}{\mu}$. Hence, there is no biological equilibrium when $H > \frac{s}{\mu}$.

Define the function $\psi$ on the interval $[0, \frac{s}{\mu}]$ by

$$\begin{aligned}
\psi(H) = {} & a\beta\eta_1\eta_2\eta_3 f\big(H, \frac{\eta_1(s-\mu H)}{\delta}, \frac{a\eta_1\eta_2\eta_3\beta(s-\mu H)}{c\delta(\beta+\delta)}\big)\\
&+ c(\beta+\delta)\eta_1 g(H, \frac{\eta_1(s-\mu H)}{\delta}) - c\delta(\beta+\delta).
\end{aligned}$$

Clearly, $\psi(0) = -c\delta(\beta+\delta) < 0$, $\psi(\frac{s}{\mu}) = c\delta(\beta+\delta)(\mathcal{R}_0 - 1)$ and

$$\psi'(H) = a\beta\eta_1\eta_2\eta_3\Big(\frac{\partial f}{\partial H} - \frac{\mu\eta_1}{\delta}\frac{\partial f}{\partial I} - \frac{a\beta\mu\eta_1\eta_2\eta_3}{c\delta(\beta+\delta)}\frac{\partial f}{\partial V}\Big) + c(\beta+\delta)\eta_1\Big(\frac{\partial g}{\partial H} - \frac{\mu\eta_1}{\delta}\frac{\partial g}{\partial I}\Big) > 0.$$

Thus, if $\mathcal{R}_0 > 1$, there exists another biologically meaningful equilibrium $E^*(H^*, I^*, D^*, V^*)$ with $H^* \in (0, \frac{s}{\mu})$, $I^* > 0$, $D^* > 0$ and $V^* > 0$.

Summarizing the above discussions, we get the following theorem.

**Theorem**

*(i) When $\mathcal{R}_0 \le 1$, model (10.1) has a unique infection-free equilibrium of the form $E_f(H_0, 0, 0, 0)$, where $H_0 = \frac{s}{\mu}$.*

*(ii) When $\mathcal{R}_0 > 1$, in addition to $E_f$, model (10.1) has a unique chronic infection equilibrium of the form $E^*(H^*, I^*, D^*, V^*)$ with $H^* \in (0, \frac{s}{\mu})$, $I^* > 0$, $D^* > 0$ and $V^* > 0$.* □

## 10.3 Global Stability

In this section, we investigate the global stability of each equilibrium. First, we have the following result.

**Theorem** *The infection-free equilibrium $E_f$ is globally asymptotically stable if $\mathcal{R}_0 \le 1$, and it is unstable if $\mathcal{R}_0 > 1$.* □

*Proof* Based on the method introduced in [29], we construct a Lyapunov functional as follows

$$\begin{aligned}
L_0 = \int_\Omega \Big\{ &\frac{1}{\eta_1} I(x,t) + \frac{\beta\eta_3 f(H_0,0,0)}{c(\beta+\delta)} D(x,t) + \frac{f(H_0,0,0)}{c} V(x,t) \\
&+ \frac{1}{\eta_1}\int_0^\infty f_1(\tau)e^{-\alpha_1\tau}\int_{t-\tau}^t \big[f\big(H(x,\theta), I(x,\theta), V(x,\theta)\big)V(x,\theta) \\
&+ g\big(H(x,\theta), I(x,\theta)\big)I(x,\theta)\big]d\theta d\tau + \frac{a\beta\eta_3 f(H_0,0,0))}{c(\beta+\delta)}\int_0^\infty f_2(\tau)e^{-\alpha_2\tau}\int_{t-\tau}^t I(x,\theta)d\theta d\tau \\
&+ \frac{\beta f(H_0,0,0))}{c}\int_0^\infty f_3(\tau)e^{-\alpha_3\tau}\int_{t-\tau}^t D(x,\theta)d\theta d\tau \Big\} dx.
\end{aligned}$$

For convenience, we let $\varphi = \varphi(x,t)$ and $\varphi_\tau = \varphi(x, t-\tau)$ for any $\varphi \in \{H, I, D, V\}$. The time derivative of $L_0$ along the solution of system (10.1)–(10.3) satisfies

$$\begin{aligned}
\frac{dL_0}{dt} = \int_\Omega \Big\{ &\Big(f(H,I,V) - f(H_0,0,0)\Big)V \\
&+ \frac{\delta}{\eta_1} I\Big(\frac{a\beta\eta_1\eta_2\eta_3 f(H_0,0,0) + c(\beta+\delta)\eta_1 g(H,I)}{\delta c(\beta+\delta)} - 1\Big)\Big\} dx.
\end{aligned}$$

By (10.5), we obtain $\limsup_{t\to\infty} H(x,t) \le H_0$. This implies that all omega limit points satisfy $H(x,t) \le H_0$. Hence, it is sufficient to consider solutions for which $H(x,t) \le H_0$. By the explicit formula of $\mathcal{R}_0$ given in (10.8) and $(H_0)$–$(H_3)$, we get

$$\begin{aligned}\frac{dL_0}{dt} &\le \int_\Omega \left\{ \Big( f(H,I,V) - f(H_0,0,0) \Big) V + \frac{\delta}{\eta_1}(\mathcal{R}_0 - 1) I \right\} dx \\ &\le \int_\Omega \frac{\delta}{\eta_1}(\mathcal{R}_0 - 1) I dx.\end{aligned}$$

If follows from $\mathcal{R}_0 \le 1$ that $\frac{dL_0}{dt} \le 0$. It is easy to show that the largest invariant set in $\{(H,I,D,V) | \frac{dL_0}{dt} = 0\}$ is $\{E_0\}$. By LaSalle invariance principle [48], the infection-free equilibrium $E_f$ is globally asymptotically stable when $\mathcal{R}_0 \le 1$.

It remains to show the instability of $E_f$ when $\mathcal{R}_0 > 1$.
Let $0 = \lambda_1 < \lambda_2 < \cdots < \lambda_n < \cdots$ be the eigenvalues of the operator $-\Delta$ on $\Omega$ with the homogeneous Neumann boundary conditions, and $\mathcal{E}(\lambda_i)$ be the eigenfunction space corresponding to $\lambda_i$ in $C^1(\Omega)$. Let $\{\varphi_{ij} : j = 1, 2, \ldots, \dim \mathcal{E}(\lambda_i)\}$ be an orthonormal basis of $\mathcal{E}(\lambda_i)$, $\mathbb{Y} = [C^1(\Omega)]^4$, and $\mathbb{Y}_{ij} = \{d\varphi_{ij} : d \in \mathbb{R}^4\}$. Then

$$\mathbb{Y} = \bigoplus_{i=1}^{\infty} \mathbb{Y}_i \text{ and } \mathbb{Y}_i = \bigoplus_{j=1}^{\dim \mathcal{E}(\mu_i)} \mathbb{Y}_{ij},$$

where $\bigoplus$ denotes the direct sum of the subspaces.

Let $E_e(H_e, I_e, D_e, V_e)$ be an arbitrary equilibrium. Let $U_1(x,t) = H(x,t) - H_e$, $U_2(x,t) = I(x,t) - I_e$, $U_3(x,t) = D(x,t) - D_e$ and $U_4(x,t) = V(x,t) - V_e$. By substituting $U_i(x,t)$ into system (10.1) and linearizing, we get the following system

$$\begin{aligned}\frac{\partial U_1}{\partial t} &= -\big(\mu + \tfrac{\partial f}{\partial H} V_e + \tfrac{\partial g}{\partial H} I_e\big) U_1(x,t) - \big(\tfrac{\partial f}{\partial I} V_e + \tfrac{\partial g}{\partial I} I_e + g(H_e, I_e)\big) U_2(x,t) \\ &\quad - \big(\tfrac{\partial f}{\partial V} V_e + f(H_e, I_e, V_e)\big) U_4(x,t), \\ \frac{\partial U_2}{\partial t} &= \big(\tfrac{\partial f}{\partial H} V_e + \tfrac{\partial g}{\partial H} I_e\big) \int_0^\infty f_1(\tau) e^{-\alpha_1 \tau} U_1(x, t-\tau) d\tau \\ &\quad + \big(\tfrac{\partial f}{\partial I} V_e + \tfrac{\partial g}{\partial I} I_e + g(H_e, I_e)\big) \int_0^\infty f_1(\tau) e^{-\alpha_1 \tau} U_2(x, t-\tau) d\tau \\ &\quad + \big(\tfrac{\partial f}{\partial V} V_e + f(H_e, I_e, V_e)\big) \int_0^\infty f_1(\tau) e^{-\alpha_1 \tau} U_4(x, t-\tau) - \delta U_2(x,t), \\ \frac{\partial U_3}{\partial t} &= d_D \Delta U_3 + a \int_0^\infty f_2(\tau) e^{-\alpha_2 \tau} U_2(x, t-\tau) d\tau - (\beta + \delta) U_3(x,t), \\ \frac{\partial U_4}{\partial t} &= d_V \Delta U_4 + \beta \int_0^\infty f_3(\tau) e^{-\alpha_3 \tau} U_3(x, t-\tau) d\tau - c U_4(x,t),\end{aligned}$$

By a simple calculation, the characteristic equation of the above system at the equilibrium $E_f$ is given by

$$(\xi + \mu) g_i(\xi) = 0, \tag{10.10}$$

where

$$\begin{aligned} g_i(\xi) &= \xi^3 + \big(c + \beta + 2\delta + \lambda_i d_D + \lambda_i d_V - \overline{\eta}_1 g(H_0, 0)\big)\xi^2 \\ &+ [(\beta + 2\delta + \lambda_i d_D - \overline{\eta}_1 g(H_0, 0))(c + \lambda_i d_V) + (\beta + \delta + \lambda_i d_D)(\delta - \overline{\eta}_1 g(H_0, 0))]\xi \\ &+ \delta(\beta + \delta + \lambda_i d_D)(c + \lambda_i d_V) - a\beta\overline{\eta}_1\overline{\eta}_2\overline{\eta}_3 f(H_0, 0, 0) \\ &- (\beta + \delta + \lambda_i d_D)(c + \lambda_i d_V)\overline{\eta}_1 g(H_0, 0), \end{aligned}$$

where

$$\overline{\eta}_i = \int_0^{\infty} f_i(\tau) e^{-(\alpha_i + \xi)\tau} d\tau, \quad i = 1, 2, 3. \tag{10.11}$$

Clearly, $\xi_1 = -\mu$ is a root of (10.10). The remaining roots are the solutions of the transcendental cubic equation $g_i(\xi) = 0$. We have $\lim\limits_{\xi \to +\infty} g_i(\xi) = +\infty$. Since $\lambda_1 = 0$, we get $g_1(0) = c\delta(\beta + \delta)(1 - \mathcal{R}_0) < 0$. Consequently, the equation $g_1(\xi) = 0$ has a positive real root and so $E_f$ is unstable when $\mathcal{R}_0 > 1$. This completes the proof. ■

Finally, we establish the global stability of the chronic infection equilibrium $E^*$. To do this, we assume that $\mathcal{R}_0 > 1$ and the incidence functions $f$ and $g$ satisfy the following further hypothesis

$$\begin{cases} \left(1 - \dfrac{f(H, I, V)}{f(H, I^*, V^*)}\right)\left(\dfrac{f(H, I^*, V^*)}{f(H, I, V)} - \dfrac{V}{V^*}\right) \leq 0, \\ \left(1 - \dfrac{f(H^*, I^*, V^*)g(H, I)}{f(H, I^*, V^*)g(H^*, I^*)}\right)\left(\dfrac{f(H, I^*, V^*)g(H^*, I^*)}{f(H^*, I^*, V^*)g(H, I)} - \dfrac{I}{I^*}\right) \leq 0. \end{cases} \tag{$H_4$}$$

Thus, we have the following result.

**Theorem** *Assume that $\mathcal{R}_0 > 1$ and (H4) holds. Then the chronic infection equilibrium $E^*$ is globally asymptotically stable.* □

*Proof* Construct a Lyapunov functional as follows

$$\begin{aligned} L_1 = \int_{\Omega} \Bigg\{ & H - H^* - \int_{H^*}^{H} \frac{f(H^*, I^*, V^*)}{f(S, I^*, V^*)} dS + \frac{1}{\eta_1} I^* \Phi\left(\frac{I}{I^*}\right) \\ &+ \frac{f(H^*, I^*, V^*)V^*}{a\eta_2 I^*} D^* \Phi\left(\frac{D}{D^*}\right) + \frac{(\beta + \delta) f(H^*, I^*, V^*)V^*}{a\beta\eta_2\eta_3 I^*} V^* \Phi\left(\frac{V}{V^*}\right) \\ &+ \frac{1}{\eta_1} f(H^*, I^*, V^*)V^* \int_0^{\infty} f_1(\tau) e^{-\alpha_1 \tau} \int_{t-\tau}^{t} \Phi\left(\frac{f\big(H(x, \theta), I(x, \theta), V(x, \theta)\big)V(x, \theta)}{f(H^*, I^*, V^*)V^*}\right) d\theta d\tau \\ &+ \frac{1}{\eta_1} g(H^*, I^*)I^* \int_0^{\infty} f_1(\tau) e^{-\alpha_1 \tau} \int_{t-\tau}^{t} \Phi\left(\frac{g\big(H(x, \theta), I(x, \theta)\big)I(x, \theta)}{g(H^*, I^*)I^*}\right) d\theta d\tau \\ &+ \frac{1}{\eta_2} f(H^*, I^*, V^*)V^* \int_0^{\infty} f_2(\tau) e^{-\alpha_2 \tau} \int_{t-\tau}^{t} \Phi\left(\frac{I(x, \theta)}{I^*}\right) d\theta d\tau \\ &+ \frac{1}{\eta_3} f(H^*, I^*, V^*)V^* \int_0^{\infty} f_3(\tau) e^{-\alpha_3 \tau} \int_{t-\tau}^{t} \Phi\left(\frac{D(x, \theta)}{D^*}\right) d\theta d\tau \Bigg\} dx, \end{aligned}$$

where $\Phi(u) = u - 1 - \ln u$, $u > 0$. It is not hard to see that $\Phi(u) \geq 0$ for all $u > 0$, and $\Phi(u) = 0$ if and only if $u = 1$. The time derivative of $L_1$ along the solution of system (10.1)–(10.3) satisfies

$$
\begin{aligned}
\frac{dL_1}{dt} &= \int_{\Omega} \Bigg\{ \mu H^* \left(1 - \frac{H}{H^*}\right)\left(1 - \frac{f(H^*, I^*, V^*)}{f(H, I^*, V^*)}\right) \\
&+ f(H^*, I^*, V^*)V^* \left(-1 - \frac{V}{V^*} + \frac{f(H, I^*, V^*)}{f(H, I, V)} + \frac{f(H, I, V)V}{f(H, I^*, V^*)V^*}\right) \\
&+ g(H^*, I^*)I^* \left(-1 - \frac{I}{I^*} + \frac{f(H, I^*, V^*)g(H^*, I^*)}{f(H^*, I^*, V^*)g(H, I)} + \frac{f(H^*, I^*, V^*)g(H, I)I}{f(H, I^*, V^*)g(H^*, I^*)I^*}\right) \\
&- \frac{1}{\eta_1} f(H^*, I^*, V^*)V^* \int_0^{\infty} f_1(\tau)e^{-\alpha_1 \tau} \left[\Phi\left(\frac{f(H^*, I^*, V^*)}{f(H, I^*, V^*)}\right) + \Phi\left(\frac{f(H_\tau, I_\tau, V_\tau)V_\tau I^*}{f(H^*, I^*, V^*)V^* I}\right)\right. \\
&\left. + \Phi\left(\frac{f(H, I^*, V^*)}{f(H, I, V)}\right)\right] d\tau - \frac{1}{\eta_1} g(H^*, I^*)I^* \int_0^{\infty} f_1(\tau)e^{-\alpha_1 \tau} \left[\Phi\left(\frac{f(H^*, I^*, V^*)}{f(H, I^*, V^*)}\right)\right. \\
&\left. + \Phi\left(\frac{g(H_\tau, I_\tau)I_\tau}{g(H^*, I^*)I}\right) + \Phi\left(\frac{f(H, I^*, V^*)g(H^*, I^*)}{f(H^*, I^*, V^*)g(H, I)}\right)\right] d\tau \\
&- \frac{1}{\eta_2} f(H^*, I^*, V^*)V^* \int_0^{\infty} f_2(\tau)e^{-\alpha_2 \tau} \Phi\left(\frac{D^* I_\tau}{DI^*}\right) d\tau \\
&- \frac{1}{\eta_3} f(H^*, I^*, V^*)V^* \int_0^{\infty} f_3(\tau)e^{-\alpha_3 \tau} \Phi\left(\frac{V^* D_\tau}{VD^*}\right) d\tau \Bigg\} dx \\
&- \frac{f(H^*, I^*, V^*)V^*}{\delta + \beta} d_D \int_{\Omega} \frac{|\nabla D|^2}{D^2} dx - \frac{f(H^*, I^*, V^*)V^*}{c} d_V \int_{\Omega} \frac{|\nabla V|^2}{V^2} dx.
\end{aligned}
$$

Since the function $f(H, I, V)$ is strictly monotonically increasing with respect to $H$, we have

$$
\left(1 - \frac{H}{H^*}\right)\left(1 - \frac{f(H^*, I^*, V^*)}{f(H, I^*, V^*)}\right) \leq 0.
$$

Based on the hypothesis (H4), we have

$$
-1 - \frac{V}{V^*} + \frac{f(H,I^*,V^*)}{f(H,I,V)} + \frac{V}{V^*}\frac{f(H,I,V)}{f(H,I^*,V^*)} = \left(1 - \frac{f(H,I,V)}{f(H,I^*,V^*)}\right)\left(\frac{f(H,I^*,V^*)}{f(H,I,V)} - \frac{V}{V^*}\right) \leq 0.
$$

and

$$
\begin{aligned}
&-1 - \frac{I}{I^*} + \frac{f(H,I^*,V^*)g(H^*,I^*)}{f(H^*,I^*,V^*)g(H,I)} + \frac{f(H^*,I^*,V^*)g(H,I)I}{f(H,I^*,V^*)g(H^*,I^*)I^*} \\
&= \left(1 - \frac{f(H^*,I^*,V^*)g(H,I)}{f(H,I^*,V^*)g(H^*,I^*)}\right)\left(\frac{f(H,I^*,V^*)g(H^*,I^*)}{f(H^*,I^*,V^*)g(H,I)} - \frac{I}{I^*}\right) \leq 0.
\end{aligned}
$$

Since $\Phi(u) \geq 0$ for $u > 0$, we have $\frac{dL_1}{dt} \leq 0$. Further, the largest compact invariant set in $\{(H, I, D, V)|\frac{dL_1}{dt} = 0\}$ is the singleton $\{E^*\}$. It follows from LaSalle invariance principle that $E^*$ is globally asymptotically stable when $\mathcal{R}_0 > 1$. ■

Now, choose the incidence function $f(H, I, V)$ as follows:

$$
\begin{cases} \dfrac{kH\varrho(V)}{V}, & V \neq 0, \\ kH\varrho'(0), & V = 0, \end{cases} \tag{10.12}
$$

with $\varrho(0) = 0, \varrho'(V) > 0$ and $\varrho''(V) \leq 0$. From the Mean Value Theorem, we deduce that

$$\varrho'(V)V \leq \varrho(V) \leq \varrho'(0)V.$$

It is clear to see that $f(H, I, V)V = kH\varrho(V)$ for all $H, I, V \geq 0$. By a simple computation, we can easily show that the function $f(H, I, V)$ given by (10.12) satisfies the four hypotheses $(H_1)$–$(H_4)$. Therefore, the PDE model and results presented by Geng et al. [32] are improved and generalized. In [32], the authors considered only two discrete delays and they did not investigate the instability of the infection-free equilibrium $E_f$ in the case where $\mathcal{R}_0 > 1$.

## 10.4 Application

In this section, we apply our theoretical results obtained in the preceding sections to the following model:

$$\begin{aligned}
\frac{\partial H}{\partial t} &= s - \mu H(x,t) - \frac{k_1 H(x,t)V(x,t)}{1+b_1 V(x,t)} - \frac{k_2 H(x,t)I(x,t)}{1+b_2 I(x,t)},\\
\frac{\partial I}{\partial t} &= \int_0^{\infty} f_1(\tau)e^{-\alpha_1\tau}\left[\frac{k_1 H(x,t-\tau)V(x,t-\tau)}{1+b_1 V(x,t-\tau)} + \frac{k_2 H(x,t-\tau)I(x,t-\tau)}{1+b_2 I(x,t-\tau)}\right]d\tau - \delta I(x,t),\\
\frac{\partial D}{\partial t} &= d_D\Delta D + a\int_0^{\infty} f_2(\tau)e^{-\alpha_2\tau} I(x,t-\tau)d\tau - (\beta+\delta)D(x,t),\\
\frac{\partial V}{\partial t} &= d_V\Delta V + \beta\int_0^{\infty} f_3(\tau)e^{-\alpha_3\tau} D(x,t-\tau)d\tau - cV(x,t),
\end{aligned} \tag{10.13}$$

where $k_1$ and $k_2$ denote the virus-to-cell infection and the cell-to-cell transmission rates. The non-negative constants $b_1$ and $b_2$ measure the saturation effect. The other state variables and parameters have the same biological meanings as in system (10.1). As before, we consider model (10.13) with initial conditions

$$\begin{aligned}
&H(x,\theta) = \phi_1(x,\theta) \geq 0, \quad I(x,\theta) = \phi_2(x,\theta) \geq 0,\\
&D(x,\theta) = \phi_3(x,\theta) \geq 0, \quad V(x,\theta) = \phi_4(x,\theta) \geq 0, \quad (x,\theta) \in \bar{\Omega} \times (-\infty, 0],
\end{aligned} \tag{10.14}$$

and Neumann boundary conditions

$$\frac{\partial D}{\partial \nu} = \frac{\partial V}{\partial \nu} = 0, \quad on\ \partial\Omega \times (0, +\infty), \tag{10.15}$$

The problem (10.13)–(10.15) is a particular case of system (10.1)–(10.3) with $f(H, I, V) = \dfrac{k_1 H}{1+b_1 V}$ and $g(H, I) = \dfrac{k_2 H}{1+b_2 I}$. Based on the previous sections, system (10.13) has one infection-free equilibrium $E_f(\frac{s}{\mu}, 0, 0)$, and a unique chronic infection equilibrium $E^*(H^*, I^*, D^*, V^*)$ when $\mathcal{R}_0 = \frac{a\beta k_1 s\eta_1\eta_2\eta_3}{\delta\mu c(\beta+\delta)} + \frac{k_2 s\eta_1}{\delta\mu} > 1$.

On the other hand, it is clear that the hypotheses $(H_0)$–$(H_3)$ are satisfied. For the fifth hypothesis, we have

$$\left(1 - \frac{f(H, I, V)}{f(H, I^*, V^*)}\right)\left(\frac{f(H, I^*, V^*)}{f(H, I, V)} - \frac{V}{V*}\right) = \frac{-b_1(V - V^*)^2}{V^*(1 + b_1V^*)(1 + b_1V)} \leq 0,$$

$$\left(1 - \frac{f(H^*, I^*, V^*)g(H, I)}{f(H, I^*, V^*)g(H^*, I^*)}\right)\left(\frac{f(H, I^*, V^*)g(H^*, I^*)}{f(H^*, I^*, V^*)g(H, I)} - \frac{I}{I^*}\right) = \frac{-b_2(I - I^*)^2}{I^*(1 + b_2I^*)(1 + b_2I)} \leq 0.$$

Hence, the last hypothesis (H4) is satisfied. From the two last Theorems we deduce the following result.

**Corollary** *(i) If $\mathcal{R}_0 \leq 1$, then the infection-free equilibrium $E_f$ of system (10.13)–(10.15) is globally asymptotically stable.*

*(ii) If $\mathcal{R}_0 > 1$, then the infection-free equilibrium $E_f$ becomes unstable and the chronic infection equilibrium $E^*$ of (10.13)–(10.15) is globally asymptotically stable.* □

## 10.5 Conclusion

In this work, we have proposed and studied the dynamical behavior of an HBV infection model with capsids and two modes of transmission that are the classical virus-to-cell infection and the direct cell-to-cell transmission. Both modes of transmission are modeled by two general incidence functions. Also in the proposed model, we have considered three distributed delays and spatial diffusion for both capsids and viruses. We have proved that the dynamical behavior of the model is completely determined by the basic reproduction number $\mathcal{R}_0$. More precisely, the infection-free equilibrium is globally asymptotically stable when $R_0 \leq 1$, which biologically means that the HBV is cleared and the infection die out. When $R_0 > 1$, the infection-free equilibrium becomes unstable and the chronic infection equilibrium is globally asymptotically stable which indicates that the HBV persists in the liver.

From the above analytical results, we deduce a strategy for controlling HBV infection by reducing the value of $\mathcal{R}_0$ to a level equal or less than one. On the other hand, Lots of HBV infection models and the corresponding results existing in the literature are generalized and improved by considering both modes of transmission and three distributed delays.

## References


1. Ribeiro RM, Lo A, Perelson AS (2002) Dynamics of hepatitis B virus infection. Microbes Infect 4(8):829–835
2. WHO (2018) Hepatitis B. https://www.who.int/news-room/fact-sheets/detail/hepatitis-b
3. Nowak MA, Bonhoeffer S, Hill AM, Boehme R, Thomas HC, McDade H (1996) Viral dynamics in hepatitis B virus infection. Proc Natl Acad Sci USA 93(9):4398–4402
4. Min L, Su Y, Kuang Y (2008) Mathematical analysis of a basic virus infection model with application to HBV infection. Rocky Mt J Math 38(5):1573–1585
5. Gourley SA, Kuang Y, Nagy JD (2008) Dynamics of a delay differential equation model of hepatitis B virus infection. J Biol Dyn 2(2):140–153
6. Li J, Wang K, Yang Y (2011) Dynamical behaviors of an HBV infection model with logistic hepatocyte growth. Math Comput Model 54(1–2):704–711
7. Eikenberry S, Hews S, Nagy JD, Kuang Y (2009) The dynamics of a delay model of hepatitis B virus infection with logistic hepatocyte growth. Math Biosci Eng 6(2):283–299
8. Wang K, Fan A, Torres A (2010) Global properties of an improved hepatitis B virus model. Nonlinear Anal: Real World Appl 11(4):3131–3138
9. Hews S, Eikenberry S, Nagy JD, Kuang Y (2010) Rich dynamics of a hepatitis B viral infection model with logistic hepatocyte growth. J Math Biol 60(4):573–590
10. Yousfi N, Hattaf K, Tridane A (2011) Modeling the adaptive immune response in HBV infection. J Math Biol 63(5):933–957
11. Pang J, Cui J, Hui J (2012) The importance of immune responses in a model of hepatitis B virus. Nonlinear Dyn 67(1):723–734
12. Manna K, Chakrabarty SP (2015) Chronic hepatitis B infection and HBV DNA-containing capsids: modeling and analysis. Commun Nonlinear Sci Numer Simul 22(1–3):383–395
13. Wang J, Tian X (2013) Global stability of a delay differential equation of hepatitis B virus infection with immune response. Electron J Differ Equ 94:1–11
14. Manna K, Chakrabarty SP (2017) Global stability of one and two discrete delay models for chronic hepatitis B infection with HBV DNA-containing capsids. Comput Appl Math 36(1):525–536
15. Manna K (2017) Global properties of a HBV infection model with HBV DNA-containing capsids and CTL immune response. Int J Appl Comput Math 3(3):2323–2338
16. Bachraoui M, Hattaf K, Yousfi N (2019) Dynamics of a fractional order HBV infection model with capsids and CTL immune response. Commun Math Biol Neurosci 6:1–15
17. Britton NF (2003) Essential mathematical biology. Springer, London
18. Funk GA, Jansen VAA, Bonhoeffer S, Killingback T (2005) Spatial models of virus-immune dynamics. J Theor Biol 233(2):221–236
19. Wang K, Wang W (2007) Propagation of HBV with spatial dependence. Math Biosci 210(1):78–95
20. Wang K, Wang W, Song S (2008) Dynamics of an HBV model with diffusion and delay. J Theor Biol 253(1):36–44
21. Gan Q, Xu R, Yang P, Wu Z (2010) Travelling waves of a hepatitis B virus infection model with spatial diffusion and time delay. IMA J Appl Math 75(3):392–417
22. Xu R, Ma Z (2009) An HBV model with diffusion and time delay. J Theor Biol 257(3):499–509
23. Chí NC, Vales EÁ, Almeida GG (2012) Analysis of a HBV model with diffusion and time delay. J Appl Math 2012:1–25
24. Zhang Y, Xu Z (2014) Dynamics of a diffusive HBV model with delayed Beddington-DeAngelis response. Nonlinear Anal: Real World Appl 15:118–139
25. Hattaf K, Yousfi N (2015) A generalized HBV model with diffusion and two delays. Comput Math Appl 69(1):31–40
26. Shaoli W, Xinlong F, Yinnian H (2011) Global asymptotical properties for a diffused HBV infection model with CTL immune response and nonlinear incidence. Acta Math Sci 31(5):1959–1967

27. Manna K, Chakrabarty SP (2015) Global stability and a non-standard finite difference scheme for a diffusion driven HBV model with capsids. J Differ Equ Appl 21(10):918–933
28. Manna K (2017) Dynamics of a diffusion-driven HBV infection model with capsids and time delay. Int J Biomath 10(5):1–18
29. Hattaf K, Yousfi N (2013) Global stability for reaction-diffusion equations in biology. Comput Math Appl 66(8):1488–1497
30. Hattaf K, Yousfi N (2015) Global dynamics of a delay reaction-diffusion model for viral infection with specific functional response. Comput Appl Math 34(3):807–818
31. Guo T, Liu H, Xu C, Yan F (2018) Global stability of a diffusive and delayed HBV infection model with HBV DNA-containing capsids and general incidence rate. Discret Contin Dyn Syst-B 23(10):4223–4242
32. Geng Y, Xu J, Hou J (2018) Discretization and dynamic consistency of a delayed and diffusive viral infection model. Appl Math Comput 316:282–295
33. Manna K, Hattaf K (2019) Spatiotemporal dynamics of a generalized HBV infection model with capsids and adaptive immunity. Int J Appl Comput Math 5(3):1–29
34. Mothes W, Sherer NM, Jin J, Zhong P (2010) Virus cell-to-cell transmission. J Virol 84:8360–8368
35. Zhong P, Agosto LM, Munro JB, Mothes W (2013) Cell-to-cell transmission of viruses. Curr Opin Virol 3:44–50
36. Sattentau Q (2008) Avoiding the void: cell-to-cell spread of human viruses. Nat Rev Microbiol 6:815–826
37. Hattaf K, Yousfi N (2016) A generalized virus dynamics model with cell-to-cell transmission and cure rate. Adv Differ Equ 2016(1):174
38. Hattaf K, Yousfi (2018) Qualitative analysis of a generalized virus dynamics model with both modes of transmission and distributed delays. Int J Differ Equ 2018:1–7
39. Hattaf K (2019) Spatiotemporal dynamics of a generalized viral infection model with distributed delays and CTL immune response. Computation 7(2):1–16
40. Hattaf K, Yousfi N (2016) A numerical method for a delayed viral infection model with general incidence rate. J King Saud Univ-Sci 28(4):368–374
41. Wang XY, Hattaf K, Huo HF, Xiang H (2016) Stability analysis of a delayed social epidemics model with general contact rate and its optimal control. J Ind Manag Optim 12(4):1267–1285
42. Travis CC, Webb GF (1974) Existence and stability for partial functional differential equations. Trans Am Math Soc 200:395–418
43. Fitzgibbon WE (1978) Semilinear functional differential equations in Banach space. J Differ Equ 29:1–14
44. Martin RH, Smith HL (1990) Abstract functional differential equations and reaction-diffusion systems. Trans Am Math Soc 321:1–44
45. Martin RH, Smith HL (1991) Reaction-diffusion systems with time delays: monotonicity, invariance, comparison and convergence. J für die reine und angew Math 413:1–35
46. Wu J (1996) Theory and applications of partial functional differential equations. Springer, New York
47. Henry D (1981) Geometric theory of semilinear parabolic equations lecture notes in mathematics, vol. 840. Springer, Berlin
48. Hale JK, Verduyn Lunel SM (1993) Introduction to functional differential equations. Springer, New York

# Chapter 11
# Discrete Mathematical Modeling and Analysis of Tumor Therapy

**Abdelaziz Chetouani**

**Abstract** A nonlinear discrete mathematical model is presented for the interactions between tumor cells and oncolytic virotherapy. Positive equilibrium points of the system are investigated and their stability analysis is examined. Moreover, the numerical simulation of the proposed model is also performed by using numerical method which preserves the theoretical properties. The uninfected tumor cells can be eliminated with time, and complete recovery is possible because of virus therapy, if suitable conditions are satisfied. The system appears to exhibit periodic cycles and chaotic behavior for some values of the system parameters.

## 11.1 Introduction

Cancer is one of the major causes of death in developing countries. In spite of the significant progress made in cancer therapies, mortality rates for most malignancies remain dramatically high. The control of cancer progression is one of the major challenges faced by modern medicine. Cancer results either due to decreased cell death or increased cell birth. Namely, decreased propensity for apoptosis contributes to tumour formation. The classical treatment of tumor therapy (radiotherapy, chemotherapy and immunotherapy) suffers with disadvantages such as narrow therapeutic index drugs that further reduces as tumour evolves drug resistance. Another paradigm of cancer therapy is the incomplete extermination of the invasive primary tumour mass or distribution of tumour cells leading to recidivism of disease.

The current goal for developing new therapies for the treatment of cancer is to design therapeutic agents that have a high potency against malignant cells with little or no toxicities to normal cells. Future treatment modalities need to be more selective and specific, allowing higher and thus effective drug doses to reach at each tumour cell. With the advent of modern biotechnology tools and better understanding of

---

A. Chetouani (✉)
Team of Operational Research and Applied Statistics, National School of Commerce and Management, University Mohamed Ier, Oujda, Morocco
e-mail: a.chetouani@ump.ac.ma



A. Boutayeb (ed.), *Disease Prevention and Health Promotion in Developing Countries*,
https://doi.org/10.1007/978-3-030-34702-4_11

cancer biology and virology, it becomes feasible to engineer viruses with increased tumour selectivity and enhanced oncolytic activity.

A connection between cancer and viruses has long been theorized and case reports of cancer regression (cervical cancer, Burkitt lymphoma, Hodgkin lymphoma) after immunization or infection with an unrelated virus appeared at the beginning of the 20th century [8]. Efforts to treat cancer through immunization or deliberate infection with a virus began in the mid 20th century [8, 13]. As the technology for creating a custom virus did not exist, all early efforts focused on finding natural oncolytic viruses.

During the 1960s, promising research involved in using poliovirus [11], adenovirus [8], Coxsackie virus [7], and others [13]. The early complications were occasional cases of uncontrolled infection, resulting in significant morbidity and mortality; the very frequent development of an immune response, while harmless to the patient [8], destroyed the virus and thus prevented it from destroying the cancer [11]. In a number of cases, cancer cells exposed to viruses have experienced extensive necrosis, which cannot be entirely accounted for by viral replication alone. Cytotoxic T-cell responses directed against virus infected cells have been identified as an important factor in tumor necrosis. However, since viruses are normal human microorganisms, they induce an immune response, which reduces the effectiveness of viruses.

All modern research on oncolytic viruses involves viruses that have been modified to be less susceptible to immune suppression, to more specifically target particular classes of cancer cells, or to express desired cancer suppressing genes. The first Oncolytic virus to be approved by a regulatory agency was a genetically modified adenovirus named H101 by Shanghai Sunway Biotech.

It gained regulatory approval in 2005 from China's State Food and Drug Administration (SFDA) for the treatment of head and neck cancer [4, 6]. Sunway's H101 and the very similar Onyx-15 have been engineered to remove a viral defense mechanism that interacts with a normal human gene p53, which is very frequently deregulated in cancer cells [6]. Onyx-015 is a adenovirus that was developed in 1987 with the function of the E1B gene knocked out, meaning cells infected with Onyx-015 are incapable of blocking p53's function. If Onyx-015 infects a normal cell, with a functioning p53 gene, it will be prevented from multiplying by the action of the p53 transcription factor. However if Onyx-015 infects a p53 deficient cell it should be able to survive and replicate, resulting in selective destruction of cancer cells [1, 9].

The interaction between the growing tumor and the replicating oncolytic virus are highly complex and nonlinear. Thus to precisely define the required conditions for successful therapy by this approach, mathematical models are needed. Several mathematical models of the evolution of tumors under viral injection were recently developed [2, 14]. Other mathematical models for tumor-virus dynamics are, mainly, spatially explicit models, described by systems of partial differential equations, the local dynamics is usually modeled by systems of equations carrying close resemblance to a basic model of virus dynamics [14]. Wu et al. modeled and compared the evolution of a tumor under different initial conditions [15]. Friedman and Tao (2003) presented a rigorous mathematical analysis of somewhat different model [5]. Artem

S. Novozhilov [10] suggested a mathematical model that describes the interaction between two types of tumor cells (the uninfected cells that are susceptible because of the cancer phenotype) with ratio dependent functional response between them. Considering a more realistic type of functional response with saturation effect of virus–cell interaction as even when a virus is oncolytic and it punches a hole in a tumor, the immune response of the individual to the virus occurs so fast that the effects are quickly wiped out and the tumor continues, a novel mathematical model is build upon the model of Artem S. Novozhilov [10] with a modified functional response between the cells. A deep discussion of the linear stability analysis of the biologically feasible equilibrium states of this model is outlined. The ranges of the system parameters for which the system has chaotic behavior is found.

Some authors discussed the problem of chaos and stability analysis of some biological models such as cancer and tumor model, genital herpes epidemic, stochastic lattice gas prey–predator model and many other models, see, for example, [3, 12]. The problem of optimal control of the unstable equilibrium states of cancer self-remission and tumor system using a feedback control approach is studied by Sarkar and Banerjee and El-Gohary [3, 12].

The main objective of present chapter is to study the interaction between growing tumor and the replicating Oncolytic virus with a functional response with saturation effect. The saturation effect accounts for the fact that the number of contacts an individual cell reaches some maximal value as our immune system evolves to stop virus just as the virus evolves to enter cells and replicate. Our model exhibits that complete elimination of tumor is possible with the help of oncolytic virus therapy in the treatment of tumor.

## 11.2 Mathematical Model (the Modified Prey Predator Model)

The model considers two types of tumor cells $x_n$ and $y_n$ growing in logistic fashion:

- $x_n$ is the size of the uninfected tumor cell population
- $y_n$ is the size of infected tumor cell population.

It is assumed that oncolytic viruses enter tumor cells and replicate. These tumor cells, infected with oncolytic viruses, further cause infection in other tumor cells. Oncolytic virus preferentially infects and lysis cancer cells both by direct destruction of the tumor cells, and, if modified, as vectors enabling genes expressing anticancer proteins to be delivered specifically to the tumor site. Based on these assumptions, the model is given by the following discrete equations :

$$x_{n+1} = x_n + \alpha_1 x_n \left(1 - \frac{x_n + y_n}{K}\right) - \frac{\beta x_n y_n}{x_n + y_n + \alpha}, \tag{11.1}$$

$$y_{n+1} = y_n + \alpha_2 y_n \left(1 - \frac{x_n + y_n}{K}\right) + \frac{\beta x_n y_n}{x_n + y_n + \alpha} - a y_n, \tag{11.2}$$

with initial conditions : $x_0 > 0$ and $y_0 > 0$. Here $\alpha_1$ and $\alpha_2$ are the maximum per capita growth rates of uninfected and infected cells respectively; $K$ is the carrying capacity, $\beta$ is the transmission rate (this parameter also includes the replication rate of the viruses); The expression $\frac{\beta x_n y_n}{x_n+y_n+\alpha}$, displays a saturation effect accounting for the fact that the number of contacts an individual cell reaches some maximal value as our immune system evolves to stop virus just as the viruses evolve to enter cells and replicate. $\alpha$ is the measure of the immune response of the individual to the viruses which prevents it from destroying the cancer and $a$ is the rate of infected cell killing by the viruses (cytotoxicity). All the parameters of the model are supposed to be positive and time independent.

## 11.3 Boundedness of Solutions

Boundedness is interpreted as a natural restriction of growth because of limited resources. To establish the biological validity of the model system, we have to show that the solutions of system (11.1) are bounded, for this we determine the region of attraction in the following theorem

**Theorem 1** *For any positive initial conditions $x_0, y_0 > 0$, the solutions of (11.1) are positive, more precisely, $x, y \in \Omega = \{(x, y) \in \mathbf{R}^2_+ \backslash 0 < x + y \leq K\}$.*

*Proof* From (11.1) we get :

$$x_{n+1} + y_{n+1} = x_n + y_n + (\alpha_1 x_n + \alpha_2 y_n)\left(1 - \frac{x_n + y_n}{K}\right) - a y_n$$

$$x_{n+1} + y_{n+1} \leq \max(\alpha_1, \alpha_2)(x_n + y_n)\left(1 - \frac{x_n + y_n}{K}\right)$$

then by usual comparison theorem, we get the following expression

$$\lim_{n\to\infty} \sup(x_n + y_n) \leq K$$

Thus, it suffices to consider solutions in the region $\Omega$. □

Solutions of the initial value problem starting in $\Omega$ and defined by (11.1) exist and are unique on a maximal interval. Since solutions remain bounded in the region $\Omega$, the maximal interval is well posed both mathematically and epidemiologically.

## 11.4 Equilibrium Points

An equilibrium point is a point at which variables of a system remain unchanged over time. The system (11.1) has the following equilibria:

$$E_0(0,0),\ E_1(K,0),\ E_2(0,\overline{y}) \text{ and } E_3(x^*,y^*),$$

where $\overline{y}=\frac{K}{r}(\alpha_2-\alpha)$ and $y^*=\frac{-M+\sqrt{M^2-4\alpha_2 N}}{2\alpha_2}=f(x)$ where $M=(2x\alpha_2+a\alpha_2-K(\alpha_2-\alpha))$ and $N=\alpha_2 x^2+x(\alpha_2 a-K(\alpha_2-\alpha)-K\beta)-Ka(\alpha_2-\alpha)$.

The existence of trivial equilibrium point $E_0(0,0)$ is obvious. This equilibrium point implies the complete elimination of tumor. Biologically, it means that both infected and uninfected tumor cells can be eliminated with time, and complete recovery is possible because of the virus therapy.

The existence of equilibrium point $E_1(K,0)$. is obvious. This equilibrium implies the failure of virus therapy. Biologically, it means that both infected and uninfected tumor cells tend to the same state, as they would have been reached without virus administration.

The equilibrium point $E_2(0,\overline{y})$ exists if $\alpha_2>\alpha$. This equilibrium implies complete infection of tumor cells and stabilization of tumor load to a finite minimal size $\overline{y}=\frac{K}{\alpha_2}(\alpha_2-\alpha)$. Biologically, it gives a real life situation in which tumor load can be reduced to lower size if tumor is detected at initial stage.

To see the existence of the interior equilibrium point $E_3(x^*,y^*)$ we note that $x^*,y^*$ are positive solutions of the system of algebraic equations given below

$$\alpha_1\left(1-\frac{x+y}{K}\right)=\frac{\beta y}{x+y+\alpha} \tag{11.3}$$

$$\alpha_2\left(1-\frac{x+y}{K}\right)=-\frac{\beta y}{x+y+\alpha}+a \tag{11.4}$$

Substituting the value of $y^*$ in Eq. (11.3), we get

$$\alpha_1\,(K-x-f(x))\,(x+f(x)+\alpha)=K\beta f(x) \tag{11.5}$$

To show existence of $x^*$, it suffices to show that Eq. (11.5) has a unique positive solution. Taking

$$G(x)=\alpha_1\,(K-x-f(x))\,(x+f(x)+\alpha)-K\beta f(x)$$

We note that

$$G(0)=\alpha_1\,(K-f(0))\,(f(0)+\alpha)-K\beta f(0)>0 \tag{11.6}$$

provided

$$\alpha_1 a - \alpha_2 \beta > 0 \text{ and } \alpha_2 - a > 0 \tag{11.7}$$

or

$$\frac{\alpha_1}{\beta} > \frac{\alpha_2}{a} > 1 \tag{11.8}$$

and

$$G(K) = -\alpha_1 f(K)(K + f(K) + \alpha) + \beta K) < 0$$

provided

$$a < \frac{\beta K}{K + \alpha} \tag{11.9}$$

Thus, there exists an $x^* \in [0, K]$ such that $G(x^*) = 0$.

For $x^*$ to be unique, we must have

$$G'(x) = -\alpha_1(1 + f'(x))(2x + 2f(x) + \alpha - K) - K\beta f'(x) < 0, \tag{11.10}$$

The corresponding value of $y^*$ is given by $y^* = f(x^*)$. For the calculus of $x^*$, the Newton method was used.

Thus if all the three conditions (11.5)–(11.7) hold, an unique interior equilibrium always exists, to calculate. However, these conditions depend upon the parameter values so they do not always hold. If both Eqs. (11.5) and (11.6) does not hold other equilibrium points of the system become locally asymptotically stable.

## 11.5 Local Stability Analysis of Equilibrium Points

To discuss the local stability of equilibrium points we compute the jacobian matrix of system (11.1). The modulus of the real parts of the eigenvalues of the variational matrix evaluated at a given equilibria determines its stability. The entries of general variational matrix are given by differentiating the right hand side of system (11.1) with respect to $x$, $y$. The matrix is given by

$$V(E) = \begin{pmatrix} A & B \\ C & D \end{pmatrix}$$

where

$$A = 1 + \alpha_1 \left(1 - \frac{x + y}{K}\right) - \frac{\alpha_1 x}{K} - \frac{\beta y}{x + y + \alpha} + \frac{\beta x y}{(x + y + \alpha)^2}$$

$$B = -\frac{\alpha_1 x}{K} - \frac{\beta x}{x + y + \alpha} + \frac{\beta x y}{(x + y + \alpha)^2}$$

$$C = -\frac{\alpha_2 y}{K} + \frac{by}{x+y+\alpha} - \frac{\beta xy}{(x+y+\alpha)^2}$$

$$D = 1 + \alpha_2\left(1 - \frac{x+y}{K}\right) - \frac{\alpha_2 y}{K} + \frac{\beta y}{x+y+\alpha} - \frac{\beta xy}{(x+y+\alpha)^2} - a$$

We denote the jacobian matrix corresponding to $E_i$ by $V(E_i), i = 0, 1, 2, 3$.

### *11.5.1 Stability Analysis of $E_0$*

To explore local stability of the trivial equilibrium point, we calculate the jacobian matrix of $E_0$. The variational matrix of equilibrium point $E_0$ is given by

$$V(E_0) = \begin{pmatrix} A & B \\ C & D \end{pmatrix} \tag{11.11}$$

**Theorem 2** *$E_0$ is an unstable equilibrium point.*

*Proof* Eigenvalues of $V(E_0)$ are given by $1 + \alpha_1$ and $1 + \alpha_2 - a$. Hence the modulus of both eigenvalues of the matrix is greater than 1. □

### *11.5.2 Stability Analysis of $E_1$*

To study the stability behavior of $E_1$, we compute the variational matrix $V(E_1)$ as follows:

$$V(E_1) = \begin{pmatrix} 1-\alpha_1 & -\alpha_1 - \frac{\beta K}{K+\alpha} \\ 0 & 1 + \frac{\beta K}{K+\alpha} - a \end{pmatrix} \tag{11.12}$$

**Theorem 3**

1. *$E_1$ is a stable equilibrium point if $\frac{bK}{K+a} < \alpha$,*
2. *$E_1$ is a saddle point if $\frac{\beta K}{K+\alpha} > a$.*

*Proof* The eigenvalues of the matrix $V(E_1)$ are given by $1-\alpha_1$ and $1 + \frac{\beta K}{K+\alpha} - a$.

Thus, the modulus of the eigenvalues of $V(E_1)$ are less than 1 and $E_1$ is a stable equilibrium point if $\frac{bK}{K+a} < \alpha$, consequently $E_1$ is a saddle point if $\frac{\beta K}{K+\alpha} > a$.

The inequality $\frac{\beta K}{K+\alpha} > a$ implies that $E_1$ is locally asymptotically stable if death rate of infected cells due to the virus attack is larger than the rate of transmission of infection from virus to the uninfected cells (measure of the immune response of the individual to the viruses is very less as compared to carrying capacity of the cells). Stability of this equilibrium point suggests that infected cells would die without having time to infect other cells and tumor grows unaffectedly. □

### 11.5.3 Stability Analysis of $E_2$

The jacobian matrix of $E_2(0, \overline{y})$ where $\overline{y} = \frac{K}{\alpha_2}(\alpha_2 - a)$ is given by

$$V(E_2) = \begin{pmatrix} 1 + \frac{\alpha_1 a}{\alpha_2} - \frac{\beta K(\alpha_2 - a)}{K(\alpha_2 - a) + \alpha\alpha_2} & 0 \\ -\alpha_2 + a + \frac{\beta K(\alpha_2 - a)}{K(\alpha_2 - a) + \alpha\alpha_2} & 1 - \alpha_2 - a \end{pmatrix} \tag{11.13}$$

**Theorem 4** *1. $E_2$ is a stable equilibrium point if $\frac{\alpha_1 a}{\alpha_2} < \frac{\beta K(\alpha_2 - a)}{K(\alpha_2 - a) + \alpha\alpha_2}$ or $\alpha < \frac{K(\alpha_2 - a)}{\alpha_1\alpha_2 a}(\beta\alpha_2 - a\alpha_1)$,*
*2. $E_2$ is a saddle point if $\alpha > \frac{K(\alpha_2 - a)}{\alpha_1\alpha_2 a}(\beta\alpha_2 - a\alpha_1)$.*

*Proof* The eigenvalues of the matrix $V(E_2)$ are given by $1 - \alpha_2 + a$ and $1 + \frac{\alpha_1 a}{\alpha_2} - \frac{\beta K(\alpha_2 - a)}{K(\alpha_2 - a) + \alpha\alpha_2}$. Thus $V(E_2)$ has eigenvalues of modulus less than 1 and $E_2$ is a stable equilibrium point if $\frac{\alpha_1 a}{\alpha_2} < \frac{\beta K(\alpha_2 - a)}{K(\alpha_2 - a) + \alpha\alpha_2}$ or $\alpha < \frac{K(\alpha_2 - a)}{\alpha_1\alpha_2 a}(\beta\alpha_2 - a\alpha_1)$, consequently $E_2$ is a saddle point if $\alpha > \frac{K(\alpha_2 - a)}{\alpha_1\alpha_2 a}(\beta\alpha_2 - a\alpha_1)$.

Local asymptotic stability of $E_2$ implies that $\beta\alpha_2 > a\alpha_1$, Since $\alpha$ is a positive parameter and it cannot be less than a negative quantity, so $E_2$ is locally asymptotically stable point if $\frac{\alpha_2}{a} > \frac{\alpha_1}{\beta}$ together with $\frac{\alpha_2}{a} > 1$ or $\frac{\alpha_2}{a} > \max\left(1, \frac{\alpha_1}{\beta}\right)$. □

Hence $E_2$ is locally asymptotically stable under any of the two situations:

1. If net growth rate of uninfected cells is less than the rate of transmission of virus infection than growth rate of infected cells must be greater than the death rate of infected cells caused by the viruses.
2. If net growth rate of uninfected cells is more than the rate of transmission of virus infection then the ratio of net growth rate of uninfected cells to the death rate of infected cells caused by the viruses is more than the ratio of net growth rate of uninfected cells to rate at which they become infective.

### 11.5.4 Stability Analysis of $E_3$

The jacobian Variational matrix of $E_3$ is given by

$$V(E_3) = \begin{pmatrix} A^* & B^* \\ C^* & D^* \end{pmatrix} \tag{11.14}$$

where

$$A^* = 1 + \alpha_1 \left(1 - \frac{x^* + y^*}{K}\right) - \frac{\alpha_1 x^*}{K} - \frac{\beta y^*}{x^* + y^* + \alpha} + \frac{\beta x^* y^*}{(x^* + y^* + \alpha)^2}$$

$$B^* = -\frac{\alpha_1 x^*}{K} - \frac{\beta x^*}{x^* + y^* + \alpha} + \frac{\beta x^* y^*}{(x^* + y^* + \alpha)^2}$$

$$C^* = -\frac{\alpha_2 y^*}{K} + \frac{\beta y^*}{x^* + y^* + \alpha} - \frac{\beta x^* y^*}{(x^* + y^* + \alpha)^2}$$

$$D^* = 1 + \alpha_2 \left(1 - \frac{x^* + y^*}{K}\right) - \frac{\alpha_2 y^*}{K} + \frac{\beta y^*}{x^* + y^* + \alpha} - \frac{\beta x^* y^*}{(x^* + y^* + \alpha)^2} - a$$

**Theorem 5** *$E_3$ is always locally asymptotically stable if it exists.*

*Proof* The eigenvalues of $V(E_3)$ are

$$1 - \frac{\alpha_1 x^* + \alpha_2 y^*}{2K} \pm \frac{1}{2}\sqrt{\left(2 - \frac{\alpha_1 x^* + \alpha_2 y^*}{K}\right)^2 - 4\left(1 + \frac{\beta x^* y^* (\alpha_1 - \alpha_2)}{(x^* + y^* + \alpha)K} + \frac{\alpha \beta^2 x^* y^*}{(x^* + y^* + \alpha)^3}\right)}.$$

The modulus of the eigenvalues are less than 1. Thus $E_3$ is always locally asymptotically stable □

## 11.6 Global Stability of Interior Equilibrium Point

An equilibrium point is globally asymptotically stable if system always approaches it regardless of its initial position.

Lyapunov functions enable to find biologically realistic conditions sufficient to ensure existence and uniqueness of a globally asymptotically stable equilibrium state. Global stability of the interior equilibrium point of system (11.1) is determined in the sequel

**Theorem 6** *If the following inequality holds*

$$\left(\frac{by^*}{\alpha(x^* + y^* + \alpha)}\right)^2 < 4\left(\frac{\alpha_1}{K} - \frac{\beta y^*}{\alpha(x^* + y^* + \alpha)}\right)\left(\frac{\alpha_2}{K} + \frac{\beta x^*}{(K + \alpha)(x^* + y^* + \alpha)}\right)$$

*then $E_3$ is globally asymptotically stable for any $x_0, y_0 \in \Omega$.*

*Proof* Consider the following positive definite function

$$W_n = x_n - x^* - x^* \ln\left(\frac{x_n}{x^*}\right) + y_n - y^* - y^* \ln\left(\frac{y_n}{y^*}\right).$$

Computing $W_{n+1}$, we get

$$W_{n+1} = x_n + \alpha_1 x_n \left(1 - \frac{x_n + y_n}{K}\right) - x^* - x^* \ln \left( \frac{x_n + \alpha_1 x_n \left(1 - \frac{x_n+y_n}{K}\right) - \frac{\beta x_n y_n}{x_n+y_n+\alpha}}{x^*} \right) +$$

$$y_n + \alpha_2 y_n \left(1 - \frac{x_n + y_n}{K}\right) - a y_n - y^* - y^* \ln \left( \frac{y_n + \alpha_2 y_n \left(1 - \frac{x_n+y_n}{K}\right) + \frac{\beta x_n y_n}{x_n+y_n+\alpha} - a y_n}{y^*} \right) =$$

$$w_n - x^* \ln \left( \frac{x_n + \alpha_1 x_n \left(1 - \frac{x_n+y_n}{K}\right) - \frac{\beta x_n y_n}{x_n+y_n+\alpha}}{x^*} \right) - y^* \ln \left( \frac{y_n + \alpha_2 y_n \left(1 - \frac{x_n+y_n}{K}\right) + \frac{\beta x_n y_n}{x_n+y_n+\alpha} - a y_n}{y^*} \right)$$

We note that $W_{n+1} < W_n$ inside $\Omega$ if

$$\left( \frac{\beta y^*}{\alpha(x^* + y^* + \alpha)} \right)^2 < 4 \left( \frac{\alpha_1}{K} - \frac{\beta y^*}{\alpha(x^* + y^* + \alpha)} \right) \left( \frac{\alpha_2}{K} + \frac{\beta x^*}{(K + \alpha)(x^* + y^* + \alpha)} \right)$$

Which completes the proof of the theorem. □

## 11.7 Numerical Simulation

To test the above theoretical results, the model is simulated numerically. The system of equations is computed using the following set of compatible parameters, which satisfy the stability conditions.

$$\alpha_1 = 20, K = 100, \alpha_2 = 1, \alpha = 0.05, b = 0.02, a = 0.003. \quad (11.15)$$

The equilibrium points for these parameters are $(0, 0)$, $(100, 0)(0, 99.7)$ and $(10.5, 89.4)$.

The conditions for local asymptotic stability of interior equilibrium point are satisfied for this set of parameter values. In Fig. 11.1 densities of tumor cells for parameter values (11.15) is shown. It is observed from the figure that infected tumor cell population first rise and then attain a constant equilibrium value whereas uninfected tumor cell population first rise abruptly and then decrease due to virus infection and cytotoxicity to attain its equilibrium value (Fig. 11.2).

In Fig. 11.1, density of tumor cells is drawn for $\alpha = 0.3$ and other parameters remaining same as in Eq. (11.15). This figure implies that the system converges to equilibrium point $E_1(100, 0)$ when death rate of infected tumor cells due to the viruses increases from 0.003 to 0.3.

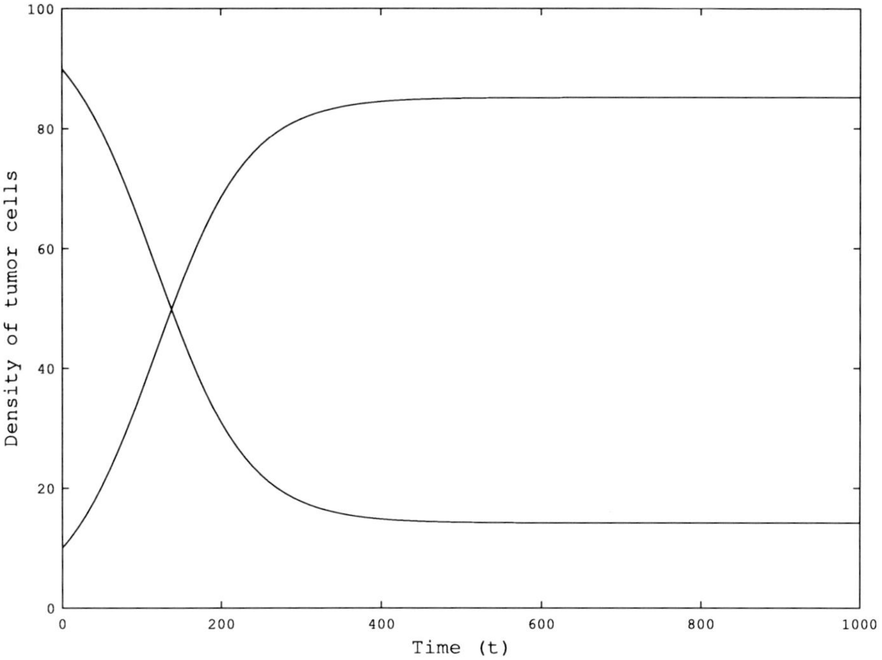


**Fig. 11.1** Densities of tumor cells for parameters given in 11.15

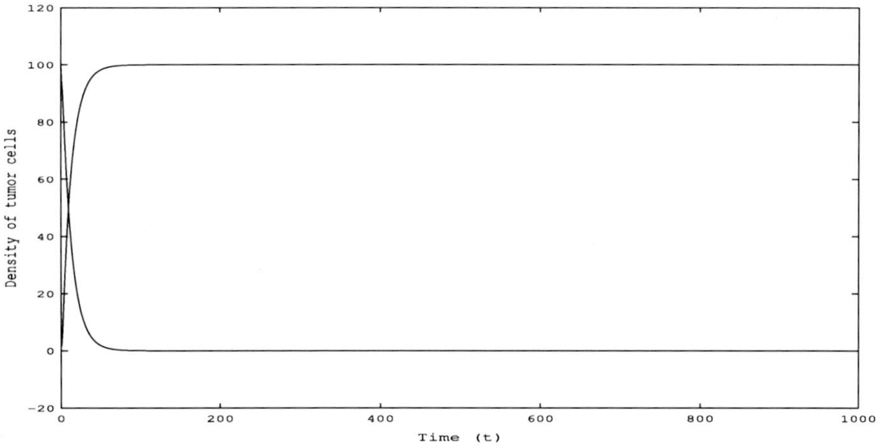


**Fig. 11.2** Convergence of the system to $E_1$, for $\alpha = 0.3$ and other parameters remaining as in Eq. 11.15

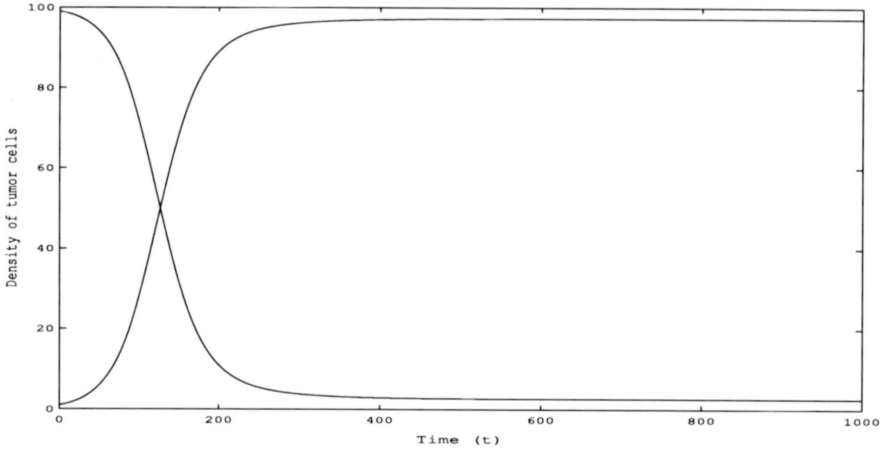


**Fig. 11.3** Convergence of the system to $E_2$, for $\beta = 0.04$ and other parameters remaining as in Eq. 11.15

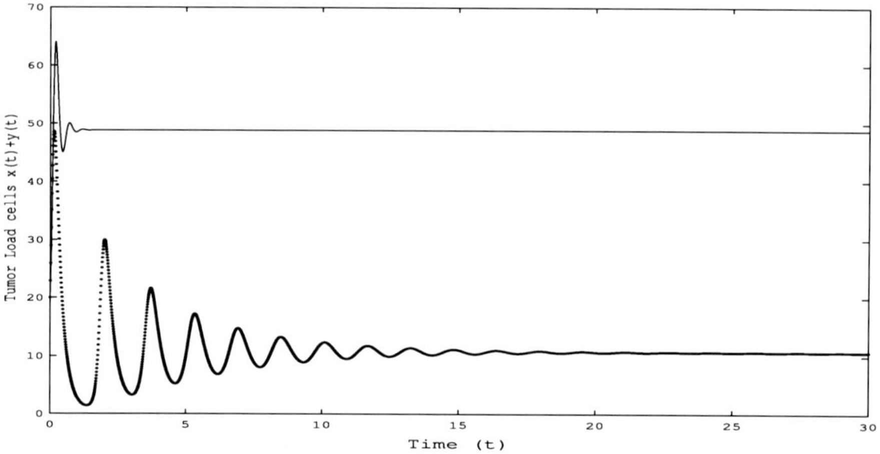


**Fig. 11.4** Variation of tumor load with time for different transmission rate of infection from virus and parameters $\alpha_1 = 40$, $K = 100$, $\alpha_2 = \alpha = 0.05$, $a = 40$, $\beta = \{30, 10\}$

Figure 11.3 shows the density of tumor cells for $\beta = 0.04$ and other parameters remaining same as in Eq. (11.15). It demonstrates the convergence of the system to equilibrium point $E_2(0, 99.8)$ for higher infectivity of the oncolytic virus. Numerically the tumor load decreases when per capita growth rate of infected cells ($\alpha_2$) is less than or equal to the death rate of infected cells due to virus $a$ for high replication rate of viruses in the cells.

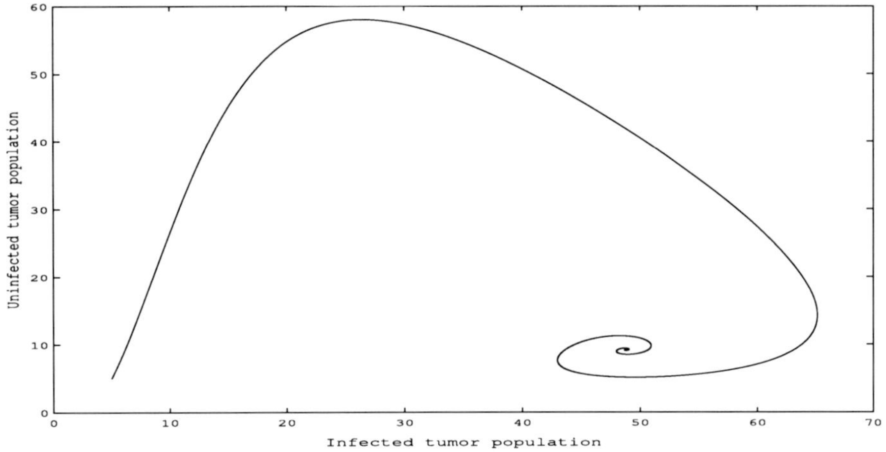


**Fig. 11.5** Stable limit cycles for parameter values $\alpha_1 = 40, K = 100, \alpha_2 = 2, \alpha = 0.05, a = 4, \beta = 20, x_0 = y_0 = 5$

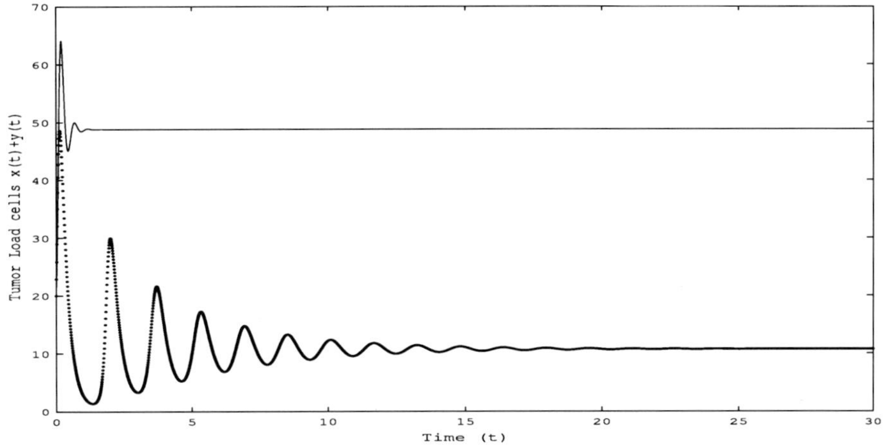


**Fig. 11.6** Variation of tumor load with time for different transmission rate of infection from virus and parameters $\alpha_1 = 40, K = 100, \alpha_2 = 2, a = 0.05, \alpha = 2$

Figure 11.4 shows variation of tumor load with time for different transmission rate of virus infection $\beta$. It is found from the graph that for $\alpha_2 = a = 2$, tumor load decreases with the increase in b for all $\beta > 1$ and decreases for $\beta \geq 30$.

Figure 11.5 displays the formation of limit cycle in the system. It is observed from numerical simulation that stable limit cycles are formed for $10 \leq \beta \leq 35$ and for $\beta > 35$ no limit cycles are formed. However, when $\alpha_2 < a$ (for parameter values $\alpha_2 = 1, a = 2$ and other parameters remaining same as (11.15), we have found that stable limit cycles are formed for $10 \leq \beta \leq 40$ (Fig. 11.6).

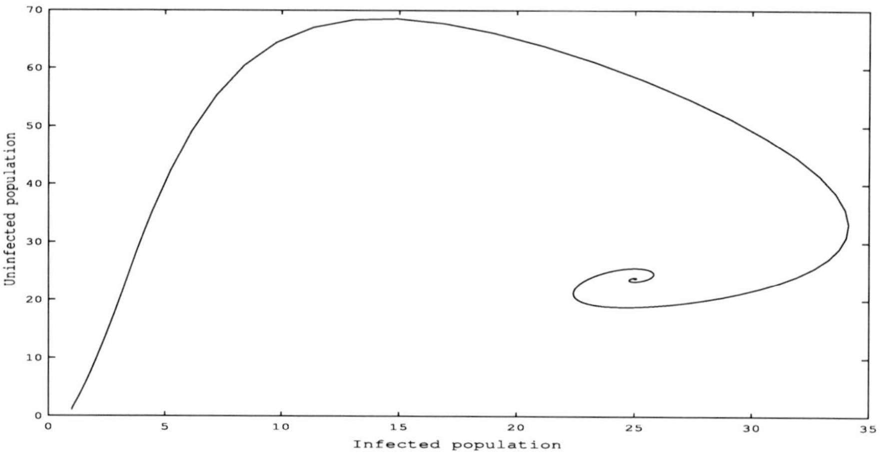


**Fig. 11.7** Stable limit cycles for parameter values $\alpha_1 = 40, K = 100, \alpha_2 = 2, a = 0.05, \alpha = 2, b = 30, x_0 = y_0 = 1$

Figure 11.7 shows stable limit cycle for $b = 30$ and keeping other parameters fixed as above. However, when $b > 40$, tumor load decreases and strange chaotic attractors are obtained.

## References

1. Barker DD, Berk AJ (1987) Adenovirus proteins from both e1b reading frames are required for transformation of rodent cells by viral infection and dna transfection. Virology 156(1):107–121
2. Dominik W, Natalia K (2005) Computational biology of cancer: lecture notes and mathematical modeling. World Scientific, Singapore
3. El-Gohary A, Al-Ruzaiza A (2007) Chaos and adaptive control in two prey, one predator system with nonlinear feedback. Chaos Solitons Fractals 34(2):443–453
4. Frew S, Sammut S, Shore A, Ramjist J, Al-Bader S, Rezaie R, Daar A, Singer P (2008) Chinese health biotech and the billion-patient market. Nat Biotechnol 26(1):37–53
5. Friedman A, Tao Y (2003) Analysis of a model of a virus that replicates selectively in tumor cells. J Math Biol 47(5):391–423
6. Garber K (2006) China approves world's first oncolytic virus therapy for cancer treatment. J Natl Cancer Inst 98(5):298–300
7. Kunin CM (1964) Cellular susceptibility to enteroviruses. Bacteriol Rev 28(4):382
8. Kuruppu D, Tanabe KK (2005) Viral oncolysis by herpes simplex virus and other viruses. Cancer Biol Ther 4(5):524–531
9. McCormick F (2003) Cancer specific viruses and the development of ONYX-015. Cancer Biol Ther 2(supl):156–159
10. Novozhilov AS, Berezovskaya FS, Koonin EV, Karev GP (2006) Mathematical modeling of tumor therapy with oncolytic viruses: regimes with complete tumor elimination within the framework of deterministic models. Biol Direct 1(1):1–18
11. Pond A, Manuelidis E (1964) Oncolytic effect of poliomyelitis virus on human epidermoid carcinoma (hela tumor) heterologously transplanted to guinea pigs. Am J Pathol 45(2):233–249

12. Sarkar RR, Banerjee S (2005) Cancer self remission and tumor stability-a stochastic approach. Math Biosci 196(1):65–81
13. Voroshilova M (1989) Potential use of nonpathogenic enteroviruses for control of human disease. Progress in Medical Virology (Fortschritte der medizinischen Virusforschung Progres en virologie medicale) 36:191–202
14. Wodarz D (2001) Viruses as antitumor weapons: defining conditions for tumor remission. Cancer Res 61(8):3501–3507
15. Wu JT, Byrne HM, Kirn DH, Wein LM (2001) Modeling and analysis of a virus that replicates selectively in tumor cells. Bull Math Biol 63(4):731

# Chapter 12
# A Model of Dengue Fever with Control

**Mohamed Derouich and Mohamed E. N. Lamlili**

**Abstract** According to the World Health Organization, incidence and prevalence of dengue has shown a dramatic increase in the last decades. Worldwide, 390 million dengue infections are diagnosed each year with a prevalence of 3.9 billion people. A total of 128 countries, are at risk of infection with dengue viruses. Unfortunately, there is no specific treatment for dengue/severe dengue. However, prevention and control namely vaccination, education campaign, use of appropriate protection... can help to avoid this disease. A mathematical model based on differential equations and optimal control theory is used to show how infected population could be reduced and epidemic outbreak slowed down. A stability analysis of equilibrium points is done and different simulations are carried out according to levels of preventions and controls. The epidemics is discussed and illustrated by figures for different values of parameters.

## 12.1 Introduction

Dengue has emerged as a worldwide problem since the 1960s. The disease is common in many popular tourist destinations in the Caribbean (including Puerto Rico), Central and South America, Southeast Asia, and the Pacific Islands. In fact, according to the world health organization (WHO) [19] and Centers for disease control and prevention (CDC) [4], 128 countries are at risk of infection with dengue viruses, with 390 million dengue infections diagnosed each year and a prevalence of 3.9 billion people. Dengue-related symptoms can be mild or severe. The mild forms of the disease are called dengue, dengue fever, dandy fever, and break-bone fever. The

M. Derouich (✉)
Laboratory of Stochastic and Deterministic Modelling (LaSDM), National School Applied Sciences (ENSA), University Mohamed Ier, Oujda, Morocco
e-mail: mderouich2011@gmail.com

M. E. N. Lamlili
Laboratory of Stochastic and Deterministic Modelling (LaSDM), Faculty of Sciences, University Mohamed Ier, Oujda, Morocco
e-mail: mohamed.lamlili@gmail.com

 
A. Boutayeb (ed.), *Disease Prevention and Health Promotion in Developing Countries*,
https://doi.org/10.1007/978-3-030-34702-4_12

severe syndromes are called hemorrhagic dengue, dengue hemorrhagic fever (DHF), dengue shock syndrome (DSS). Severe one is considered as a more serious form of the disease leading to: shock, internal bleeding, or even death. About 1 in 20 people who get sick with dengue will develop severe dengue and a people who had a dengue infection are more likely to develop severe dengue. This disease is a medical emergency and requires immediate medical attention or hospitalization.

We note that the disease is caused by four different serotypes (DEN1, DEN2, DEN3 and DEN4). A person infected by one of the four ones will never be infected again by the same serotypes. However, the lost of immunity to the three others may appear in about 12 weeks and then the infected person becomes more susceptible to develop sever dengue. Dengue viruses are spread to people through the bites of infected Aedes species mosquitoes (Ae. aegypti or Ae. albopictus). These are the same types of mosquitoes that spread Zika and chikungunya viruses. These mosquitoes typically lay eggs near standing water in containers that hold water, like buckets, bowls, animal dishes, flower pots, and vases. They bite people during the day and night, and live both indoors and outdoors near people. Mosquitoes become infected when they bite a dengue infected person. Therefore, they can spread the virus to other people through bites. Unfortunately, there is no specific treatment for dengue/severe dengue. However, prevention and control can help to avoid the disease. Currently, the main method to control or prevent the transmission of dengue virus is to fight vector mosquitoes through reducing egg-laying natural and artificial man-made habitats mainly by the disinfection of household waste and the use of appropriate insecticides and protection from bite of mosquitoes in addition to vaccination, education campaign, active monitoring and surveillance of vectors.

In order to help in the management and the reduction of this epidemic's effects, the use of mathematical models, based on ordinary differential equations as well as the optimal control theory, can be a source of information helping decision makers to develop and implement efficient strategies.

Several mathematical models have been proposed to investigate dengue epidemiology, some of which explicitly model the mosquito population [10, 15, 18], while others implicitly model it in the transmission term [1, 6, 16]. In 1975 Bailey [2] provided the basis for dengue models addressing a single serotype. Adams and Boots [1] proposed a mathematical model, including versions with seasonal variation in the oviposition rate and mosquito diapause, to examine how the reproductive number and extinction probability of the virus are related to vertical infection efficiency.

This work is adopted by [5] for modeling transmission dynamics of dengue fever in southern Taiwan where the studied population is divided into host (human), vector (pre-adult), and vector (adult female mosquito population). Generally, The basic vector–host dynamic models were composed of the Susceptible-Exposed-Infectious-Recovery (SEIR) mosquito population and the Susceptible-Infectious-Recovery (SIR) human populations [20–22]. Based on their single-serotype model [9, 11], Esteva and Vargas built a two-strain model. The vector population is subdivided into a susceptible class and two serotype-specific infectious classes. For each serotype, the host population is governed by a SIR model. Bartley et al. [14] proposed a more complex modelling structure, representing the evolution of the immune response: (1) Short-term (2–9 months) and partial cross-immunity. (2) Sub-neutralizing antibody-level inducing an increase in the infectivity in the secondary infected host and, consequently, impacting the transmission rate from host to vector. (3) Immunity to one serotype without cross-reaction with other.

Derouich and Boutayeb [7] developed a model with two subsequent infections at separate timeintervals, considering that the first epidemic ends when the second occurs. We resume and improve this work by introducing an optimal control in order to reduce the infected population and slow down the epidemic outbreak.

## 12.2 First Epidemic

### *12.2.1 Formulation of the Model and Stability Analysis*

#### 12.2.1.1 The Mathematical Model

The proposed model describes the interaction between human population denoted by $N_h$ and vector population denoted by $N_v$: the human population is divided into three classes Susceptible, Infected and Removed (Immuned) individuals, with $S_h(t)$, $I_h(t)$, $R_h(t)$ denoting their fraction in the population at time $t$ and the vector population is divided into two classes: Susceptible and Infected, no immune class exists for mosquitoes because the infected period end when the mosquitoes die, with $S_v(t)$, $I_v(t)$ denoting their fraction in the population at time $t$.

In this model death is proportional to human population (respectively vector population) size with rate constant $\mu_h$ (resp. $\mu_v$) and we assume a constant $\Lambda_h$ (resp. $\Lambda_v$) due to births and immigrations. So $\frac{dN_h}{dt} = \Lambda_h - \mu_h N_h$ (resp. $\frac{dN_v}{dt} = \Lambda_v - \mu_v N_v$).

As indicated in [7] the model supposes a homogeneous mixing of human and mosquito population so that each bite has an equal probability of being taken from any particular human. While noting $b_s$ the average biting rate of susceptible vectors, $p_{hv}$ the average transmission probability of an infectious human to a susceptible vector, the rate of exposure for vectors is given by: $(p_{hv} I_h b_s)/N_h$.

It is admitted [20] that some infections increase the number of bites by the infected mosquitoes in relation to the susceptible. Therefore, we will assume that the rate of infected mosquito bites $b_i$ is greater than the one of susceptible mosquitos $b_s$.

Noting $p_{vh}$ the average transmission probability of an infectious vector to human and $I_v$ the infectious vector number, the rate of exposure for humans is given by: $(p_{vh} I_v b_i)/N_h$ so:

- The adequate contact rate of human to vectors is given by: $C_{hv} = p_{hv} b_s$
- The adequate contact rate of vectors to human is given by: $C_{vh} = p_{vh} b_i$.

A schematic representation of the model is shown in Fig. 12.1.

The dynamics of this disease in the human and vector populations is described by the following differential equations:

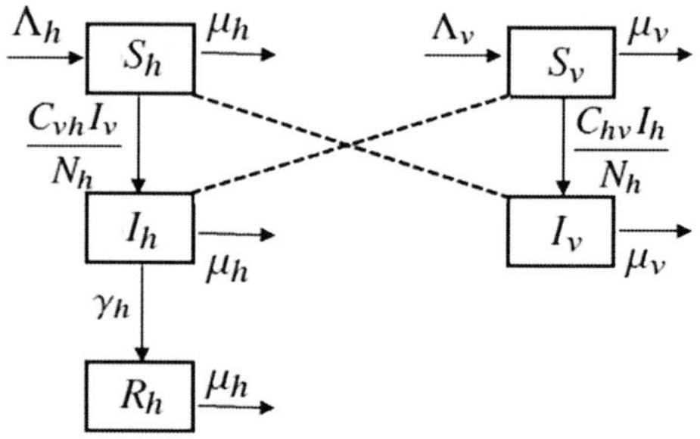


**Fig. 12.1** Compartments of human and vector populations

**Human population**

$$\begin{cases} \dfrac{dS_h}{dt} = \Lambda_h - \left(\mu_h + \dfrac{C_{vh}I_v}{N_h}\right) S_h \\ \dfrac{dI_h}{dt} = \dfrac{C_{vh}I_v}{N_h} S_h - (\mu_h + \gamma_h) I_h \\ \dfrac{dR_h}{dt} = \gamma_h I_h - \mu_h R_h \\ \dfrac{dN_h}{dt} = \Lambda_h - \mu_h N_h \end{cases}$$

**Vector population**

$$\begin{cases} \dfrac{dS_v}{dt} = \Lambda_v - \left(\mu_v + \dfrac{C_{hv}I_h}{N_h}\right) S_v \\ \dfrac{dI_v}{dt} = \left(\dfrac{C_{hv}I_h}{N_h}\right) S_v - \mu_v I_v \\ \dfrac{dN_v}{dt} = \Lambda_v - \mu_v N_v \end{cases}$$

Up to now there is no vaccine against dengue viruses but prevention and control can avoid this disease, mathematically, we introduce a control $u_1 = u_1(t)$ and $u_2 = u_2(t)$ which represent:

- Prevention denoted by $u_1$: it involves the use of repellents, cremes, mosquito nets, or wearing long clothing and covering. Moreover, it also takes into consideration the efforts made by municipalities to raise awareness of the danger of the mosquitoes and the virus.
- Vector control denoted by $u_2$: to avoid the proliferation of vector population by using:
  - Chemical control: insecticides, larvicides and genetics manipulation of producing mosquitoes refractory to infection of transmission, or sterile insects
  - Mechanical control: to reduce the number of breeding sites.

Introducing these two controls to the model above leads to the following controlled model:

$$\textbf{Human population}\begin{cases}\frac{dS_h}{dt} = \Lambda_h - \frac{C_{vh}I_v}{N_h}S_h(1-u_1) - \mu_h S_h\\ \frac{dI_h}{dt} = \frac{C_{vh}I_v}{N_h}S_h(1-u_1) - (\mu_h+\gamma_h)I_h\\ \frac{dR_h}{dt} = \gamma_h I_h - \mu_h R_h\\ \frac{dN_h}{dt} = \Lambda_h - \mu_h N_h\end{cases}$$

$$\textbf{Vector population}\begin{cases}\frac{dS_v}{dt} = \Lambda_v(1-u_2) - \frac{C_{hv}I_h}{N_h}(1-u_1)S_v - (\mu_v+u_2)S_v\\ \frac{dI_v}{dt} = \frac{C_{hv}I_h}{N_h}(1-u_1)S_v - (\mu_v+u_2)I_v\\ \frac{dN_v}{dt} = \Lambda_v(1-u_2) - (u_2+\mu_v)N_v\end{cases}$$

Since $R_h = N_h - S_h - I_h$ and $S_v = N_v - I_v$ the two previous systems become:

$$\begin{cases}\frac{dS_h}{dt} = \Lambda_h - \frac{C_{vh}I_v}{N_h}S_h(1-u_1) - \mu_h S_h\\ \frac{dI_h}{dt} = \frac{C_{vh}I_v}{N_h}S_h(1-u_1) - (\mu_h+\gamma_h)I_h\\ \frac{dN_h}{dt} = \Lambda_h - \mu_h N_h\\ \frac{dI_v}{dt} = \frac{C_{hv}I_h}{N_h}(1-u_1)(N_v - I_v) - (\mu_v+u_2)I_v\\ \frac{dN_v}{dt} = \Lambda_v(1-u_2) - (u_2+\mu_v)N_v\end{cases} \tag{12.1}$$

#### 12.2.1.2 Stability Analysis

**Equilibrium Points and $R_0$**

For the model above, equilibrium points are defined such that there is no variations in $S_h$, $I_h$, $R_h$, $S_v$, $N_h$ with respect to t:

$$\Lambda_h - \frac{C_{vh}I_v}{N_h}S_h(1-u_1) - \mu_h S_h = 0 \tag{12.2}$$

$$\frac{C_{vh}I_v}{N_h}S_h(1-u_1) - (\gamma_h+\mu_h)I_h = 0 \tag{12.3}$$

$$\Lambda_h - \mu_h N_h = 0 \tag{12.4}$$

$$\frac{C_{hv}I_h}{N_h}(1-u_1)(N_v - I_v) - (\mu_v+u_2)I_v = 0 \tag{12.5}$$

$$\Lambda_v(1-u_2) - (u_2+\mu_v)N_v = 0 \tag{12.6}$$

For any values of the parameters, the disease-free equilibrium is given by

$$E_1 = (N_h*, 0, N_h^*, 0, N_v^*) \text{ and } E_2 = (S_h^*, I_h^*, N_h^*, I_v^*, N_v^*)$$

where :

$$N_h^* = \frac{\Lambda_h}{\mu_h}$$

$$S_h^* = \frac{\Lambda_h}{\mu_h} \frac{\mu_h C_{vh}(1-u1) + (\gamma_h + \mu_h)(\mu_v + u_2)}{(\gamma_h + \mu_h) R_0^2 + \frac{\mu_h}{\mu_v + u_2} C_{vh}(1-u_1)}$$

$$I_h^* = \frac{\Lambda_h (R_0^2 - 1)}{(\gamma_h + \mu_h) R_0^2 + \frac{\mu_h}{\mu_v + u_2} C_{vh}(1-u_1)}$$

$$I_v^* = \frac{\mu_h C_{hv}(1-u_1) N_v (R_0^2 - 1)}{\mu_h C_{hv}(1-u_1)(R_0^2 - 1) + (\gamma_h + \mu_h)(\mu_v + u_2) R_0^2 + \mu_h C_{vh}(1-u_1)}$$

$$N_v^* = \frac{\Lambda_v (1-u_2)}{\mu_v + u_2}$$

The basic reproduction number for the model is (see Appendix A.1):

$$R_0^2 = \frac{\mu_h C_{hv} C_{vh} (1-u_1)^2 N_v}{\Lambda_h (\gamma_h + \mu_h)(\mu_v + u_2)}$$

**Theorem 7** *The system admits two equilibrium*

- *If $R_0 < 1$ the system admits a trivial equilibrium $E_1 = (\frac{\Lambda_h}{\mu_h}, 0, \frac{\Lambda_h}{\mu_h}, 0, \frac{\Lambda_h(1-u_2}{\mu_v+u_2})$*
- *If $R_0 > 1$ then there exists an endemic equilibrium $E_2 = (S_h^*, I_h^*, N_h^*, I_v^*, N_v^*)$.*

*Proof* See Appendix A.2.

**Local Stability of the Equilibria**

**Theorem 8** *If $R_0 < 1$, then $E_1$ is locally asymptotically stable*

*Proof* The local stability analysis based on variational principle is used. The Jacobian of the system (1) at point $E_1 = (N_h*, 0, N_h^*, 0, N_v^*)$ is written as:

$$J(E_1) = \begin{pmatrix} -\mu_h & 0 & -C_{vh}(1-u_1) & 0 & 0 \\ 0 & -(\gamma_h + \mu_h) & C_{vh}(1-u_1) & 0 & 0 \\ 0 & \frac{\mu_h C_{hv}(1-u_1)}{\Lambda_h} N_v^* & -(\mu_v + u_2) & 0 & 0 \\ 0 & 0 & 0 & -\mu_h & 0 \\ 0 & 0 & 0 & 0 & -(\mu_v + u_2) \end{pmatrix}$$

Then the characteristic polynomial is given by:

$$P(\lambda) = (\mu_h + \lambda)^2((\mu_h + u_2) - \lambda) \begin{vmatrix} -(\gamma_h + \mu_h) - \lambda & C_{vh}(1-u_1) \\ \frac{\mu_h C_{hv}(1-u_1)}{\Lambda_h} N_v^* & -(\mu_v + u_2) - \lambda \end{vmatrix}$$

$$= (\mu_h + \lambda)^2\big((\mu_h + u_2) - \lambda\big)\bigg(\lambda^2 + (\gamma_h + \mu_h + \mu_v + u_2)\lambda$$

$$+ (\gamma_h + \mu_h)(\mu_v + u_2) - \frac{\mu_h C_{vh} C_{hc}(1-u_1)^2}{\Lambda_h} N_v\bigg)$$

$$= (\mu_h + \lambda)^2((\mu_h + u_2) - \lambda)\big(\lambda^2 + (\gamma_h + \mu_h + \mu_v + u_2)\lambda$$
$$+ (\gamma_h + \mu_h)(\mu_v + u_2)(1 - R_0^2)\big)$$

Consequently $E_1$ is stable if and only if the coefficients of $\lambda^2 + (\gamma_h + \mu_h + \mu_v + u_2)\lambda^2 + (\gamma_h + \mu_h)(\mu_v + u_2)$ are positive which implies $\Rightarrow E_1$ is stable if and only if $R_0 < 1$.

**Theorem 9** *If $R_0 > 1$, then $E_2$ is locally asymptotically stable.*

*Proof* See Appendix A.3.

### Global Stability of the Equilibria

**Theorem 10** *$E_1$ is globally asymptotically stable.*

*Proof* Since asymptotic behavior of $E_1$ will be studied, $N_h$ is substituted by $N_h^*$ and $N_v$ by $N_v^*$ because $\lim N_h \to N_h^*$ and $\lim N_v \to N_v^*$.

Let $V = \frac{C_{vh}(1-u_1)}{\mu_v+u_2} I_v + I_h$ be a linear Lyapunov function.

So

$$
\begin{aligned}
\dot{V} &= \frac{C_{vh}(1-u_1)}{\mu_v+u_2}\frac{dI_v}{dt} + \frac{dI_h}{dt} \\
&= \frac{C_{vh}C_{hv}(1-u_1)}{N_h^*(\mu_v+u_2)} I_h(N_v^* - I_v) - C_{vh}(1-u_1)I_v + \frac{C_{vh}(1-u_1)S_h}{N_h^*} I_v - (\mu_h+\gamma_h)I_h \\
&= -\frac{C_{vh}(1-u_1)}{N_h^*}(N_h^* - S_h)I_v - (\gamma_h+\mu_h)\left(1 - \frac{C_{vh}C_{hv}(1-u_1)}{N_h^*(\mu_h+\gamma_h)(\mu_v+u_2)}(N_v^* - I_v)\right) I_h \\
&= -\frac{C_{vh}(1-u_1)}{N_h^*}(N_h^* - S_h)I_v - (\gamma_h+\mu_h)\left(1 - R_0^2\left(1 - \frac{I_v}{N_v^*}\right)\right) I_h \\
&= -\frac{C_{vh}(1-u_1)}{N_h^*}(N_h^* - S_h)I_v - (\gamma_h+\mu_h)\left(1 - R_0^2 + R_0^2\frac{I_v}{N_v^*}\right) I_h
\end{aligned}
$$

So for $R_0^2 \le 1$ and as $S_h \le N_h^*$ we obtain: $\dot{V} \le 0$ on the other hand $\dot{V} = 0 \Rightarrow (N_h^* - S_h)I_v = 0$ and $I_h = 0$ then $S_h = N_h^*$ or $I_v = 0$ and $I_h = 0$.

Therefore $E_1$ is globally asymptotically stable.

#### 12.2.1.3 Impact of Control

The effect of prevention and vector control is measured by considering their impact on the reproduction number $R_0$. Thus, this effect is determined by differentiating $R_0$ with respect to $u_1$ (respectively $u_2$)

$$
\frac{\partial R_0}{\partial u_1} = -\sqrt{\frac{C_{hv}C_{vh}N_v}{N_h(\mu_h+\gamma_h)(\mu_v+u_2)}} \le 0 \tag{12.7}
$$

$$
\frac{\partial R_0}{\partial u_2} = -\frac{1}{2}\frac{(1-u_1)\,C_{hv}C_{vh}N_v}{N_h\,(\mu_h+\gamma_h)\,(\mu_v+u_2)^2}\frac{1}{\sqrt{\frac{C_{hv}C_{vh}N_v}{N_h(\mu_h+\gamma_h)(\mu_v+u_2)}}} \le 0 \tag{12.8}
$$

Since $\frac{\partial R_0}{\partial u_1}$ (resp. $\frac{\partial R_0}{\partial u_2}$) is negative, it implies that $R_0$ is a decreasing function of $u_1$ (resp. $u_2$), this indicates that the control $u_1$ (resp. $u_2$) has a negative impact on $R_0$ and will lead to reduction in this disease burden.

## 12.3 Second Epidemic

In the same way as in the previous section we suppose the onset of a second epidemic with another virus. But in this case, we may assume that a proportion of the population of susceptibles is globally immunized against the four serotypes or partially immunized against one, two or three viruses.

But in this model we suppose that the human population is divided into two categories:

- A subpopulation that has been infected once by serotype 2
- A subpopulation $SN_h$ that has been infected twice: the first by the serotype 1 an the second by the serotyp 2, this subpopulation is derived only from the removed from the first epidemic (serotype 1) that are exposed to DHF ($SN_h(t_0) = SS_h(t_0) = R_h^*$.)

Therefore the model is given by the following equations:

$$
\textbf{Human population}\quad\left\{\begin{array}{lcl}
\frac{dS_h}{dt} &=& \Lambda_h - \mu_h S_h - \frac{C_{vh} I_v}{N_h} S_h \\
\frac{dI_h}{dt} &=& \frac{C_{vh} I_v}{N_h} S_h - (\mu_h + \gamma_h) I_h \\
\frac{dR_h}{dt} &=& \gamma_h I_h - \mu_h R_h \\
\frac{dN_h}{dt} &=& \Lambda_h - \mu_h N_h - \alpha_h SI_h \\
\frac{dSS_h}{dt} &=& -\mu_h SS_h - \frac{C_{vh} I_N}{N_h} SS_h \\
\frac{dSI_h}{dt} &=& \frac{C_{vh} I_v}{N_h} SS_h - (\mu_h + \gamma_h + \alpha_h) SI_h \\
\frac{dSR_h}{dt} &=& \gamma_h SI_h - \mu_h SR_h \\
\frac{dSN_h}{dt} &=& -\mu_h SN_h - \alpha_h SI_h
\end{array}\right.
$$

$$
\textbf{Vector population}\quad\left\{\begin{array}{lcl}
\frac{dS_v}{dt} &=& \Lambda_v - \frac{C_{vh}}{N_h}(I_h + SI_h) S_v - \mu_v S_v \\
\frac{dI_v}{dt} &=& \frac{C_{hv}}{N_h}(I_h + SI_h)(N_v + I_v) - \mu_v I_v \\
\frac{dN_v}{dt} &=& \Lambda_v - \mu_v N_v
\end{array}\right.
$$

where $\alpha_h$ is mortality rate due to dengue hemorrhagic fever (DHF), and dengue shock syndrome (DSS).

With the conditions $S_h + I_h + R_h + SS_h + SI_h + SR_h = N_h$, $SS_h + SI_h + SR_h = SN_h$ and $S_v + I_v = N_v$, so: $R_h = N_h - S_h - I_h - SN_h$, $S_v = N_v - I_v$ and

$SR_h = SN_h - SS_h - SI_h$ then

$$\begin{cases} \dfrac{dS_h}{dt} = & \Lambda_h - \dfrac{C_{vh}I_v}{N_h}S_h - \mu_h S_h \\ \dfrac{dI_h}{dt} = & \dfrac{C_{vh}I_v}{N_h}S_h - (\mu_h + \gamma_h)I_h \\ \dfrac{dN_h}{dt} = & \Lambda_h - \mu_h N_h - \alpha_h SI_h \\ \dfrac{dI_v}{dt} = & \dfrac{C_{hv}}{N_h}SI_h(N_v - I_v) - \mu_v I_v \\ \dfrac{dN_v}{dt} = & \Lambda_v - \mu_v N_v \\ \dfrac{dSS_h}{dt} = & -\dfrac{C_{vh}I_v}{N_h}SS_h - \mu_h SS_h \\ \dfrac{dSI_h}{dt} = & \dfrac{C_{vh}I_v}{N_h}SS_h - (\mu_h + \gamma_h + \alpha_h)SI_h \\ \dfrac{dSN_h}{dt} = & -\mu_h SN_h - \alpha_h SI_h \end{cases}$$

The controlled model is given by the following system

$$\begin{cases} \dfrac{dS_h}{dt} = & \Lambda_h - \dfrac{C_{vh}(1-u_1)I_v}{N_h}S_h - \mu_h S_h \\ \dfrac{dI_h}{dt} = & \dfrac{C_{vh}(1-u_1)I_v}{N_h}S_h - (\mu_h + \gamma_h)I_h \\ \dfrac{dN_h}{dt} = & \Lambda_h - \mu_h N_h - \alpha_h SI_h \\ \dfrac{dI_v}{dt} = & \dfrac{C_{hv}}{N_h}(I_h(1-u_1) + SI_h(1-u_3))(N_v - I_v) - (\mu_v + u_2)I_v \\ \dfrac{dN_v}{dt} = & \Lambda_v(1-u_2) - (\mu_v + u_2)N_v \\ \dfrac{dSS_h}{dt} = & -\dfrac{C_{vh}(1-u_3)I_v}{N_h}SS_h - \mu_h SS_h \\ \dfrac{dSI_h}{dt} = & \dfrac{C_{vh}(1-u_3)I_v}{N_h}SS_h - (\mu_h + \gamma_h + \alpha_h)SI_h \\ \dfrac{dSN_h}{dt} = & -\mu_h SN_h - \alpha_h SI_h \end{cases} \quad (12.9)$$

where $u_1$, $u_2$ and $u_3$ are controls.

The objective functions is defined as

$$\mathcal{J}(u_1, u_2, u_3) = \int_0^T \left( I_h + SI_h + N_v + \frac{A}{2}u_1^2(t) + \frac{B}{2}u_2^2(t) + \frac{C}{2}u_3^2(t) \right) dt$$

where:

- the first three terms in the functional objective represent benefit of $I_h$, $SI_h$ and $N_v$ populations that we wish to reduce
- $A$, $B$ and $C$ are positive weights that balance the size of the terms.
- $U$ is the control set defined by
  $U = \{(u_1, u_2, u_3)/u_i$ is measurable, $0 \le u_i(t) \le 1, t \in [0, T]$ for $i = 1, 2, 3\}$.

The objective is to characterize an optimal control $(u_1^*, u_2^*, u_3^*) \in U$ satisfying

$$\mathcal{J}((u_1^*, u_2^*, u_3^*)) = \min_{(u_1,u_2,u_3)\in U} \mathcal{J}(u_1, u_2, u_3)$$

## 12.3.1 Analysis of the Optimal Control Problem

We first show the existence of solutions of the system, thereafter we will prove the existence of optimal control.

### 12.3.1.1 Existence and Positivity of Solutions

**Theorem 11**
*The set* $\Omega = \{(S_h, I_h, N_h, I_v, N_v, SS_h, SI_h, SN_h) \in \mathbb{R}^8/0 \leq S_h, I_h, N_h, I_v, N_v, SS_h, SI_h, SN_h \leq \frac{\Lambda_h}{\mu}, 0 \leq I_v, N_v \leq \frac{\Lambda_v}{\mu_v}\}$ *is positively invariant under system (12.9).*

*Proof* See Appendix B.1.

**Theorem 12**
*The controlled system (12.9) that satisfies a given initial conditions* $\big(S_h(0), I_h(0), N_h(0), I_v(0), N_v(0), SS_h(0), SI_h(0)\big) \in \omega$ *has a unique solution.*

*Proof* See Appendix B.2.

### 12.3.1.2 Existence of an Optimal Control

**Theorem 13**
*Consider the control problem with system (12.9). There exists an optimal control* $(u_1^*, u_2^*, u_3^*) \in U$ *such that*

$$\mathcal{J}((u_1^*, u_2^*, u_3^*)) = \min_{(u_1,u_2,u_3)\in U} \mathcal{J}(u_1, u_2, u_3)$$

*Proof* The existence of the optimal control can be obtained using a result by Fleming and Rishel [12]. Note that:

- From Theorems 11 and 12 it follows that the set of controls and corresponding state variables is nonempty. (see [12], Theorem. 9.2.1)].)
- $\mathcal{J}(u_1, u_2, u_3) = \displaystyle\int_0^T \left( I_h + SI_h + N_v + \frac{A}{2}u_1^2(t) + \frac{B}{2}u_2^2(t) + \frac{C}{2}u_3^2(t) \right) dt$ is convex in $u_1$, $u_2$ and $u_3$.
- The control space $U = \{(u_1, u_2, u_3)/u_1, u_2$ and $u_3$ are measurable, $0 \leq u_1(t), u_2(t), u_3(t) \leq 1, t \in [0, T]\}$ is convex and closed by definition.
- All the right hand sides of equations of system (12.9) are continuous, bounded above by a sum of bounded control and state, and can be written as a bilinear function of $u_1(t)$, $u_2(t)$ and $u_3(t)$ with coefficients depending on time and state.

- The integrand in the objective functional, $I_h + SI_h + N_v + \frac{A}{2}u_1^2(t) + \frac{B}{2}u_2^2(t) + \frac{C}{2}u_3^2(t)$ is clearly convex on $U$.
- Let $\alpha_1 = 1/3 \inf_{t\in[0,T]} (I_h(t), SI_h(t), N_v(t)), \alpha_2 = \inf(A, B, C)$ and $\alpha = 2$ (because, the state variables are bounded)

$$\text{then} \quad I_h + SI_h + N_v + \frac{A}{2}u_1^2(t) + \frac{B}{2}u_2^2(t) + \frac{C}{2}u_3^2(t) \geq \alpha_1 + \alpha_2(|u_1|^2 + |u_2|^2 + |u_2|^2)$$

The conditions of Theorem III. 4.1 from [12] are satisfied then we conclude that there exists an optimal control.

#### 12.3.1.3 Characterization of the Optimal Control

The necessary conditions for the optimal control arise from the Pontryagin's maximum principle [17].

**Theorem 14** *Given an optimal control* $(u_1^*, u_2^*, u_3^*)$ *and solutions* $S_h^*$, $I_h^*$, $I_v^*$, $N_v^*$, $SS_h^*$, $SI_h^*$ *and* $SN_h^*$ *of the corresponding state system, there exist adjoint variables* $\lambda_1, \lambda_2, \lambda_3, \lambda_4, \lambda_5, \lambda_5, \lambda_7$ *and* $\lambda_8$ *satisfying*

$$\begin{cases} \lambda_1' = (\lambda_1 - \lambda_2)\frac{C_{vh}(1-u_1)I_v}{N_h} + \mu_h\lambda_1 \\ \lambda_2' = -1 + (\mu_h + \gamma_h)\lambda_2 + \frac{C_{vh}}{N_h}(1-u_1)(N_v - I_v)\lambda_4 \\ \lambda_3' = \frac{C_{vh}(1-u_1)I_v}{N_h^2} S_h(\lambda_2 - \lambda_1) + \mu_h\lambda_3 + \frac{C_{hv}}{N_h^2}(I_h(1-u_1) \\ \quad +SI_h(1-u_3))(N_v - I_v)\lambda_4 + \frac{C_{vh}(1-u_3)I_v}{N_h^2} SS_h(\lambda_7 - \lambda_6) \\ \lambda_4' = \frac{C_{vh}(1-u_1)}{N_h} S_h(\lambda_1 - \lambda_2) + \left[\frac{C_{hv}}{N_h}(I_h(1-u_1) + SI_h(1-u_3)) + (\mu_v + u_2)\right]\lambda_4 \\ \quad + \frac{C_{vh}(1-u_3)}{N_h} SS_h(\lambda_6 - \lambda_7) \\ \lambda_5' = -1 - \frac{C_{hv}}{N_h}(I_h(1-u_1) + SI_h(1-u_3))\lambda_4 + (\mu_v + u_2)\lambda_5 \\ \lambda_6' = (\lambda_6 - \lambda_7)\frac{C_{vh}(1-u_3)I_v}{N_h} + \mu_h\lambda_6 \\ \lambda_7' = -1 - \frac{C_{hv}}{N_h}(1-u_3)(N_v - I_v)\lambda_4 + \alpha_h\lambda_3 + \lambda_7(\mu_h + \gamma_h + \alpha_h) + \lambda_8\alpha_h \\ \lambda_8' = \lambda_8\mu_h \end{cases}$$

*With transversality conditions:* $\lambda_1(T) = \lambda_2(T) = \lambda_3(T) = \lambda_4(T) = \lambda_4(T) = \lambda_5(T) = \lambda_6(T) = \lambda_7(T) = \lambda_8(T) = 0.$

*Moreover the optimal control is given by*

$$u_1^* = min\left(1, max\left(0, \frac{1}{A}\left[(\lambda_2 - \lambda_1)\frac{C_{vh}I_v^*}{N_h^*}S_h^* + \lambda_4\frac{C_{hv}I_h^*}{N_h^*}(N_v^* - I_v^*)\right]\right)\right)$$

$$u_2^* = min\left(1, max\left(0, \frac{1}{B}\left[\lambda_4 I_v^* + \lambda_5(\Lambda_v + N_v^*)\right]\right)\right)$$

$$u_3^* = min\left(1, max\left(0, \frac{1}{C}\left[(\lambda_7 - \lambda_6)\frac{C_{vh}I_v^*}{N_h^*}SS_h^* + \lambda_4\frac{C_{hv}SI_h^*}{N_h^*}(N_v^* - I_v^*)\right]\right)\right)$$

*Proof* Appendix B.3.

## 12.4 Numerical Simulation

To solve the system (12.9) numerically we will use the Gauss-Seidel-like implicit finite-difference method developed by Gumel et al. [13] and denoted by GSS1 method.

The time interval $[t_0, T]$ is discretized with a step $h$ (time step size) such that
$t_i = t_0 + ih$
$i = 0, 1, \ldots, n$ and $t_n = T$
So at each point $t_i$ we will note $S_h^i = S_h(t_i)$, $I_h^i = I_h(t_i)$,
$N_h^i = N_h(t_i)$, $I_v^i = I_v(t_i)$, $N_v^i = N_v(t_i)$, $SS_h^i = SS_h(t_i)$,
$SI_h^i = SI_h(t_i)$, $SN_hh^i = SN_h(t_i)$,
$\lambda_1^i = \lambda_1(t_i)$, $\lambda_2^i = \lambda_2(t_i)$, $\lambda_3^i = \lambda_3(t_i)$, $\lambda_4^i = \lambda_4(t_i)$, $\lambda_5^i = \lambda_5(t_i)$, $\lambda_6^i = \lambda_6(t_i)$, $\lambda_7^i = \lambda_7(t_i)$, $\lambda_8^i = \lambda_8(t_i)$, $u_1^i = u_1(t_i)$, $u_2^i = u_2(t_i)$ et $u_3^i = u_3(t_i)$

For the approximation of the derivative we used simultaneously forward difference for $\frac{dS_h(t)}{dt}$, $\frac{dI_h(t)}{dt}$, $\frac{dN_h(t)}{dt}$, $\frac{dI_v(t)}{dt}$, $\frac{dN_v(t)}{dt}$, $\frac{dSS_h(t)}{dt}$, $\frac{dSI_h(t)}{dt}$ and $\frac{dSN_h(t)}{dt}$ and backward difference for $\frac{d\lambda_1(t)}{dt}$, $\frac{d\lambda_2(t)}{dt}$, $\frac{d\lambda_3(t)}{dt}$, $\frac{d\lambda_4(t)}{dt}$, $\frac{d\lambda_5(t)}{dt}$, $\frac{d\lambda_6(t)}{dt}$, $\frac{d\lambda_7(t)}{dt}$ and $\frac{d\lambda_8(t)}{dt}$.

So the derivatives are approached by the following finite differences:

$$\frac{\partial S_h^i}{\partial t} \approx \frac{S_h^i - S_h^{i-1}}{k}, \quad \frac{\partial I_h^i}{\partial t} \approx \frac{I_h^i - I_h^{i-1}}{k}, \quad \frac{\partial N_h^i}{\partial t} \approx \frac{N_h^i - N_h^{i-1}}{k},$$

$$\frac{\partial I_v^i}{\partial t} \approx \frac{I_v^i - I_v^{i-1}}{k}, \quad \frac{\partial N_v^i}{\partial t} \approx \frac{N_v^i - N_v^{i-1}}{k},$$

$$\frac{\partial SS_h^i}{\partial t} \approx \frac{SS_h^i - SS_h^{i-1}}{k}, \quad \frac{\partial SI_h^i}{\partial t} \approx \frac{SI_h^i - SI_h^{i-1}}{k}, \quad \frac{\partial SN_h^i}{\partial t} \approx \frac{SN_h^i - SN_h^{i-1}}{k}.$$

for $i = 1, \ldots, n$. Where $k = t_{i+1} - t_i$

$$\frac{\partial \lambda_1^{n-i}}{\partial t} \approx \frac{\lambda_1^{n-i} - \lambda_1^{n-i-1}}{k}, \quad \frac{\partial \lambda_2^{n-i}}{\partial t} \approx \frac{\lambda_2^{n-i} - \lambda_2^{n-i-1}}{h}, \quad \frac{\partial \lambda_3^{n-i}}{\partial t} \approx \frac{\lambda_3^{n-i} - \lambda_3^{n-i-1}}{h},$$

$$\frac{\partial \lambda_4^{n-i}}{\partial t} \approx \frac{\lambda_4^{n-i} - \lambda_4^{n-i-1}}{k}, \quad \frac{\partial \lambda_5^{n-i}}{\partial t} \approx \frac{\lambda_5^{n-i} - \lambda_5^{n-i-1}}{h}, \quad \frac{\partial \lambda_6^{n-i}}{\partial t} \approx \frac{\lambda_6^{n-i} - \lambda_6^{n-i-1}}{k},$$

$$\frac{\partial \lambda_7^{n-i}}{\partial t} \approx \frac{\lambda_7^{n-i} - \lambda_7^{n-i-1}}{h}, \quad \frac{\partial \lambda_8^{n-i}}{\partial t} \approx \frac{\lambda_8^{n-i} - \lambda_8^{n-i-1}}{k}.$$

for $i = 0, \ldots, n-1$. Where $k = t_{i+1} - t_i$

Hence the problem is given by the following numerical scheme: for $i = 1, \dots, n$

$$
\begin{cases}
\dfrac{S_h^{i+1} - S_h^i}{k} = \Lambda_h - \dfrac{C_{vh}(1 - u_1^i)I_v^i}{N_h^i} S_h^{i+1} - \mu_h S_h^{i+1} \\
\dfrac{I_h^{i+1} - I_h^i}{k} = \dfrac{C_{vh}(1 - u_1^i)I_v^i}{N_h^i} S_h^{i+1} - (\mu_h + \gamma_h) I_h^{i+1} \\
\dfrac{N_h^{i+1} - N_h^i}{k} = \Lambda_h - \mu_h N_h^{i+1} - \alpha_h S I_h^i \\
\dfrac{I_v^{i+1} - I_v^i}{k} = \dfrac{C_{hv}}{N_h^{i+1}} (I_h^{i+1}(1 - u_1^i) + S I_h^i (1 - u_3^i))(N_v^i - I_v^{i+1}) - (\mu_v + u_2^i) I_v^{i+1} \\
\dfrac{N_v^{i+1} - N_v^i}{k} = \Lambda_v (1 - u_1^i) - (\mu_v + u_2^i) N_v^{i+1} \\
\dfrac{SS_h^{i+1} - SS_h^i}{k} = -\dfrac{C_{vh}(1 - u_3^i) I_v^{i+1}}{N_h^{i+1}} SS_h^{i+1} - \mu_h SS_h^{i+1} \\
\dfrac{SI_h^{i+1} - SI_h^i}{k} = \dfrac{C_{vh}(1 - u_3^i) I_v^{i+1}}{N_h^{i+1}} SS_h^{i+1} - (\mu_h + \gamma_h + \alpha_h) SI_h^{i+1} \\
\dfrac{SN_h^{i+1} - SN_h^i}{k} = -\mu_h SN_h^{i+1} - \alpha_h SI_h^{i+1} \\
\dfrac{\lambda_1^{n-i} - \lambda_1^{n-i-1}}{k} = (\lambda_1^{n-i-1} - \lambda_2^{n-i}) \dfrac{C_{vh}(1 - u_1^i) I_v^{i+1}}{N_h^{i+1}} + \mu \lambda_1^{n-i-1} \\
\dfrac{\lambda_2^{n-i} - \lambda_2^{n-i-1}}{k} = -1 + (\mu_h + \gamma_h) \lambda_3^{n-i} + \dfrac{C_{hv}}{N_h^{i+1}} (1 - u_1^i)(N_v^{i+1} - I_v^{i+1}) \lambda_4^{n-i} \\
\dfrac{\lambda_3^{n-i} - \lambda_3^{n-i-1}}{k} = \dfrac{C_{vh}(1 - u_1^i) I_v^{i+1}}{(N_h^{i+1})^2} S_h^{i+1} (\lambda_2^{n-i-1} - \lambda_1^{n-i-1}) + \mu_h \lambda_3^{n-i-1} \\
\qquad + \dfrac{C_{hv}}{(N_h^{i+1})^2} (I_h^{i+1}(1 - u_1^i) + S I_h^{i+1}(1 - u_3^i))(N_v^{i+1} - I_v^{i+1}) \lambda_4^{n-i} \\
\qquad + \dfrac{C_{vh}(1 - u_3^i) I_v^{i+1}}{(N_h^{i+1})^2} SS_h^{i+1} (\lambda_7^{n-i} - \lambda_6^{n-i}) \\
\dfrac{\lambda_4^{n-i} - \lambda_4^{n-i-1}}{k} = \dfrac{C_{vh}(1 - u_1^i)}{N_h^{i+1}} S_h^{i+1} (\lambda_1^{n-i-1} - \lambda_2^{n-i-1}) \\
\qquad + \left[ \dfrac{C_{hv}}{N_h^{i+1}} (I_h^{i+1}(1 - u_1^i) + S I_h^{i+1}(1 - u_3^i)) + (\mu_v + u_1^i) \right] \lambda_4^{n-i-1} \\
\qquad + \dfrac{C_{vh}(1 - u_3^i)}{N_h^{i+1}} SS_h^{i+1} (\lambda_6^{n-i} - \lambda_7^{n-i}) \\
\dfrac{\lambda_5^{n-i} - \lambda_5^{n-i-1}}{k} = -1 - \dfrac{C_{hv}}{N_h^{i+1}} (I_h^{i+1}(1 - u_1^i) + S I_h^{i+1}(1 - u_3^i)) \lambda_4^{n-i-1} + (\mu_v + u_2^i) \lambda_5^{n-i-1} \\
\dfrac{\lambda_6^{n-i} - \lambda_6^{n-i-1}}{k} = (\lambda_6^{n-i-1} - \lambda_7^{n-i}) \dfrac{C_{vh}(1 - u_3^i) I_v^{i+1}}{N_h^{i+1}} + \mu_h \lambda_6^{n-i} \\
\dfrac{\lambda_7^{n-i} - \lambda_7^{n-i-1}}{k} = -1 - \dfrac{C_{hv}}{N_h^{i+1}} (1 - u_3^i)(N_v^{i+1} - I_v^{i+1}) \lambda_4^{n-i-1} + \alpha_h \lambda_3^{n-i-1} \\
\qquad + \lambda_7^{n-i-1} (\mu_h + \gamma_h + \alpha_h) + \lambda_8^{n-i} \alpha_h \\
\dfrac{\lambda_8^{n-i} - \lambda_8^{n-i-1}}{k} = \lambda_8^{n-i-1} \mu_h
\end{cases}
$$

Then we consider:
$S_h^0 = S_h(0),\ I_h^0 = I_h(0),\ N_h^0 = N_h(0),\ I_v^0 = I_v(0),\ N_v^0 = N_v(0),\ SS_h^0 = SS_h(0),$
$SI_h^0 = SI_h(0),\ SN_h^0 = SN_h(0),\ u_1^0 = 0, u_2^0 = 0, u_3^0 = 0$
$\lambda_1^n(T) = \lambda_2^n(T) = \lambda_3^n(T) = \lambda_4^n(T) = \lambda_5^n(T) = \lambda_6^n(T) = \lambda_7^n(T) = 0$ and $\lambda_8^n = 0$

So for $i = 0, \dots, n-1$

$$
\begin{cases}
S_h^{i+1} &= N_h^i \dfrac{k\Lambda_h + S_h^i}{N_h^i + kC_{vh}(1-u_1^i)I_v^i + k\mu_h N_h^i}\\
I_h^{i+1} &= \dfrac{kC_{vh}(1-u_1^i)I_v^i S_h^{i+1} + I_h^i N_h^i}{N_h^i(1+k(\mu_h+\gamma_h))}\\
N_h^{i+1} &= \dfrac{k\Lambda_h + N_h^i - k\alpha_h SI_h^i}{1+k\mu_h}\\
I_v^{i+1} &= \dfrac{kC_{hv}N_v^i(I_h^{i+1}(1-u_1^i) + SI_h^i(1-u_3^i)) + I_v^i N_h^{i+1}}{N_h^{i+1}(1+k(\mu_v+u_2^i)) + kC_{hv}(I_h^{i+1}(1-u_1^i) + SI_h^i(1-u_3^i))}\\
N_v^{i+1} &= \dfrac{N_v^i + \Lambda_v(1-u_2^i)k}{1+k(\mu_v+u_2^i)}\\
SS_h^{i+1} &= \dfrac{N_h^{i+1}SS_h^i}{N_h^{i+1} + kC_{vh}(1-u_3^i)I_v^{i+1} + kN_h^{i+1}\mu_h}\\
SI_h^{i+1} &= \dfrac{N_h^{i+1}SI_h^i + kC_{vh}(1-u_3^i)I_v^{i+1}SS_h^{i+1}}{N_h^{i+1} + k(\mu_h+\gamma_h+\alpha_h)N_h^{i+1}}\\
SN_h^{i+1} &= \dfrac{SN_h^i - k\alpha_h SI_h^{i+1}}{1+k\mu_h}\\
\lambda_1^{n-i-1} &= \dfrac{\lambda_1^{n-i}N_h^{i+1} + \lambda_2^{n-i}kC_{vh}(1-u_1^i)I_v^{i+1}}{kC_{vh}(1-u_1^i)I_v^{i+1} + (1+k\mu_h)N_h^{i+1}}\\
\lambda_2^{n-i-1} &= \dfrac{1}{1+k(\mu_h+\gamma_h)}\left[\lambda_2^{n-i} + k + k(\mu_h+\gamma_h)\lambda_2^{n-i} + k\dfrac{C_{hv}}{N_h^{i+1}}(1-u_1^i)(N_v^{i+1} - I_v^{i+1})\lambda_4^{n-i}\right]\\
\lambda_3^{n-i-1} &= \dfrac{kC_{vh}I_v^{i+1}}{(N_h^{i+1})^2(1+k\mu_h)}\left[S_h^{i+1}(1-u_1^i)(\lambda_1^{n-i-1} - \lambda_2^{n-i-1})\right.\\
&\quad \left. + SS_h^{i+1}(1-u_3^i)(\lambda_6^{n-i} - \lambda_7^{n-i})\right] + \dfrac{\lambda_3^{n-i}}{1+k\mu_h}\\
&\quad - \dfrac{kC_{hv}}{(N_h^{i+1})^2(1+k\mu_h)}\left[I_h^{i+1}(1-u_1^i) + SI_h^{i+1}(1-u_3^i)\right](N_v^{i+1} - I_v^{i+1})\lambda_4^{n-i}\\
\lambda_4^{n-i-1} &= \dfrac{N_h^{i+1}\lambda_4^{n-1} + kC_{vh}(1-u_1)S_h^{i+1}(\lambda_2^{n-i-1} - \lambda_1^{n-i-1}) + kC_{vh}(1-u_3^i)SS_h(\lambda_7^{n-i} - \lambda_6^{n-i})}{N_h^{i+1}(1+k(\mu_v+u_2^i)) + kC_{hv}(I_h^{i+1}(1-u_1^i) + SI_h^{i+1}(1-u_3^i))}\\
\lambda_5^{n-i-1} &= \dfrac{1}{1+k(\mu_v+u_2^i)}\left[k + \dfrac{kC_{hv}}{N_h^{i+1}}(I_h^{i+1}(1-u_1^i) + SI_h^{i+1}(1-u_3^i))\lambda_4^{n-i-1} + \lambda_5^{n-i}\right]\\
\lambda_6^{n-i-1} &= \dfrac{\lambda_6^{n-i}N_h^{i+1} + kC_{vh}(1-u_3^i)I_v^{i+1}\lambda_7^{n-i}}{N_h^{i+1}(1+k\mu_h) + kC_{vh}(1-u_3^i)I_v^{i+1}}\\
\lambda_7^{n-i-1} &= \dfrac{1}{1+k(\mu_h+\gamma_h+\alpha_h)}\left[\lambda_7^{n-i} + k + \dfrac{kC_{hv}}{N_h^{i+1}}(1-u_3^i)(N_v^{i+1} - I_v^{i+1})\lambda_4^{n-i-1} - k\alpha_h\lambda_3^{n-i-1}\right]\\
&\quad - \dfrac{k\lambda_8^{n-i}\alpha_h}{1+k(\mu_h+\gamma_h+\alpha_h)}\\
\lambda_8^{n-i-1} &= \dfrac{\lambda_8^{n-i}}{1+k\mu_h}
\end{cases}
$$

$$\begin{cases} M_1^{i+1} &= \frac{1}{A}\left[(\lambda_2^{n-i-1}-\lambda_1^{n-i-1})\frac{C_{vh}I_v^{i+1}}{N_h^{i+1}}S_h^{i+1}+\lambda_4^{n-i-1}\frac{C_{hv}I_h^{i+1}}{N_h^{i+1}}(N_v^{i+1}-I_v^{i+1})\right] \\ M_2^{i+1} &= \frac{1}{B}\left[\lambda_4^{n-i-1}I_v^{i+1}-\lambda_5^{n-i-1}(\Lambda_v-N_v^{i+1})\right] \\ M_3^{i+1} &= \frac{1}{C}\left[(\lambda_7^{n-i-1}-\lambda_6^{n-i-1})\frac{C_{vh}I_v^{i+1}}{N_h^{i+1}}SS_h^{i+1}+\lambda_4^{n-i-1}\frac{C_{hv}SI_h^{i+1}}{N_h^{i+1}}(N_v^{i+1}-I_v^{i+1})\right] \\ u_1^{i+1} &= \min(1,\max(0,M_1^{i+1})) \\ u_2^{i+1} &= \min(1,\max(0,M_2^{i+1})) \\ u_3^{i+1} &= \min(1,\max(0,M_3^{i+1})) \end{cases}$$

Simulations are performed by taking parameters in (Table 12.1) [7].

In order to illustrate the impact of the control on the basic reproduction number, we consider two scenarios depending on initial value of $R_0$

**Table 12.1** Input parameters of the dengue vector–host model

| Symbol | Meaning | Value |
|---|---|---|
| $p_{hv}$ | Transmission probability of vector to human | 0.75 |
| $p_{vh}$ | Transmission probability of human to vector | 0.75 |
| $b_s$ | Bites per susceptible mosquito per day | 0.5 |
| $b_i$ | Bites per infectious mosquito per day | 1.0 |
| $C_{hv}$ | Effective contact rate, human to vector | 0.375 |
| $C_{vh}$ | Effective contact rate, vector to human | 0.75 |
| $\frac{1}{\mu_h}$ | Human life span | 25000 days |
| $\frac{1}{\mu_v}$ | Vector life span | 4 days |
| $\frac{1}{\mu_h+\gamma_h}$ | Host infection duration | 3 days |

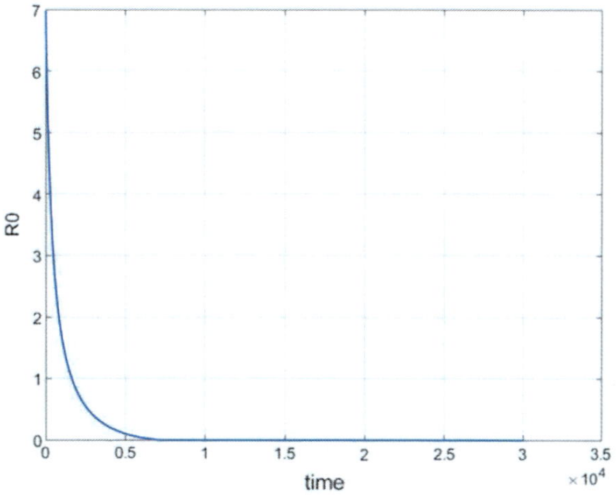


**Fig. 12.2** Basic reproduction number with control $u_1, u_2, u_3 \in [0, 1]$, initial value of $R_0 > 1$

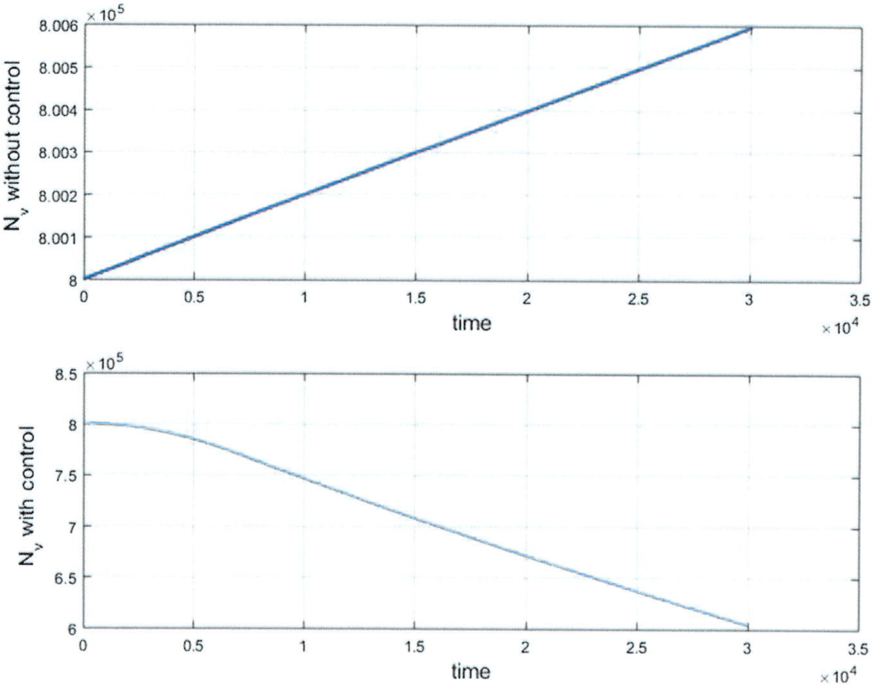


**Fig. 12.3** Vector population, (Top) without control, (Bottom) with control $u_1, u_2, u_3 \in [0, 1]$, initial value of $R_0 > 1$

$R_0 > 1$ The basic reproduction number $R_0$ can be controlled and reduced to $R_0 < 1$ (Fig. 12.2) by using control $u_1, u_2, u_3 \in [0, 1]$ (Fig. 12.6), which leads to a reduction in population of vector (Fig. 12.3), in infected human (Fig. 12.4) and in infected vector (Fig. 12.5).

$R_0 < 1$ The vector population and the infected vector can be exterminated (Figs. 12.7, 12.8 and 12.10) by using control $u_1, u_2, u_3 \in [0, 1]$ (Fig. 12.11), and reducing significantly the number of infected human (Fig. 12.9).

## 12.5 Conclusion

Our proposed model ensures a better understanding of the impact of prevention and control on the basic reproduction number $R_0$.

A comparison of the model with and without optimal control is done to analyze the efficiency of optimal control. It is shown that optimal control allows an interesting reduction of the number of infected individuals. In order to illustrate the global picture of the epidemic, the numbers of infected individuals under the optimal control and without control are presented in figures.

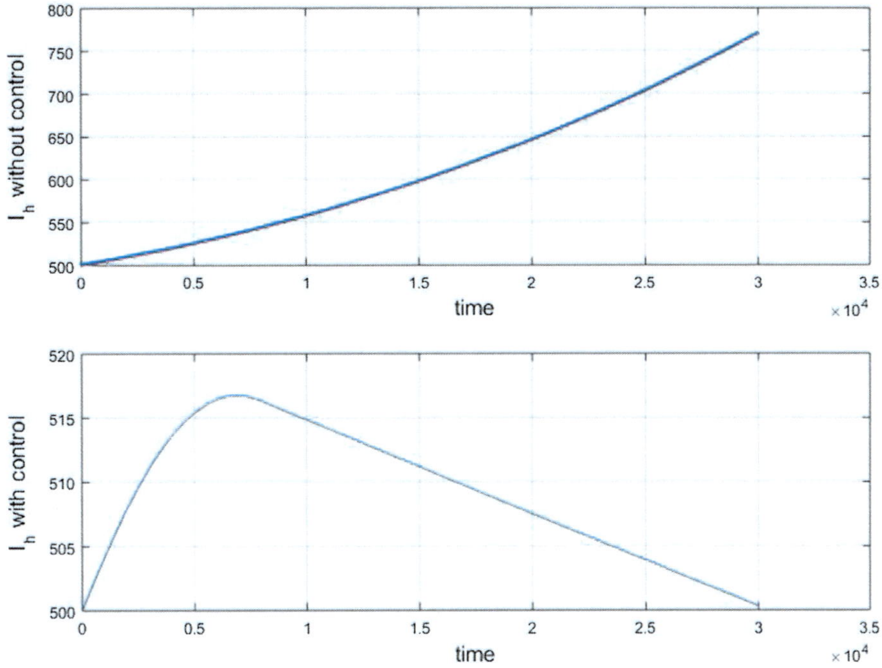


**Fig. 12.4** Number of infected host, (Top) without control, (Bottom) with control $u_1, u_2, u_3 \in [0, 1]$, initial value of $R_0 > 1$

# Appendix A

## *1. Reproduction Number*

Using notations in [8], the matrices $F$ and $V$ and their Jacobian matrices for the new infection terms and the remaining transfer term evaluated at the disease free equilibrium are respectively given by;

$$F = \begin{pmatrix} \frac{C_{vh} I_v}{N_h} S_h(1-u_1) \\ \frac{C_{hv} I_h}{N_h}(1-u_1)(N_v - I_v) \end{pmatrix}; V = \begin{pmatrix} (\mu_h + \gamma_h) I_h \\ (\mu_v + u_2) I_v \end{pmatrix}$$

$$J_F = \begin{pmatrix} 0 & \frac{C_{vh} S_h}{N_h}(1-u_1) \\ \frac{C_{hv}(1-u_1)}{N_h}(N_v - I_v) & -\frac{C_{hv} I_h}{N_h}(1-u_1) \end{pmatrix}$$

$$J_v = \begin{pmatrix} \mu_h + \gamma_h & 0 \\ 0 & \mu_v + u_2 \end{pmatrix} \Rightarrow J_v^{-1} = \begin{pmatrix} \frac{1}{\mu_h + \gamma_h} & 0 \\ 0 & \frac{1}{\mu_v + u_2} \end{pmatrix}$$

$$J_F J_v^{-1} = \begin{pmatrix} 0 & \frac{C_{vh} S_h (1-u_1)}{N_h(\mu_v + u_2)} \\ \frac{C_{hv}(1-u_1)(N_v - I_v)}{N_h(\mu_h + \gamma_h)} & -\frac{C_{hv} I_h (1-u_1)}{N_h(\mu_v + u_2} \end{pmatrix}$$

For $S_h = N_h \; I_h = R_h = 0 \; S_v = N_v \; I_v = 0$

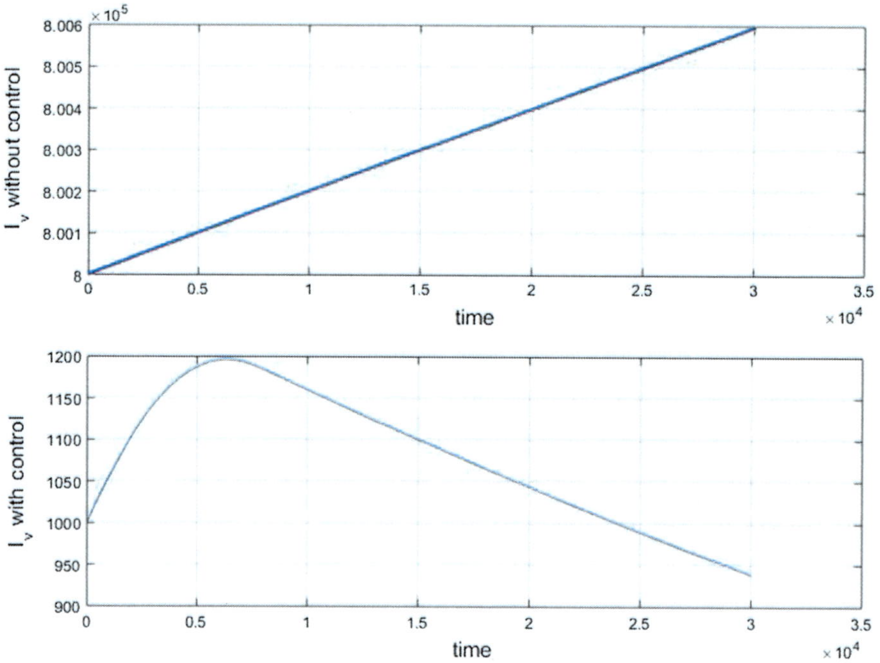


**Fig. 12.5** Number of infected vector, (Top) without control, (Bottom) with control $u_1, u_2, u_3 \in [0, 1]$, initial value of $R_0 > 1$

**Fig. 12.6** Evolution of the control, initial value of $R_0 > 1$

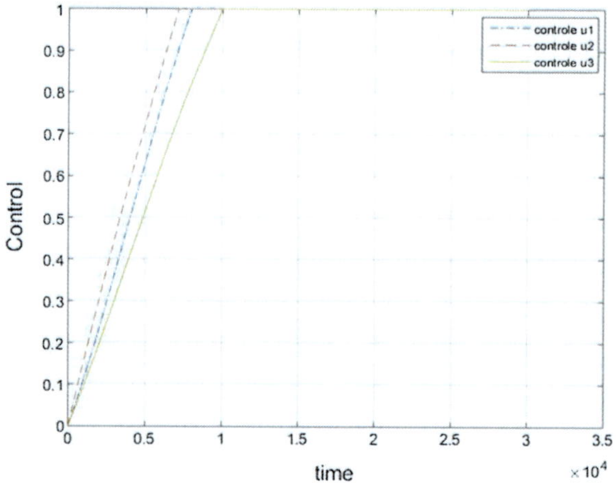

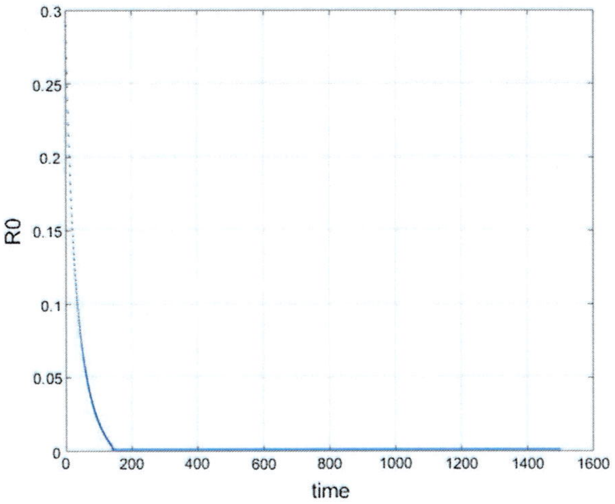


**Fig. 12.7** Basic reproduction number with control $u_1, u_2, u_3 \in [0, 1]$, initial value of $R_0 < 1$

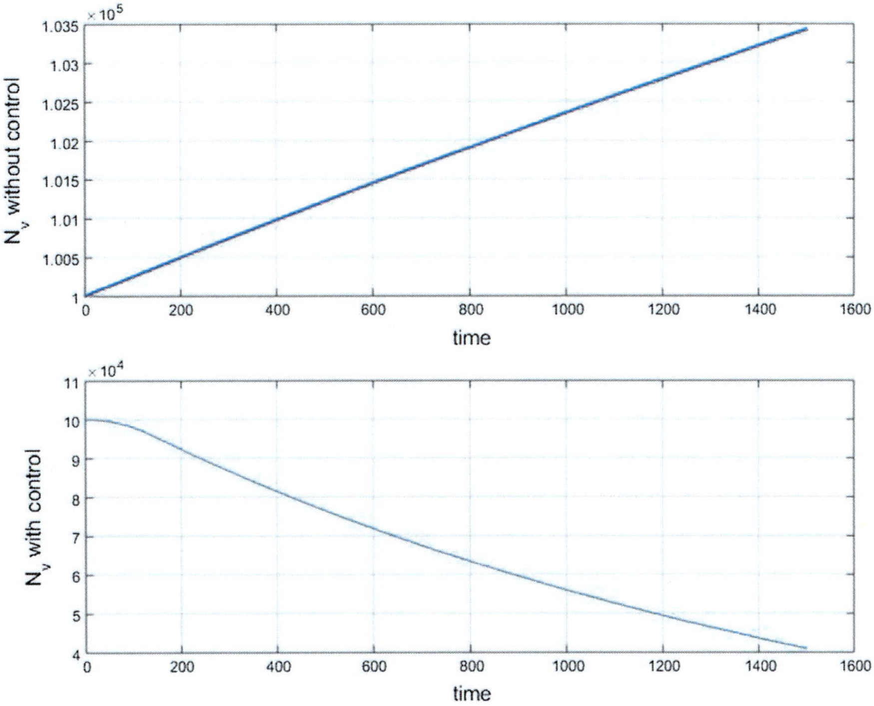


**Fig. 12.8** Vector population, (Top) without control, (Bottom) with control $u_1, u_2, u_3 \in [0, 1]$, initial value of $R_0 < 1$

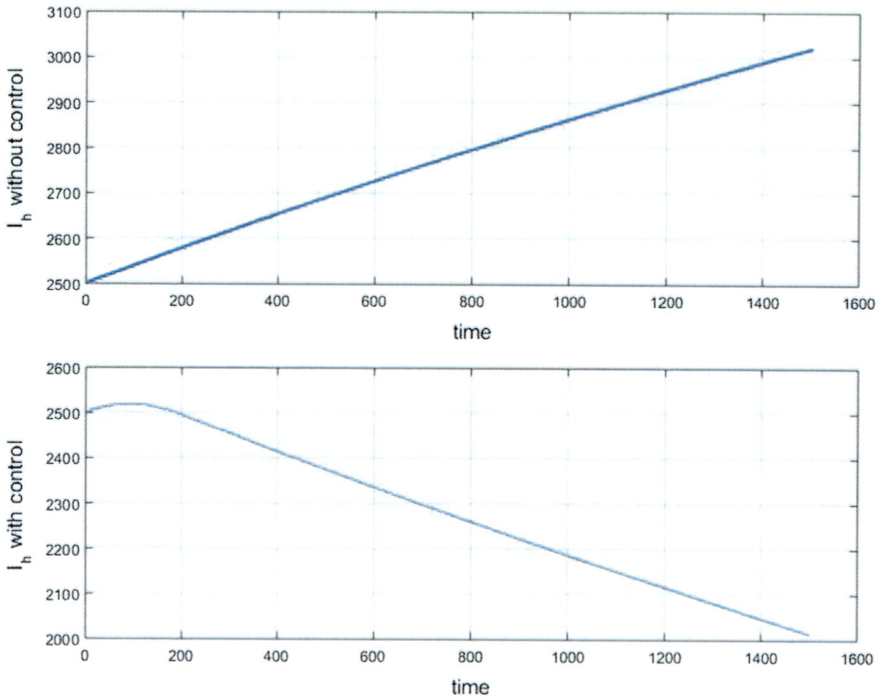


**Fig. 12.9** Number of infected host, (Top) without control, (Bottom) with control $u_1, u_2, u_3 \in [0, 1]$, initial value of $R_0 < 1$

Thus

$$J_F J_v^{-1} = \begin{pmatrix} 0 & \frac{C_{vh}(1-u_1)}{(\mu_v+u_2)} \\ \frac{C_{hv}(1-u_1)N_v}{N_h(\mu_h+\gamma_h)} & 0 \end{pmatrix}$$

It follows that the basic reproduction, denoted by $R_0$, is given by

$$R_0 = \rho(J_F J_v^{-1}) = (1 - u_1)\sqrt{\frac{C_{hv}C_{vh}N_v}{N_h(\mu_h + \gamma_h)(\mu_v + u_2)}}$$

## 2. *Proof of Theorem 1*

From (12.5) we obtain:

$$\frac{C_{hv}I_h}{N_h}(N_v - I_v)(1 - u_1) - (\mu_v + u_2)I_v = 0 \tag{12.10}$$

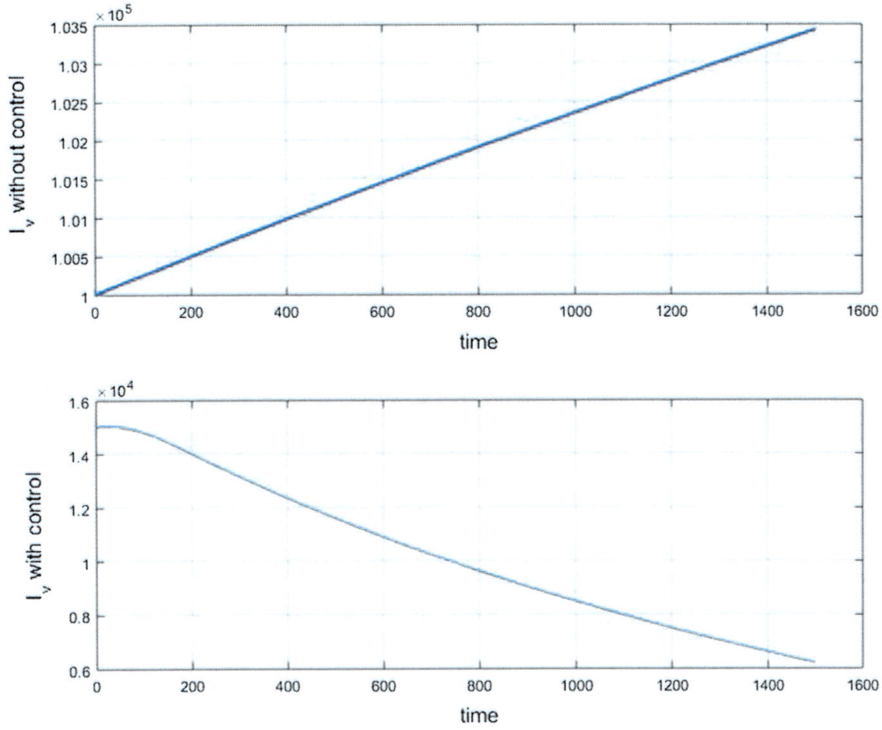


**Fig. 12.10** Number of infected vector, (Top) without control, (Bottom) with control $u_1, u_2, u_3 \in [0, 1]$, initial value of $R_0 < 1$

**Fig. 12.11** Evolution of the control, initial value of $R_0 < 1$

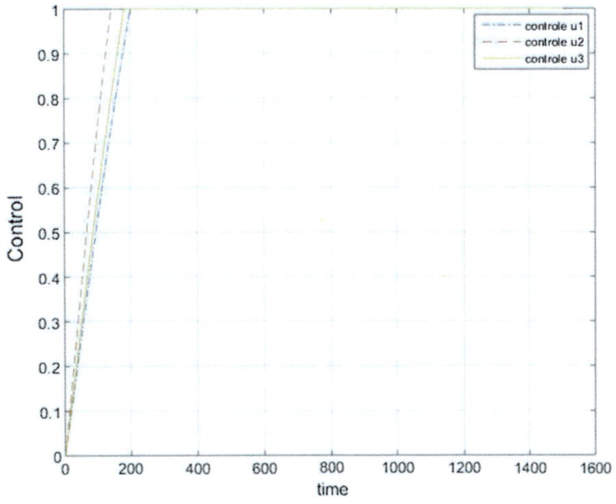

⇒

$$I_v = \frac{C_{hv} I_h N_v (1-u_1)}{C_{hv} I_h (1-u_1) + (\mu_v + u_2) N_h} \tag{12.11}$$

From (12.6) we obtain: $N_h = \dfrac{\Lambda_h}{\mu_h}$

Therefore

$$I_v = \frac{\mu_h C_{hv} N_v (1-u_1) I_h}{\mu_h C_{hv} (1-u_1) I_h + \Lambda_h (\mu_v + u_2)}$$

From (12.2) we obtain

$$\Lambda_h - \frac{C_{vh} I_v}{N_h} S_h (1-u_1) - \mu_h S_h = 0$$

⇒

$$\frac{C_{vh} I_v}{N_h} S_h (1-u_1) = \Lambda_h - \mu_h S_h$$

From (12.3) we obtain

$$\frac{C_{vh} I_v}{N_h} S_h (1-u_1) = (\gamma_h + \mu_h) I_h$$

⇒

$$\Lambda_h - \mu_h S_h = (\gamma_h + \mu_h) I_h$$

⇒

$$S_h = \frac{\Lambda_h - (\gamma_h + \mu_h) I_h}{\mu_h}$$

In the Eq. (12.3) we substitute $N_h$, $S_h$ and $I_v$, therefore

$$C_{vh} \frac{1}{N_h} I_v S_h (1-u_1) - (\gamma_h + \mu_h) I_h = 0$$

⇒

$$\frac{\mu_h C_{vh} C_{hv} N_v (1-u_1)^2 [\Lambda_h I_h - (\gamma_h + \mu_h) I_h^2]}{\Lambda_h [\mu_h C_{vh} (1-u_1) I_h + \Lambda_h (\mu_v + u_2)]} - (\gamma_h + \mu_h) I_h = 0$$

$\Rightarrow$

$$\frac{\mu_h C_{vh} C_{hv} N_v (1-u_1)^2 [\Lambda_h I_h - (\gamma_h + \mu_h) I_h^2] - \Lambda_h (\mu_h C_{vh} (1-u_1)(\mu_h + \gamma_h)) I_h^2}{[\mu_h C_{hv} (1-u_1)] \Lambda_h I_h + \Lambda_h^2 (\mu_v + u_2)} - \frac{\Lambda_h^2 (\gamma_h + \mu_h)(\mu_v + u_2) I_h}{[\mu_h C_{hv} (1-u_1)] \Lambda_h I_h + \Lambda_h^2 (\mu_v + u_2)} = 0$$

$\Rightarrow$

$$I_h [\Lambda_h \mu_h C_{hv} C_{vh} (1-u_1)^2 N_v - \Lambda_h^2 (\gamma_h + \mu_h)(\mu_v + u_2) - (\gamma_h + \mu_h) \mu_h C_{vh} (1-u_1)(C_{hv}(1-u_1) N_v + \Lambda_h) I_h] = 0 \quad (12.12)$$

So $I_h = 0$ or

$$I_h = \frac{\Lambda_h \mu_h C_{hv} C_{vh} (1-u_1)^2 N_v - \Lambda_h^2 (\gamma_h + \mu_h)(\mu_v + u_2)}{(\gamma_h + \mu_h) \mu_h C_{vh} (1-u_1)(C_{hv}(1-u_1) N_v + \Lambda_h)} \quad (12.13)$$

$$I_h = \frac{\Lambda_h^2 (\gamma_h + \mu_h)(\mu_v + u_2) \left[ \frac{\Lambda_h \mu_h C_{hv} C_{vh} (1-u_1)^2 N_v}{\Lambda_h^2 (\gamma_h + \mu_h)(\mu_v + u_2)} - 1 \right]}{\mu_h (\gamma_h + \mu_h) C_{hv} C_{vh} (1-u_1)^2 N_v + \Lambda_h \mu_h (\gamma_h + \mu_h) C_{vh} (1-u_1)} \quad (12.14)$$

$$I_h = \frac{\Lambda_h (R_0 - 1)}{\frac{\mu_h (\gamma_h + \mu_h) C_{hv} C_{vh} (1-u_1)^2 N_v}{\Lambda_h (\gamma_h + \mu_h)(\mu_v + u_2)} + \frac{\Lambda_h \mu_h (\gamma_h + \mu_h) C_{vh} (1-u_1)}{\Lambda_h (\gamma_h + \mu_h)(\mu_v + u_2)}} \quad (12.15)$$

$$I_h^* = \frac{\Lambda_h (R_0^2 - 1)}{(\gamma_h + \mu_h) R_0^2 + \frac{\mu_h}{\mu_v + u_2} C_{vh} (1-u_1)} \quad (12.16)$$

with $R_0^2 = \dfrac{u_h C_{vh} C_{hv} (1-u_1)^2 N_v}{\Lambda_h (\gamma_h + \mu_h)(\mu_v + u_2)}$
and we have

$$\begin{aligned} S_h &= \frac{\Lambda_h - (\gamma + \mu_h) I_h}{\mu_h} \\ &= \frac{1}{\mu_h} \left( \Lambda_h - \frac{\Lambda_h (\gamma_h + \mu_h)(R_0^2 - 1)}{(\gamma_h + \mu_h) R_0^2 + \frac{\mu_h}{\mu_v + u_2} C_{vh} (1-u_1)} \right) \\ &= \frac{1}{\mu_h} \frac{\Lambda_h (\gamma_h + \mu_h) R_0^2 + \frac{\mu_h \Lambda_h}{\mu_v + u_2} C_{vh} (1-u_1) - \Lambda_h (\gamma_h + \mu_h)(R_0^2 - 1)}{(\gamma_h + \mu_h) R_0^2 + \frac{\mu_h}{\mu_v + u_2} C_{vh} (1-u_1)} \end{aligned}$$

$$= \frac{\Lambda_h}{\mu_h} \frac{\frac{\mu_h}{\mu_v+u_2} C_{vh}(1-u_1) + (\gamma_h+\mu_h)}{(\gamma_h+\mu_h)R_0^2 + \frac{\mu_h}{\mu_v+u_2} C_{vh}(1-u_1)}$$

$$S_h^* = \frac{\Lambda_h}{\mu_h} \frac{\mu_h C_{vh}(1-u_1) + (\gamma_h+\mu_h)(\mu_v+u_2)}{(\gamma_h+\mu_h)(\mu_v+u_2)R_0^2 + \mu_h C_{vh}(1-u_1)}$$

$$I_v = \frac{\mu_h C_{hv}(1-u_1) N_v I_h}{\mu_h C_{hv}(1-u_1) I_h + \Lambda_h(\mu_v+u_2)}$$

$$= \frac{\dfrac{\mu_h C_{hv}(1-u_1) N_v \Lambda_h (R_0^2-1)}{(\gamma_h+\mu_h)R_0^2 + \frac{\mu_h}{\mu_v+u_2} C_{vh}(1-u_1}}{\dfrac{\mu_h C_{hv}(1-u_1)\Lambda_h(R_0^2-1) + \Lambda_h(\mu_v+u_2)[(\gamma_h+\mu_h)R_0^2 + \frac{\mu_h}{\mu_v+u_2} C_{vh}(1-u_1)]}{(\gamma_h+\mu_h)R_0^2 + \frac{\mu_h}{\mu_v+u_2} C_{vh}(1-u_1)}}$$

$$I_v^* = \frac{\mu_h C_{hv}(1-u_1) N_v (R_0^2-1)}{\mu_h C_{hv}(1-u_1)(R_0^2-1) + (\gamma_h+\mu_h)(\mu_v+u_2)R_0^2 + \mu_h C_{vh}(1-u_1)}$$

Form the Eq. (12.6) we have $\Lambda_v(1-u_2) - (\mu_v+u_2)N_v^* = 0$

$$\Rightarrow N_v^* = \frac{\Lambda_h(1-u_2)}{\mu_v+u_2}$$

Thus

- If $R_0 < 1$ the system admits a trivial equilibrium $E_1 = (\frac{\Lambda_h}{\mu_h}, 0, \frac{\Lambda_h}{\mu_h}, 0, \frac{\Lambda_h(1-u_2)}{\mu_v+u_2})$
- If $R_0 > 1$ then there exists an endemic equilibrium $E_2 = (S_h^*, I_h^*, N_h^*, I_v^*, N_v^*)$.

## 3. *Proof of Theorem 3*

The local stability analysis based on variational principle is used. The Jacobian of the system (12.1) at point $E_2$ is written as:

$$J(E_2) = \begin{pmatrix} -\frac{C_{vh}(1-u_1)I_v^*}{N_h^*} - \mu_h & 0 & -\frac{C_{vh}(1-u_1)S_h^*}{N_h^*} & E & 0 \\ \frac{C_{vh}(1-u_1)I_v^*}{N_h^*} & -(\gamma_h+\mu_h) & \frac{C_{vh}(1-u_1)S_h^*}{N_h^*} & -E & 0 \\ 0 & \frac{C_{hv}(1-u_1)(N_v^*-I_h^*)}{N_h^*} & D & F & \frac{C_{hv}(1-u_1)I_h^*}{N_h^*} \\ 0 & 0 & 0 & -\mu_h & 0 \\ 0 & 0 & 0 & 0 & -(\mu_v+u_2) \end{pmatrix}$$

with $D = -\frac{C_{hv}(1-u_1)}{N_h^*} I_h^* - (\mu_v+u_2)$, $E = \frac{C_{vh}(1-u_1)S_h^* I_v^*}{N_h^2}$ and $F = -\frac{C_{hv}(1-u_1)(N_v^*-I_v^*)I_h^*}{N_h^{*2}}$

Therefore $P(\lambda) = (\mu_h+\lambda)(\mu_v+u_2+\lambda)Q(\lambda)$ with

$$Q(\lambda) = \begin{vmatrix} -\frac{C_{vh}(1-u_1)I_v^*}{N_h^*} - \mu_h - \lambda & 0 & -\frac{C_{vh}(1-u_1)S_h^*}{N_h^*} \\ \frac{C_{vh}(1-u_1)I_v^*}{N_h^*} & -(\gamma_h+\mu_h) - \lambda & \frac{C_{vh}(1-u_1)S_h^*}{N_h^*} \\ 0 & \frac{C_{hv}(1-u_1)(N_v^*-I_h^*)}{N_h^*} & -\frac{C_{hv}(1-u_1)}{N_h^*} - (\mu_v+u_2) - \lambda \end{vmatrix}$$

$$= \left(\frac{C_{vh}(1-u_1)I_v^*}{N_h^*} - \mu_h - \lambda\right)\left[(\gamma_h + \mu_h + \lambda)\left(\frac{C_{vh}(1-u_1)I_h^*}{N_h^*} + (\mu_v + u_2) + \lambda\right) - \frac{C_{vh}C_{hv}(1-u_1)^2 S_h^*}{N_h^{*2}}(N_v - I_v^*)\right] - \left[\frac{C_{vh}(1-u_1)I_v^*}{N_h^*}\frac{C_{vh}C_{hv}(1-u_1)^2}{N_h^{*2}}S_h^*(N_v^* - I_v^*)\right]$$

We have

$$\begin{aligned}
&\Lambda_h - \frac{C_{vh}(1-u_1)I_v^*}{N_h^*}S_h^* - \mu_h S_h^* = 0 && \Rightarrow \frac{C_{vh}(1-u_1)I_v^*}{N_h^*} + \mu = \frac{\Lambda_h}{S_h^*}\\
&\frac{C_{vh}(1-u_1)I_v^*}{N_h^*}S_h^* - (\gamma_h + \mu_h)I_h^* = 0 && \Rightarrow \gamma_h + \mu_h = \frac{C_{vh}(1-u_1)I_v^* S_h^*}{N_h^* I_h^*}\\
&\frac{C_{hv}I_h^*(1-u_1)(N_v - I_v^*)}{N_h^*} - (\mu_v + u_2)I_v^* = 0 && \Rightarrow \frac{C_{hv}(1-u_1)I_h^*}{N_h^*} + (\mu_v + u_2) = \frac{C_{hv}(1-u_1)I_h^* N_h^*}{N_h^* I_v^*}
\end{aligned}$$

which implies:

$$Q(\lambda) = -\left[\lambda^3 + \left(\frac{\Lambda_h}{S_h^*} + \frac{C_{vh}(1-u_1)S_h^* I_v^*}{N_h^* I_h^*} + \frac{C_{hv}(1-u_1)I_h^* N_v^*}{N_h^* I_v^*}\right)\lambda^2 + \left(\frac{C_{vh}C_{hv}(1-u_1)^2 S_h^* I_v^*}{N_h^{*2}} + \frac{\Lambda C_{vh}(1-u_1)I_v^*}{N_h^* I_h^*} + \frac{\Lambda C_{hv}(1-u_1)I_h^* N_v^*}{N_h^* S_h^* I v}\right)\lambda + \frac{\Lambda_h C_{vh} C_{hv}(1-u_1)^2}{N_h^{*2}}N_v - \frac{C_{vh}C_{hv}(1-u_1)^2 \mu_h S_h^*(N_v^* - I_v^*)}{N_h^{*2}}\right]$$

We put

$$\begin{aligned}
A &= \frac{\Lambda_h}{S_h^*} + \frac{C_{vh}(1-u_1)S_h^* I_v^*}{N_h^* I_h^*} + \frac{C_{hv}(1-u_1)I_h^* N_v^*}{N_h^* I_v^*}\\
B &= \frac{C_{vh}C_{hv}(1-u_1)^2 S_h^* I_v^*}{N_h^{*2}} + \frac{\Lambda_h C_{vh}(1-u_1)I_v^*}{N_h^* I_h^*} + \frac{\Lambda_h C_{hv}(1-u_1)I_h^* N_v^*}{N_h^* S_h^* I_v^*}\\
C &= \frac{\Lambda_h C_{vh} C_{hv}(1-u_1)^2}{N_h^{*2}}N_v^* - \frac{C_{vh}C_{hv}(1-u_1)^2 \mu_h S_h^*(N_v^* - I_v^*)}{N_h^{*2}}
\end{aligned}$$

We find $AB \geq \dfrac{\Lambda_h C_{vh} C_{hv} 1 - u_1)^2}{N_h^{*2}}(N_v^* + I_v^*)$ and we have $I_v^* \leq N_v^*$ so $A>0$, $B > 0$ and $C > 0$, thus $AB > C$.

Using Routh–Hurwitz stability criterion, it can be concluded that $E_2$ is locally asymptotically stable.

# Appendix B

## *1. Proof of Theorem 5*

From

$$\frac{dN_h}{dt} = \Lambda_h - \mu_h N_h - \alpha_h S I_h$$

$$\begin{aligned}
\frac{dN_h}{dt} &= \Lambda_h - \mu_h N_h - \alpha_h S I_h\\
&\geq -(\mu_h + \alpha_h)N_h \quad \text{(because } I_h \leq N_h \text{ and } \alpha_h \geq 0)
\end{aligned}$$

Then using Gronwall's inequality $N_h(t) \geq N_h(0)e^{\left(-\int_0^T(\mu_h+\alpha_h)dt\right)}$
$\Longrightarrow N_h(t) > 0$
From

$$\frac{dN_v}{dt} = \Lambda_v - \mu_v N_v$$

$$\frac{dN_v}{dt} = \Lambda_v - \mu_v N_v$$

$$\geq -\mu_v N_v$$

Then using Gronwall's inequality $N_v(t) \geq N_v(0)e^{\left(-\int_0^T \mu_v dt\right)}$
$\Longrightarrow N_v(t) > 0$ on the other hand we have:

$$\frac{dI_h}{dt} = \frac{C_{vh}(1-u_1)I_v}{N_h}S_h - (\mu_h + \gamma_h)I_h$$

Assume that there exists some time $t_* > 0$ such that $I_h(t_*) = 0$, other variables $(S_h, N_h, I_v, N_v, SS_h, SN_h)$ are positive and $I_h(t) > 0$ for $t \in [0, t_*[$.

So we have

$$\begin{aligned} \frac{dI_h(t)e^{(\mu_h+\gamma_h)t}}{dt} &= (\mu_h+\gamma_h)e^{(\mu_h+\gamma_h)t}I_h + e^{(\mu_h+\gamma_h)t}\left[\frac{C_{vh}(1-u_1)I_v}{N_h}S_h - (\mu_h+\gamma_h)I_h\right] \\ &= e^{(\mu_h+\gamma_h)t}\left[\frac{C_{vh}(1-u_1)I_v}{N_h}S_h\right] \end{aligned}$$

Integrating this equation from 0 to $t_*$ we have

$$\int_0^{t_*} \frac{dI_h(t)e^{(\mu_h+\gamma_h)t}}{dt}dt = \int_0^{t_*} e^{(\mu_h+\gamma_h)t}\left[\frac{C_{vh}(1-u_1)I_v}{N_h}S_h\right]dt$$

then

$$I_h(t_*) = e^{-(\mu_h+\gamma_h)t_*}I_h(0) + e^{-(\mu_h+\gamma_h)t_*}\int_0^{t_*} e^{(\mu_h+\gamma_h)t}\frac{C_{vh}(1-u_1)I_v}{N_h}S_h dt > 0$$

which contradicts $I_h(t_*) = 0$. Consequently, $I_h(t) > 0 \ \forall t \in [0, T]$.
in the same way

$$\frac{dSI_h}{dt} = \frac{C_{vh}(1-u_3)I_v}{N_h}SS_h - (\mu_h + \gamma_h + \alpha_h)SI_h$$

Assume that there exists some time $t_* > 0$ such that $SI_h(t_*) = 0$ , other variables $(S_h, I_h, N_h, I_v, N_v, SS_h, SI_h, SN_h)$ are positive and $SI_h(t) > 0$ for $t \in [0, t_*[$.

So we have

$$\begin{aligned}\frac{dSI_h(t)e^{(\mu_h+\gamma_h+\alpha_h)t}}{dt} &= (\mu_h+\alpha_h+\delta_h)e^{(\mu_h+\gamma_h+\alpha_h)t}SI_h \\ &+e^{(\mu_h+\gamma_h+\alpha_h)t}\left[\frac{C_{vh}(1-u_1)I_v}{N_h}SS_h-(\mu_h+\gamma_h+\alpha_h)SI_h\right] \\ &= e^{(\mu_h+\gamma_h+\alpha_h)t}\left[\frac{C_{vh}(1-u_1)I_v}{N_h}SS_h\right]\end{aligned}$$

Integrating this equation from 0 to $t_*$ we have

$$\int_0^{t_*}\frac{dSI_h(t)e^{(\mu_h+\gamma_h+\alpha_h)t}}{dt}dt=\int_0^{t_*}e^{(\mu_h+\gamma_h+\alpha_h)t}\left[\frac{C_{vh}(1-u_1)I_v}{N_h}SS_h\right]dt$$

then

$$SI_h(t_*)=e^{-(\mu_h+\gamma_h+\alpha_h)t_*}SI_h(0)+e^{-(\mu_h+\gamma_h+\alpha_h)t_*}\int_0^{t_*}e^{(\mu_h+\gamma_h+\alpha_h)t}\frac{C_{vh}(1-u_1)I_v}{N_h}SS_hdt>0$$

which contradicts $SI_h(t_*)=0$. Consequently, $SI_h(t)>0\ \ \forall t\in[0,T]$.

From

$$\begin{aligned}\frac{dI_v}{dt} &= \frac{C_{vh}}{N_h}(I_h(1-u_1)+SI_h(1-u_3))(N_v-I_v)-(\mu_v+u_2)I_v \\ &\geq -(\mu_v+u_2)I_v\end{aligned}$$

(because $I_h(t)\geq 0$, $SI_h(t)\geq 0$, $N_h(t)\geq 0$ and $N_v(t)-I_v(t)\geq 0$).

Then using Gronwall's inequality $I_v(t)\geq I_v(0)e^{\left(-\int_0^t(\mu_v+u_2)ds\right)}$
$\Longrightarrow I_v(t)>0$
From

$$\begin{aligned}\frac{dS_h}{dt} &= \Lambda_h-\frac{C_{vh}(1-u_1)I_v}{N_h}S_h-\mu S_h \\ &\geq -\left(\frac{C_{vh}(1-u_1)I_v(t)}{N_h(t)}+\mu\right)S_h(t)\end{aligned}$$

Then using Gronwall's inequality $S_h(t) \geq S_h(0)\exp\left(-\int_0^t \left(\frac{C_{vh}(1-u_1)I_v(s)}{N_h(s)}+\mu\right) ds\right)$

$\Longrightarrow S_h(t) > 0$

From

$$\frac{dSS_h}{dt} = -\frac{C_{vh}(1-u_1)I_v}{N_h}SS_h - \mu SS_h$$

$$= -\left(\frac{C_{vh}(1-u_1)I_v}{N_h} + \mu\right) SS_h(t)$$

$$\Longrightarrow SS_h(t) = SS_h(0)\exp\left(-\int_0^t \left(\frac{C_{vh}(1-u_1)I_v(s)}{N_h(s)} + \mu\right) ds\right) > 0.$$

On the other hand $\frac{dN_h(t)}{dt} = \Lambda_h - \mu N_h(t) - \alpha_h I_h(t) \leq \Lambda_h - \mu_h N_h(t)$

So $N_h(t) \leq \frac{\Lambda_h}{\mu_h} - \left(\frac{\Lambda_h}{\mu_h} - N_h(0)\right) e^{-\mu_h t} \Longrightarrow N_h(t) \leq \frac{\Lambda_h}{\mu_h}$

for initial value $N_h(0) \leq \frac{\Lambda_h}{\mu_h}$

and in the same way $\frac{dN_v(t)}{dt} = \Lambda_v - (\mu_v + u_2)N_v(t)$

So $N_v(t) = \frac{\Lambda_v}{\mu_v+u_2} - \left(\frac{\Lambda_v}{\mu_v+u_2} - N_v(0)\right) e^{-(\mu_v+u_2)t}$

$\Longrightarrow N_v(t) \leq \frac{\Lambda_v}{\mu_v+u_2} \leq \frac{\Lambda_v}{\mu_v}$ for initial value $N_v(0) \leq \frac{\Lambda_v}{\mu_v+u_2}$

## 2. *Proof of Theorem 6*

Let $X = \begin{pmatrix} S_h \\ I_h \\ N_h \\ I_v \\ N_v \\ SS_h \\ SI_h \\ SN_h \end{pmatrix}$ and $\partial(X) = X_t = \begin{pmatrix} \frac{dS_h(t)}{dt} \\ \frac{dI_h(t)}{dt} \\ \frac{dN_h(t)}{dt} \\ \frac{dI_v(t)}{dt} \\ \frac{dN_v(t)}{dt} \\ \frac{dSS_h(t)}{dt} \\ \frac{dSI_h(t)}{dt} \\ \frac{dSN_h(t)}{dt} \end{pmatrix}$

so the system (12.9) is rewriting in the following form: $\partial(X) = X_t = AX + F(X)$ where

$$A = \begin{pmatrix} -\mu_h & 0 & 0 & 0 & 0 & 0 & 0 & 0 \\ 0 & -(\mu_h+\gamma_h) & 0 & 0 & 0 & 0 & 0 & 0 \\ 0 & 0 & -\mu_h & 0 & 0 & 0 & -\alpha_h & 0 \\ 0 & 0 & 0 & -(\mu_v+\gamma_v) & 0 & 0 & 0 & 0 \\ 0 & 0 & 0 & 0 & -\mu_v & 0 & 0 & 0 \\ 0 & 0 & 0 & 0 & 0 & -\mu_h & 0 & 0 \\ 0 & 0 & 0 & 0 & 0 & 0 & -(\mu_h+\gamma_h) & 0 \\ 0 & 0 & 0 & 0 & 0 & 0 & -\alpha_h & -\mu_h \end{pmatrix}$$

$$\text{and } F(X) = \begin{pmatrix} \Lambda_h - \dfrac{C_{vh}(1-u_1)I_v}{N_h} S_h \\ \dfrac{C_{vh}(1-u_1)I_v}{N_h} S_h \\ \Lambda_h \\ \dfrac{C_{vh}}{N_h}(I_h(1-u_1) + SI_h(1-u_3))(N_v - I_v) \\ \Lambda_v(1-u_2) \\ -\dfrac{C_{vh}(1-u_3)I_v}{N_h} SS_h \\ \dfrac{C_{vh}(1-u_3)I_v}{N_h} SS_h \\ 0 \end{pmatrix}$$

$$F(X_1) - F(X_2) = \begin{pmatrix} \frac{C_{vh}}{N_{h1}N_{h2}} \left[(1-u_1)I_{v2}N_{h1}S_{h2} - (1-u_1')I_{v1}N_{h2}S_{h1}\right] \\ \frac{C_{vh}}{N_{h1}N_{h2}} \left[(1-u_1)I_{v1}N_{h2}S_{h1} - (1-u_1')I_{v2}N_{h1}S_{h2}\right] \\ 0 \\ \dfrac{C_{hv}}{N_{h1}N_{h2}} \psi_0 \\ \Lambda_v(u_2' - u_2) \\ \frac{C_{vh}}{N_{h1}N_{h2}} \left[(1-u_3)I_{v2}N_{h1}SS_h - (1-u_3')I_{v1}N_{h2}SS_{h1}\right] \\ \frac{C_{vh}}{N_{h1}N_{h2}} \left[(1-u_3)I_{v1}N_{h2}SS_{h1} - (1-u_3')I_{v2}N_{h1}SS_{h2}\right] \\ 0 \end{pmatrix}$$

with

$$\psi_0 = (I_{h1}N_{h2}(1-u_1) + SI_{h1}N_{h2}(1-u_3))(N_{v1} - I_{v1}) \\ - (I_{h2}N_{h1}(1-u_1') + SI_{h2}N_{h1}(1-u_3'))(N_{v2} - I_{v2})$$

then

$$\begin{aligned} \|F(X_1) - F(X_2)\| = {} & 2\frac{C_{vh}}{N_{h1}N_{h2}} \left|(1-u_1)I_{v2}N_{h1}S_{h2} - (1-u_1')I_{v1}N_{h2}S_{h1}\right| \\ & + \frac{C_{hv}}{N_{h1}N_{h2}} |\psi_0| + \left|\Lambda_v(u_2' - u_2)\right| \\ & + 2\frac{C_{vh}}{N_{h1}N_{h2}} \left|(1-u_3)I_{v1}N_{h2}SS_{h1} - (1-u_3')I_{v2}N_{h1}SS_{h2}\right| \end{aligned}$$

Let

$$
\begin{aligned}
\psi_1 &= 2\frac{C_{vh}}{N_{h1}N_{h2}}\left|(1-u_1)I_{v2}N_{h1}S_{h2} - (1-u_1')I_{v1}N_{h2}S_{h1}\right| \\
\psi_2 &= \frac{C_{hv}}{N_{h1}N_{h2}}|\psi_0| + \Lambda_v\left|u_2' - u_2\right| \\
&= \frac{C_{hv}}{N_{h1}N_{h2}}|(I_{h1}N_{h2}(1-u_1) + SI_{h1}N_{h2}(1-u_3))(N_{v1} - I_{v1}) \\
&\qquad -(I_{h2}N_{h1}(1-u_1') + SI_{h2}N_{h1}(1-u_3'))(N_{v2} - I_{v2})| + \left|\Lambda_v(u_2' - u_2)\right| \\
\psi_3 &= 2\frac{C_{vh}}{N_{h1}N_{h2}}\left|(1-u_3)I_{v1}N_{h2}SS_{h1} - (1-u_3')I_{v2}N_{h1}SS_{h2}\right|
\end{aligned}
$$

So

$$
\begin{aligned}
\psi_1 &= \frac{C_{vh}}{N_{h1}N_{h2}}\left|(1-u_1)I_{v2}N_{h1}S_{h2} - (1-u_1')I_{v1}N_{h2}S_{h1}\right| \\
&= \frac{C_{vh}}{N_{h1}N_{h2}}|I_{v2}N_{h1}S_{h2} - u_1I_{v2}N_{h2}S_{h2} - I_{v1}N_{h2}S_{h1} + u_1'I_{v1}N_{h2}S_{h1}| \\
&= \frac{C_{vh}}{N_{h1}N_{h2}}|I_{v2}N_{h1}S_{h2} - I_{v1}N_{h1}S_{h2} + I_{v1}N_{h1}S_{h2} - I_{v1}N_{h2}S_{h2} + I_{v1}N_{h2}S_{h2} - I_{v1}N_{h2}S_{h1} \\
&+u_1'I_{v1}N_{h2}S_{h1} - u_1I_{v1}N_{h2}S_{h1} + u_1I_{v1}N_{h2}S_{h1} - u_1I_{v2}N_{h2}S_{h1} + u_1I_{v2}N_{h2}S_{h1} - u_1I_{v2}N_{h2}S_{h2}| \\
&\le \frac{C_{vh}}{N_{h1}N_{h2}}|N_{h1}S_{h2}(I_{v2} - I_{v1}) + I_{v1}S_{h2}(N_{h1} - N_{h2}) + I_{v1}N_{h2}(S_{h2} - S_{h1})| \\
&\quad + \frac{C_{vh}}{N_{h1}N_{h2}}|I_{v1}N_{h2}S_{h1}(u_1' - u_1) + u_1N_{h2}S_{h1}(I_{v1} - I_{v2}) + u_1I_{v2}N_{h2}(S_{h1} - S_{h2})| \\
&\le C_{vh}\left(\frac{N_{h1}S_{h2}}{N_{h1}N_{h2}}|I_{v2} - I_{v1}| + \frac{I_{v1}S_{h2}}{N_{h1}N_{h2}}|N_{h1} - N_{h2}| + \frac{I_{v1}N_{h2}}{N_{h1}N_{h2}}|S_{h2} - S_{h1}|\right) \\
&\quad + C_{vh}\left(\frac{N_{h2}S_{h1}}{N_{h1}N_{h2}}I_{v1}|u_1' - u_1| + u_1\frac{N_{h2}S_{h1}}{N_{h1}N_{h2}}|I_{v1} - I_{v2}| + u_1\frac{I_{v2}N_{h2}}{N_{h1}N_{h2}}|S_{h1} - S_{h2}|\right) \\
&\le C_{vh}\left(|I_{v2} - I_{v1}| + \frac{I_{v1}}{N_{h1}}|N_{h1} - N_{h2}| + \frac{I_{v1}}{N_{h1}}|S_{h2} - S_{h1}|\right) \\
&\quad + C_{vh}\left(I_{v1}|u_1' - u_1| + u_1|I_{v1} - I_{v2}| + u_1\frac{I_{v2}}{N_{h1}}|S_{h1} - S_{h2}|\right)
\end{aligned}
$$

it is easy to see from $\dfrac{dN_h(t)}{dt} = \Lambda_h - \mu N_h(t) - \alpha_h I_h(t) \ge \Lambda_h - (\mu + \alpha_h)N_h(t)$ that $N_h(t) \ge \frac{\Lambda_h}{\mu_h+\alpha_h} - \left(\frac{\Lambda_h}{\mu_h+\alpha_h} - N_h(0)\right)e^{-(\mu_h+\alpha_h)t} \ge N_h(0)e^{-(\mu_h+\alpha_h)t}$
So $\frac{1}{N_h(t)} \le \frac{e^{(\mu_h+\alpha_h)t}}{N_h(0)} \le \frac{e^{(\mu_h+\alpha_h)T}}{N_h(0)} = \omega_T$
from $S_v + I_v = N_v \le \frac{\Lambda_v}{\mu_v}$ we have $I_{v1} \le \frac{\Lambda_v}{\mu_v}$ and $I_{v2} \le \frac{\Lambda_v}{\mu_v}$
Therefore

$$
\begin{aligned}
\psi_1 &\le 2C_{vh}\left(|I_{v2} - I_{v1}| + \frac{\omega_T\Lambda_v}{\mu_v}|N_{h1} - N_{h2}| + \frac{\omega_T\Lambda_v}{\mu_v}|S_{h2} - S_{h1}|\right) \\
&\quad + C_{vh}\left(\frac{\Lambda_v}{\mu_v}|u_1' - u_1| + u_1|I_{v1} - I_{v2}| + u_1\frac{\omega_T\Lambda_v}{\mu_v}|S_{h1} - S_{h2}|\right)
\end{aligned}
$$

$$\leq C_{vh}\left(2|I_{v2}-I_{v1}|+\frac{\omega_T\Lambda_v}{\mu_v}|N_{h1}-N_{h2}|+2\frac{\omega_T\Lambda_v}{\mu_v}|S_{h2}-S_{h1}|+\frac{\Lambda_v}{\mu_v}|u_1'-u_1|\right)$$
$$\leq M_1\left(|I_{v2}-I_{v1}|+|N_{h1}-N_{h2}|+|S_{h2}-S_{h1}|+|u_1'-u_1|\right)$$

where $M_1=\max\left(4C_{vh},4C_{vh}\frac{\omega_T\Lambda_v}{\mu_v},2C_{vh}\frac{\Lambda_v}{\mu_v}\right)$
Similarly

$$\psi_2 \leq M_2\left(|I_{h2}-I_{h1}|+|N_{v2}-N_{v1}|+|I_{v2}-I_{v1}|+|N_{h1}-N_{h2}|+|SI_{h2}-SI_{h1}|\right.$$
$$\left.+|u_1'-u_1|+|u_2'-u_2|+|u_3'-u_3|\right)$$

where $M_2=\max\left(4C_{hv},7C_{hv}\frac{\omega_T\Lambda_v}{\mu_v},4C_{hv}\frac{\omega_T\Lambda_h}{\mu_h},2C_{hv}\frac{\Lambda_v}{\mu_v},\Lambda_v\right)$

$$\psi_3\leq C_{vh}\left(2|I_{v2}-I_{v1}|+\frac{\omega_T\Lambda_v}{\mu_v}|N_{h1}-N_{h2}|+2\frac{\omega_T\Lambda_v}{\mu_v}|SS_{h2}-SS_{h1}|+\frac{\Lambda_v}{\mu_v}|u_3'-u_3|\right)$$
$$\leq M_3\left(|I_{v2}-I_{v1}|+|N_{h1}-N_{h2}|+|SS_{h2}-SS_{h1}|+|u_3'-u_3|\right)$$

where $M_3=M_1=\max\left(4C_{vh},4C_{vh}\frac{\omega_T\Lambda_v}{\mu_v},2C_{vh}\frac{\Lambda_v}{\mu_v}\right)$
$\Longrightarrow \|F((X_1,U))-F((X_2,U'))\|\leq M(\|X_2-X_1\|+\|U'-U\|)$
where $M=\max(M_1,M_2)$, let $L=\|A\|<+\infty$

Also, we have

$$\|\partial((X_1,U))-\partial((X_2,U'))\|\leq (M+L)(\|X_2-X_1\|+\|U'-U\|)$$

where $M+L<+\infty$.

It follows that the function $\partial$ is uniformly Lipschitz continuous. So from the definition of the control $u(t)$ and the restriction on $S_h(t)\geq 0$, $I_h(t)\geq 0$, $N_h(t)\geq 0$, $I_v(t)\geq 0$, $N_v(t)\geq 0$, $SS_h(t)\geq 0$, $SI_h(t)\geq 0$ and $SN_h(t)\geq 0$, we see that a solution of the system (12.9) exists [3].

## 3. *Proof of Theorem 8*

The Hamiltonian is defined as follows:

$$H=I_h+SI_h+N_v+\frac{A}{2}u_1^2(t)+\frac{B}{2}u_2^2(t)+\frac{C}{2}u_3^2(t)+\lambda_1 f_1(X^*)+\lambda_2 f_2(X^*)+\lambda_3 f_3(X^*)$$
$$+\lambda_4 f_4(X^*)+\lambda_5 f_5(X^*)+\lambda_6 f_6(X^*)+\lambda_7 f_7(X^*)+\lambda_8 f_8(X^*)$$

where
$X^*=(S_h,I_h,N_h,I_v,N_v,SS_h,SI_h,SN_h)$
$f_1(X^*)=\Lambda_h-\frac{C_{vh}(1-u_1)I_v}{N_h}S_h-\mu_h S_h$

$$
\begin{aligned}
f_2(X^*) &= \frac{C_{vh}(1-u_1)I_v}{N_h}S_h - (\mu_h + \gamma_h)I_h\\
f_3(X^*) &= \Lambda_h - \mu_h N_h - \alpha_h SI_h\\
f_4(X^*) &= \frac{C_{hv}}{N_h}(I_h(1-u_1) + SI_h(1-u_3))(N_v - I_v) - (\mu_v + u_2)I_v\\
f_5(X^*) &= \Lambda_v(1-u_2) - (\mu_v + u_2)N_v\\
f_6(X^*) &= -\frac{C_{vh}(1-u_3)I_v}{N_h}SS_h - \mu_h SS_h\\
f_7(X^*) &= \frac{C_{vh}(1-u_3)I_v}{N_h}SS_h - (\mu_h + \gamma_h + \alpha_h)SI_h\\
f_8(X^*) &= -\mu_h SN_h - \alpha_h SI_h
\end{aligned}
$$

The adjoint variables $\lambda_1, \lambda_2, \lambda_3, \lambda_4, \lambda_5, \lambda_6, \lambda_7$ and $\lambda_8$ are obtained by the following system:

$$
\lambda_1' = -\frac{\partial H}{\partial S_h} \quad \lambda_2' = -\frac{\partial H}{\partial I_h} \quad \lambda_3' = -\frac{\partial H}{\partial N_h}
$$

$$
\lambda_4' = -\frac{\partial H}{\partial I_v} \quad \lambda_5' = -\frac{\partial H}{\partial N_v} \quad \lambda_6' = -\frac{\partial H}{\partial SS_h}
$$

$$
\lambda_7' = -\frac{\partial H}{\partial SI_h} \quad \lambda_8' = -\frac{\partial H}{\partial SN_h}
$$

$$
\lambda_1(T) = \lambda_2(T) = \lambda_3(T) = \lambda_4(T) = \lambda_5(T) = \lambda_6(T) = \lambda_7(T) = \lambda_8(T) = 0
$$

$$
\begin{cases}
\lambda_1' &= -\frac{\partial H}{\partial S_h}\\
&= (\lambda_1 - \lambda_2)\dfrac{C_{vh}(1-u_1)I_v}{N_h} + \mu_h\lambda_1\\
\lambda_2' &= -\frac{\partial H}{\partial I_h}\\
&= -1 + (\mu_h + \gamma_h)\lambda_2 - \frac{C_{hv}}{N_h}(1-u_1)(N_v - I_v)\lambda_4\\
\lambda_3' &= -\frac{\partial H}{\partial N_h}\\
&= \dfrac{C_{vh}(1-u_1)I_v}{N_h^2}S_h(\lambda_2 - \lambda_1) + \mu_h\lambda_3 + \Big[\frac{C_{hv}}{N_h^2}(I_h(1-u_1)\\
&\quad +SI_h(1-u_3))(N_v - I_v)\Big]\lambda_4 + \dfrac{C_{vh}(1-u_3)I_v}{N_h^2}SS_h(\lambda_7 - \lambda_6)\\
\lambda_4' &= -\frac{\partial H}{\partial I_v}\\
&= \dfrac{C_{vh}(1-u_1)}{N_h}S_h(\lambda_1 - \lambda_2) + \frac{C_{hv}}{N_h}(I_h(1-u_1) + SI_h(1-u_3)) + (\mu_v + u_2)\lambda_4\\
&\quad + \dfrac{C_{vh}(1-u_3)}{N_h}SS_h(\lambda_6 - \lambda_7)\\
\lambda_5' &= -\frac{\partial H}{\partial N_v}\\
&= -1 - \frac{C_{hv}}{N_h}(I_h(1-u_1) + SI_h(1-u_3))\lambda_4 + (\mu_v + u_2)\lambda_5\\
\lambda_6' &= -\frac{\partial H}{\partial SS_h}\\
&= (\lambda_6 - \lambda_7)\dfrac{C_{vh}(1-u_3)I_v}{N_h} + \mu_h\lambda_6\\
\lambda_7' &= -\frac{\partial H}{\partial SI_h}\\
&= -1 - \frac{C_{hv}}{N_h}(1-u_3)(N_v - I_v)\lambda_4 + \alpha_h\lambda_3 + \lambda_7(\mu_h + \gamma_h + \alpha_h) + \lambda_8\alpha_h\\
\lambda_8' &= -\frac{\partial H}{\partial SN_h}\\
&= \lambda_8\mu_h\\
\lambda_1(T) &= \lambda_2(T) = \lambda_3(T) = \lambda_4(T) = \lambda_5(T) = \lambda_6(T) = \lambda_7(T) = \lambda_8(T) = 0
\end{cases}
$$

Therefore

$$
\begin{cases}
\lambda_1' &= (\lambda_1 - \lambda_2)\dfrac{C_{vh}(1-u_1)I_v}{N_h} + \mu_h\lambda_1 \\
\lambda_2' &= -1 + (\mu_h + \gamma_h)\lambda_2 - \frac{C_{hv}}{N_h}(1-u_1)(N_v - I_v)\lambda_4 \\
\lambda_3' &= \dfrac{C_{vh}(1-u_1)I_v}{N_h^2} S_h(\lambda_2 - \lambda_1) + \mu_h\lambda_3 + \frac{C_{hv}}{N_h^2}(I_h(1-u_1) \\
&\quad +SI_h(1-u_3))(N_v - I_v)\lambda_4 + \dfrac{C_{vh}(1-u_3)I_v}{N_h^2} SS_h(\lambda_7 - \lambda_6) \\
\lambda_4' &= \dfrac{C_{vh}(1-u_1)}{N_h} S_h(\lambda_1 - \lambda_2) + \left[\frac{C_{hv}}{N_h}(I_h(1-u_1) + SI_h(1-u_3)) + (\mu_v + u_2)\right]\lambda_4 \\
&\quad +\dfrac{C_{vh}(1-u_3)}{N_h} SS_h(\lambda_6 - \lambda_7) \\
\lambda_5' &= -1 - \frac{C_{hv}}{N_h}(I_h(1-u_1) + SI_h(1-u_3))\lambda_4 + (\mu_v + u_2)\lambda_5 \\
\lambda_6' &= (\lambda_6 - \lambda_7)\dfrac{C_{vh}(1-u_3)I_v}{N_h} + \mu_h\lambda_6 \\
\lambda_7' &= -1 - \frac{C_{hv}}{N_h}(1-u_3)(N_v - I_v)\lambda_4 + \alpha_h\lambda_3 + \lambda_7(\mu_h + \gamma_h + \alpha_h) + \lambda_8\alpha_h \\
\lambda_8' &= \lambda_8\mu_h \\
\lambda_1(T) &= \lambda_2(T) = \lambda_3(T) = \lambda_4(T) = \lambda_5(T) = \lambda_6(T) = \lambda_7(T) = \lambda_8(T) = 0
\end{cases}
$$

The optimal control can be determined from the optimality condition:

$$\frac{\partial H}{\partial u_1} = 0 \Longrightarrow Au_1 + (\lambda_1 - \lambda_2)\frac{C_{vh}I_v}{N_h}S_h - \lambda_4\frac{C_{hv}I_h}{N_h}(N_v - I_v) = 0$$

$$\Longrightarrow u_1^* = \frac{1}{A}\left[(\lambda_2 - \lambda_1)\frac{C_{vh}I_v}{N_h}S_h + \lambda_4\frac{C_{hv}I_h}{N_h}(N_v - I_v)\right]$$

$$\frac{\partial H}{\partial u_2} = 0 \Longrightarrow Bu_2 - \lambda_4 I_v - \lambda_5(\Lambda_v - \mu_v) = 0$$

$$\Longrightarrow u_2^* = \frac{1}{B}\left[\lambda_4 I_v + \lambda_5(\Lambda_v + N_v)\right]$$

$$\frac{\partial H}{\partial u_3} = 0 \Longrightarrow Cu_3 + (\lambda_1 - \lambda_2)\frac{C_{vh}I_v}{N_h}S_h - \lambda_4\frac{C_{hv}I_h}{N_h}(N_v - I_v) = 0$$

$$\Longrightarrow u_3^* = \frac{1}{C}\left[(\lambda_7 - \lambda_6)\frac{C_{vh}I_v}{N_h}SS_h + \lambda_4\frac{C_{hv}SI_h}{N_h}(N_v - I_v)\right].$$

## References

1. Adams B, Holmes E, Zhang C, Mammen M, Nimmannitya S, Kalayanarooj S, Boots M (2006) Cross-protective immunity can account for the alternating epidemic pattern of dengue virus serotypes circulating in bangkok. Proc Natl Acad Sci 103(38):14234–14239
2. Bailey NT et al (1975) The mathematical theory of infectious diseases and its applications, 2nd edn. Charles Griffin & Company Ltd, 5a Crendon Street, High Wycombe, Bucks HP13 6
3. Birkhoff G, Rota G (eds) (1989) Ordinary differential equations. Wiley, New York
4. Centers for disease control and prevention (2019) Dengue. https://www.cdc.gov/dengue/index.html. Accessed 13 April 2019
5. Chen SC, Hsieh MH (2012) Modeling the transmission dynamics of dengue fever: implications of temperature effects. Sci Total Environ 431:385–391
6. Cummings DA, Schwartz IB, Billings L, Shaw LB, Burke DS (2005) Dynamic effects of antibody-dependent enhancement on the fitness of viruses. Proc Natl Acad Sci 102(42):15259–15264
7. Derouich M, Boutayeb A (2006) Dengue fever: mathematical modelling and computer simulation. Appl Math Comput 177(2):528–544
8. Van den Driessche P, Watmough J (2002) Reproduction numbers and sub-threshold endemic equilibria for compartmental models of disease transmission. Math Biosci 180(1–2):29–48

9. Esteva L, Vargas C (1998) Analysis of a dengue disease transmission model. Math Biosci 150(2):131–151
10. Esteva L, Vargas C (2000) Influence of vertical and mechanical transmission on the dynamics of dengue disease. Math Biosci 167(1):51–64
11. Esteva L, Vargas C (2003) Coexistence of different serotypes of dengue virus. J Math Biol 46(1):31–47
12. Fleming W, Rishel R (1975) Deterministic and stochastic optimal control. Springer, Berlin
13. Gumel A, Shivakumar P, Sahai B (2001) A mathematical model for the dynamics of hiv-1 during the typical course of infection. Nonlinear Anal Theory Methods Appl 47(3):1773–1783
14. Hartley L, Donnelly C, Garnett G (2002) The seasonal pattern of dengue in endemic areas: mathematical models of mechanisms. Trans R Soc Trop Med Hyg 96(4):387–397
15. Medlock J, Luz PM, Struchiner CJ, Galvani AP (2009) The impact of transgenic mosquitoes on dengue virulence to humans and mosquitoes. Am Nat 174(4):565–577
16. Nagao Y, Koelle K (2008) Decreases in dengue transmission may act to increase the incidence of dengue hemorrhagic fever. Proc Natl Acad Sci 105(6):2238–2243
17. Pontryagin LS, Mishchenko E, Boltyanskii V, Gamkrelidze R (1962) The mathematical theory of optimal processes. Wiley, New York
18. Wearing HJ, Rohani P (2006) Ecological and immunological determinants of dengue epidemics. Proc Natl Acad Sci 103(31):11802–11807
19. World Health Organization (2019) Dengue and severe dengue. https://www.who.int/newsroom/fact-sheets/detail/dengue-and-severe-dengue. Accessed 13 April 2019
20. Yang H, Macoris M, Galvani K, Andrighetti M, Wanderley D (2009a) Assessing the effects of temperature on dengue transmission. Epidemiol Infect 137(8):1179–1187
21. Yang H, Macoris MdLdG, Galvani K, Andrighetti M, Wanderley D (2009b) Assessing the effects of temperature on the population of aedes aegypti, the vector of dengue. Epidemiol Infect 137(8):1188–1202
22. Yang HM, da Graça Macoris MdL, Galvani KC, Andrighetti MTM (2011) Follow up estimation of aedes aegypti entomological parameters and mathematical modellings. Biosystems 103(3):360–371

# Chapter 13
# Numerical Treatment of Multidimensional Stochastic, Competitive and Evolutionary Models

**Mostafa Zahri**

**Abstract** In this chapter, we present a computational study of multi-dimensional stochastic systems of differential equations. Especially competitive and evolutionary models. In these types of models, a certain number of uncertainties are causing side effects as random excitations and interactions. To numerically solve the considered systems, we propose the Itô-Taylor family schemes for multi-dimensional stochastic differential equations. Either for systems driven by one white noise or for systems having more than one source of excitations. A first-order accuracy is ensured in the approximation of double Itô integrals by using a truncation in the Fourier series expansion. To verify the accuracy of the proposed method, we consider a system of two stochastic differential equations with known analytical solution. Numerical results are presented for a reduced prototype system of the prebiotic evolutionary model.

## 13.1 Introduction

After the discovery of the catalytic process of some RNA-like molecules (ribozymes) [7], the formation of prebiotic material has been subject of many theoretical an experimental studies, see [4] among others. These RNA-like molecules (also referred to as replicators) with unspecific catalytic capabilities could have formed ensemble of species, the so-called catalytic networks. It should be pointed out that, although the evolution of these catalytic networks has been extensively studied from a theoretical point of view over the last decades, most of the work has been focused on the analysis of their dynamics under deterministic input conditions [11]. Less attention has been given to the role of stochastic excitations on the behavior of these prebiotic models. However, it is well known that stochastic forces may play an important role on the dy-

M. Zahri (✉)
College of Sciences, University of Sharjah, Sharjah, UAE
e-mail: mzahri@sharjah.ac.ae



A. Boutayeb (ed.), *Disease Prevention and Health Promotion in Developing Countries*,
https://doi.org/10.1007/978-3-030-34702-4_13

namics of the biochemical systems. For instance, the stochastic forces may probably occur in the reaction medium known by the prebiotic soup, see [8, 9] for more details. Therefore, it ought to be taken into account in the mathematical equations governing these models. In this chapter, we consider the problem of prebiotic evolution in one of the theoretical models proposed to study the behavior of catalytic networks [15]. This model is a closed system (only energy can be interchanged with the surroundings) where activated material (nucleotides) react to build up self-replicative units following preestablished rules. These energy rich monomers are regenerated from the by-product of the reaction (obtained mainly as the result of the hydrolysis of self-replicative species) by means of a recycle mechanism (basically due to an external energy source, for example sunlight). The closure of the system directly imposes a selection pressure on the population. All these biochemical features can be mathematically modeled by a multi-dimensional system of deterministic ordinary differential equations with nonlinear kinetic reactions, see for example [9, 15]. The spatial effects can also be incorporated into this model by introducing the diffusion operator in the ordinary differential equations resulting in a set of reaction-diffusion equations, compare [4]. To stabilize these partial differential equations, authors in [36, 44, 46] have added an additive noise into the system. In the present work, we propose a new technique to account for excitations from the prebiotic medium. The key idea is to introduce a stochastic diffusion matrix in the system of ordinary differential equations and transform this model to a system of stochastic differential equations. Here, we consider a drift term driven by both additive and multiplicative noises and it can be raised from uncertainties in catalytic coefficients or simply by excitations from the prebiotic medium. The main advantage of such approach comes from the fact that features of interest in random dynamics (i.e. random fixed points, random bifurcation, random attractors, etc.) are harder to describe in the framework of stochastic calculus than in the framework of classical deterministic calculus.

To numerically approximate the solutions of the proposed systems, we apply a generalized Milstein method [20–22, 26]. The basic ingredients of this approach are the piecewise linear approximation by the Itô-Taylor expansion of the vector fields and the numerical integration of the resulting linear equation. Fourier series expansions are used to approximate double Itô integrals. In the case of stochastic differential equations, the Milstein method has been restricted either to the class of equations with additive noise terms or scalar equations with multiplicative noise. Therefore, the application of the Milstein method to cover wider classes of stochastic differential equations is an appealing challenge. In particular, the current study focuses in the class of stochastic differential equations driven by multiplicative noise. Numerical results are presented for a prototype system of four catalyzed self-replicator species along with activated and inactivated residues. Phase-space portraits and strange attractors are also displayed. In the same context, Stochastic partial differential equations (SPDEs) are essentially partial differential equations with additive or multiplicative noise and random forcing parameters. Generally, solving SPDEs either analytically or numerically is not an easy task. However, in the last few years there was a growing interest to model interesting applications in hydrodynamics, quantum field theory, engineering and statistical mechanics by using time-space evolutionary models with non deterministic excitations [2, 5, 12]. Recently, the numerical approximation of sample solutions of such stochastic models has attracted more attention in several studies [18, 27, 28, 46, 47]. The presence of different sources of uncertainties in the form of dependent and independent stochastic processes brings more complexity to this topic. For instance, the fluid transport phenomena occurs through several physical and chemical combinations of reactions, diffusions and advections. It demonstrates a significant part of oceanography and involves an interesting interpretation of the geochemical distributions in the water [3, 6]. All these factors contain some levels of random excitations, their numerical treatment leads to the space time integration of SPDEs [13, 31]. The treatment, separation or distillation of these homogeneous or nonhomogeneous substance concentration could be a challenge for an engineering work.

In the works [29, 35, 36], we were focused more on implementing deterministic techniques for stochastic time-space integration of different SPDEs with different physical or biological meanings. For instance, we studied the stochastic method of lines for solving boundary value problems [46, 47]. In [24], we analyzed and implemented the Wick-product techniques for solving reaction-diffusion problems. However, the common point that we have remarked was, on the one hand the expensive computational cost and on the other hand the non trivial construction of effective high order methods. Where approximation of multiple stochastic integrals in the Itô sense are required. In the present work, we combine three methods, namely the method of lines (MOL) [37, 41, 42], the domain-decomposition method (DDM) for non-overlapping subdomains [23, 25, 33, 34] and the Itô-Taylor schemes for stochastic differential equation [20–22]. Moreover, we have to mention that the major difficulties in using the domain-decomposition methods is the determination of the interface solution and connecting it with the interior solution into an accurate approximation. It is side effect of dividing the problem into subproblems, so one can approximate the parts of the solution with significant independence of the other parts either by using overlapping or non-overlapping subdomains. To complete the suggested method, we introduce the barycenter interpolation method (BIM) for approximating the missing concentration values on the interfaces connecting the subdomains. The treatment of the non local behaviors of physical and biological systems are reasonable motivations for the use of DDM, which are characterized by the referred parallelization advantages or the discretization of domains with complex geometries [14, 38–40].

Although in the last years several theoretical techniques for the numerical and computational treatment for SPDEs has been developed [1, 30]. However, implementing high order accurate methods is still an interesting and relevant task. It is important to note that there exists no explicit Itô-Taylor formula for SPDEs [18]. Therefore, the use of deterministic classical methods for solving SPDEs is generally non-trivial, for more details see [45].

## 13.2 Stochastic Model for Prebiotic Evolution

The model we consider in this paper consists on the replication of $N$ reacting species $I_1, I_2, \ldots, I_N$ using activated monomers $A$ and inactivated residues $B$ according to the following reactions:

$$I_i + A \xrightarrow{\quad \alpha_i \quad} 2I_i, \qquad \text{(R1)}$$

$$I_i + I_j + A \xrightarrow{\quad k_{ji} \quad} 2I_i + I_j, \qquad \text{(R2)}$$

$$I_i \xrightarrow{\quad \delta_i \quad} B, \qquad \text{(R3)}$$

$$B \xrightarrow{\quad \gamma \quad} A. \qquad \text{(R4)}$$

These reaction steps have been used in pattern formation in a model proposed to study the behavior of catalytic networks in the RNA-like molecules, compare [4, 11, 32] among others. This notation is intended to be similar to that used in traditional chemistry for which the steps (R1)–(R2) mean:

(R1) Each specie $I_i$ $(i = 1, \ldots, N)$, in the presence of the substrate $A$, selfreplicates noncatalytically with a rate $\alpha_i$.
(R2) Specie $I_j$ $(j \neq i)$ catalyzes the selfreplication of the species $I_i$ with a rate $k_{ji}$ in the presence of the substrate $A$.
(R3) Specie $I_i$ degrades in $B$ with a rate $\delta_i$.
(R4) The product of the degradation $B$ is recyclated in energy-high substrate $A$ with a rate $\gamma$.

For more details on biochemical aspects of the considered model we refer the reader to [4, 11, 32] and further references are cited therein. The above set of reactions can be mathematically formulated based on deterministic ordinary differential equations (ODE). Thus, if we use the notation $x_i$, $y$ and $z$ to denote respectively, the concentrations of the selfreplicator species $I_i$, the activated monomers $A$ and the inactivated residues $B$ then the reactions (R1)–(R4) are modelled by the following deterministic system of ODE

$$\begin{aligned}
\frac{dx_j}{dt} &= x_j \left( y \left( \alpha_j + \sum_{i=1}^{N} k_{ij} x_i \right) - \delta_j \right), \qquad j = 1, \ldots, N, \\
\frac{dy}{dt} &= \gamma z - \left( y \left( \sum_{i=1}^{N} \alpha_i x_i + \sum_{i=1}^{N} \sum_{j=1}^{N} k_{ij} x_i x_j \right) \right), \\
\frac{dz}{dt} &= \sum_{i=1}^{N} \delta_i x_i - \gamma z,
\end{aligned} \qquad (13.1)$$

where the concentrations $x_j(t)$, $y(t)$ and $z(t)$ are functions of time variable in a time interval $[t_0, T]$ with $t_0$ and $T$ are the initial and final times, respectively. It is easy to remark that the system (13.1) verifies

$$\sum_{j=1}^{N} x_j + y + z = c,$$

with $c$ being the total concentration of the prebiotic model. The deterministic system (13.1) has been analyzed in [32] and numerical simulations are included therein. In this reference, no effects from the prebiotic medium have been accounted for in the governing equations. However, medium effects can strongly interact with kinetic reactions and neglecting medium effects may have significant consequences in the overall predictions. In order to incorporate the medium effects in the system (13.1), the authors in [4] have introduce the spatial dependence of the concentrations $x_i$, $y$ and $z$. Thus, the ODE system (13.1) is transformed to a deterministic system of partial differential equations (PDE) of reaction-diffusion type. A stochastic counterpart of this PDE system was also investigated in [36, 44].

In the present study, to account for medium effects in the prebiotic evolution model we propose random perturbations in the kinetic reactions (13.1). Hence, the system (13.1) is transformed to a set of stochastic differential equations (SDE) of the following form

$$\begin{aligned}
dx_j &= \left(x_j\left(y\left(\alpha_j + \sum_{i=1}^{N} k_{ij}x_i\right) - \delta_j\right)\right) dt + \sigma_j dW_j, \qquad j = 1, \ldots, N,\\
dy &= \left(\gamma z - \left(y\left(\sum_{i=1}^{N} \alpha_i x_i + \sum_{i=1}^{N}\sum_{j=1}^{N} k_{ij}x_i x_j\right)\right)\right) dt + \sigma dW, \qquad (13.2)\\
dz &= \left(\sum_{i=1}^{N} \delta_i x_i - \gamma z\right) dt + \sigma dW,
\end{aligned}$$

where $\sigma_j = \sigma_j(x_1, \ldots, x_N, y, z)$ and $\sigma = \sigma(x_1, \ldots, x_N, y, z)$ are perturbation coefficients, $W_i$ and $W$ are Wiener processes. Note that $\sigma_j$ and $\sigma$ may be interpreted as a dimensional parameter that scales the diffusion process. In the framework of stochastic differential equations, the Eqs. (13.2) should be interpreted as

$$d\mathbf{X}(t) = \mathcal{F}(t, \mathbf{X}(t))dt + \mathcal{G}(t, \mathbf{X}(t))d\mathbf{W}(t), \qquad \mathbf{X}(t_0) = \mathbf{X}_0, \qquad (13.3)$$

where $\mathbf{X} = (x_1, \ldots, x_N, y, z)^T$ is the $(N+2)$-vector of the unknown concentrations, $\mathcal{F}(t, \mathbf{X}(t))$ is the $(N+2)$-vector of the kinetic reactions known as drift vector, $\mathcal{G}(t, \mathbf{X}(t))$ is the $(N+2) \times d$-matrix known by diffusion matrix, $\mathbf{W}(t)$ is a $d$-vector

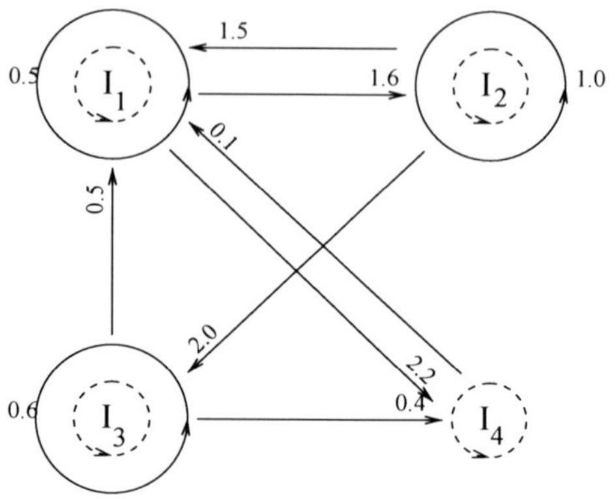


**Fig. 13.1** The reduced prototype system used for numerical simulations

Wiener process, and $\mathbf{X}_0$ is a $(N+2)$-vector of the initial conditions given at time $t_0$. Here, each entry of the $d$-vector $\mathbf{W}(t)$ forms a Brownian motion which is independent of the other elements.

Note that the model (13.2) is formed by $(N+2)$ coupled SDE with nonlinear reaction terms and stochastic excitations caused by the prebiotic medium. In our numerical results, we have used a reduced prototype system of four catalyzed selfreplicator species along with activated and inactivated residues depicted in Fig. 13.1. The numbers shown in the arrows of this figure refer to the catalytic rates $k_{ji}$, $1 \le i, j \le 4$ appeared in (13.2).

## 13.3 Itô Taylor Scheme for Multi-dimensional Stochastic Systems

One of the main concerns of the Stochastic Calculus is the new concept of differentiability. For instance, we know that the path of a Brownian motion is continuous but nowhere differentiable and in order to define a stochastic differential equation and integrals, we have to introduce the notion of stochastic differentiability. The central result is the Itô-Formula, which leads to a new definition of differential equation and a new concept of Taylor expansion.

### *13.3.1 Higher Order Itô-Formula for Stochastic Differentiation*

A process satisfying a stochastic differential equation (SDE) in the sense of Itô, see [16, 17], will be called an Itô process.

**Definition 13.1** Let $(W_t)_{t\in\mathbb{T}}$ be an $m$-dimensional Brownian motion defined on a $(\Omega, \mathfrak{A})^m$ with right continuous augmented filtration $\mathfrak{F} = (\mathfrak{F}_t)_{t\in\mathbb{T}}$. The process $(X_t^1 \ldots, X_t^d)$ is called Itô Processes, if and only if it has the following form

$$X_t^i = X_{t_0}^i + \int_{t_0}^t a_s^i ds + \sum_{j=1}^m \int_{t_0}^t b_s^{i,j} dW_s^j; \qquad i = 1, \ldots, d; \quad j = 1, \ldots, m \tag{13.4}$$

where for all $i$, $j$; $(a_t^i)_{t\in\mathbb{T}}$, $(b_t^{i,j})_{t\in\mathbb{T}}$ are $\mathfrak{F}_t$ adapted, $\int_{t_0}^T a_s^i ds < \infty$ and $\int_{t_0}^T (b_s^{i,j})^2 ds < \infty$ a.s. □

**Lemma 13.1** *Consider a one dimensional Brownian motion and a non-necessary uniform time discretization* $t_k = k\frac{T-t_0}{2^n}$ *of the interval* $[t_0, T]$*. Then we have,*

$$(1).\ \lim_{n\to\infty}\sum_{k=0}^{2^n-1}(\Delta t_k)^2 = \lim_{n\to\infty}\sum_{k=0}^{2^n-1}\Delta t_k \Delta W_{t_k} = \lim_{n\to\infty}\sum_{k=0}^{2^n-1}\Delta W_{t_k}\Delta t_k = 0.$$

$$(2).\ \lim_{n\to\infty}\sum_{k=0}^{2^n-1}(\Delta W_{t_k})^2 = \int_{t_0}^T ds = (T - t_0). \qquad (\textit{Convergence in } L^2)$$

*where* $\Delta t_k = t_{k+1} - t_k$ *and* $\Delta W_{t_k} = W_{t_{k+1}} - W_{t_k}$. □

*Proof* The proof for (1). follows from the construction bellow:

$$\lim_{n\to\infty}\sum_{k=0}^{2^n-1}(\Delta t_k)^2 \le \lim_{n\to\infty}\max_k(\Delta t_k)\sum_{k=0}^{2^n-1}\Delta t_k = \lim_{n\to\infty}\max_k(\Delta t_k)\int_{t_0}^T dt = 0$$

For the term (2). with the Brownian motion, we have

$$0 = \lim_{n\to\infty}\min_k(\Delta t_k)\int_{t_0}^T dW_s \le \lim_{n\to\infty}\sum_{k=0}^{2^n-1}\Delta t_k \Delta W_{t_k} \le \lim_{n\to\infty}\max_k(\Delta t_k)\int_{t_0}^T dW_s = 0 = 0.$$

Since $\Delta W_{t_k}$ are i.i.d and normally distributed with mean zero and variance $\Delta t_k$ and by using the strong law of large numbers the following convergence in $L^2$ is true:

$$\lim_{n\to\infty}\sum_{k=0}^{2^n-1}(\Delta W_{t_k})^2 = \left(\lim_{n\to\infty}\sum_{k=0}^{2^n-1}\Delta t_k\right) = \int_{t_0}^T ds = (T - t_0).$$

**Lemma 13.2** *Let us consider the functional* $f : [t_0, T] \times I\!R^d \to I\!R$ *with continuous partial derivatives* $\frac{\partial f}{\partial t}, \frac{\partial f}{\partial x^i}$ *and* $\frac{\partial^2 f}{\partial x^i \partial x^j}$ *for* $i = 1, \ldots, d$ *and a one dimensional Itô Process* $(X_t)_{t\in\mathbb{T}}$*. For any time discretization* $t_k = k\frac{T - t_0}{2^n}$ *of the interval* $[t_0, T]$*. then we have,*

$$(1).\ \lim_{n\to\infty}\sum_{k=0}^{2^n-1}\frac{\partial f}{\partial t}\Delta t_k = \int_{t_0}^{t}\frac{\partial f}{\partial t}ds$$

$$(2).\ \lim_{n\to\infty}\sum_{k=0}^{2^n-1}\frac{\partial f}{\partial x}\Delta X_{t_k} = \int_{t_0}^{t}\frac{\partial f}{\partial x}dX_s = \int_{t_0}^{t}\frac{\partial f}{\partial x}a_s ds + \int_{t_0}^{t}\frac{\partial f}{\partial x}b_s dW_s.$$

$$(3).\ \lim_{n\to\infty}\sum_{k=0}^{2^n-1}\frac{\partial^2 f}{\partial t^2}(\Delta t_k)^2 = 0\cdot\int_{t_0}^{t}\frac{\partial^2 f}{\partial t^2}ds = 0.$$

$$(4).\ \lim_{n\to\infty}\sum_{k=0}^{2^n-1}\frac{\partial^2 f}{\partial x^2}(\Delta X_{t_k})^2 = \int_{t_0}^{t}\frac{\partial^2 f}{\partial x^2}b_s^2 ds.$$

*where* $\Delta t_k = t_{k+1} - t_k$ *and* $\Delta X_{t_k} = X_{t_{k+1}} - X_{t_k}$. □

*Proof* The result (1). is trivial. The proof for (2).

$$\lim_{n\to\infty}\sum_{k=0}^{2^n-1}\frac{\partial f}{\partial x}\Delta X_{t_k} = \int_{t_0}^{t}\frac{\partial f}{\partial x}dX_s = \int_{t_0}^{t}\frac{\partial f}{\partial x}(a_s ds + b_s dW_s) = \int_{t_0}^{t}\frac{\partial f}{\partial x}a_s ds + \int_{t_0}^{t}\frac{\partial f}{\partial x}b_s dW_s.$$

The proof for (3). consider a uniform time discretization $\Delta t$ of the interval $[t_0, T]$, then we have

$$\lim_{n\to\infty}\sum_{k=0}^{2^n-1}\frac{\partial^2 f}{\partial t^2}(\Delta t_k)^2 = \lim_{n\to\infty}\underbrace{(\Delta t)}_{\to 0}\cdot\underbrace{\int_{t_0}^{t}\frac{\partial^2 f}{\partial t^2}ds}_{bounded} = 0$$

The proof for (4).

$$\begin{aligned}\lim_{n\longrightarrow\infty}\sum_{k=0}^{2^n-1}\frac{\partial^2 f}{\partial x^2}(\Delta X_{t_k})^2 &= \lim_{n\longrightarrow\infty}\sum_{k=0}^{2^n-1}\frac{\partial^2 f}{\partial x^2}b_{t_k}^2\Delta W_{t_k}^2\\ &+ \underbrace{\lim_{n\longrightarrow\infty}\sum_{k=0}^{2^n-1}\frac{\partial^2 f}{\partial x^2}a_{t_k}^2\Delta t_k{}^2}_{\longrightarrow 0\ (lemma\ 3.1)}\\ &+ \lim_{n\longrightarrow\infty}2\underbrace{\sum_{k=0}^{2^n-1}\frac{\partial^2 f}{\partial x^2}a_{t_k}b_{t_k}^2\Delta t_k\Delta W_{t_k}}_{\longrightarrow 0}\quad\left(\text{applying Itôisometry in}\quad L^2\right)\\ &= \int_{t_0}^{t}\frac{\partial^2 f}{\partial x^2}b_s^2 ds.\qquad\left(\text{in}\quad L^2\right)\end{aligned}$$

**Lemma 13.3** *Under the assumption of the lemmas above, the one dimensional case $d = m = 1$ of the Itô-Formula is given as*

$$f(t, X_t) = f(t_0, X_{t_0}) + \int_{t_0}^{t} \left\{ \frac{\partial f}{\partial s}(s, X_s) + a_s \frac{\partial f}{\partial x}(s, X_s) + \frac{1}{2} b_s^2 \frac{\partial^2 f}{\partial x^2}(s, X_s) \right\} ds \tag{13.5}$$
$$+ \int_{t_0}^{t} b_s \frac{\partial f}{\partial x}(s, X_s) dW_s.$$

*Proof* For a given discretization of the time interval $[t_0, T]$ by $t_k = k\frac{(T-t_0)}{2^n}$, define $\Delta t_k = t_{k+1} - t_k$; $\Delta X_{t_k} = X_{t_{k+1}} - X_{t_k}$ and $\Delta W_{t_k} = W_{t_{k+1}} - W_{t_k}$. By using the Taylor expansion of order two, we get

$$f(t, X_t) = f(t_0, X_{t_0}) + \sum_{k=0}^{2^n-1} \Delta f(t_k, X_{t_k})$$
$$= f(t_0, X_{t_0}) + \sum_{k=0}^{2^n-1} \frac{\partial f}{\partial t} \Delta t_k + \sum_{k=0}^{2^n-1} \frac{\partial f}{\partial x} \Delta X_{t_k} + \frac{1}{2} \sum_{k=0}^{2^n-1} \frac{\partial^2 f}{\partial x^2} (\Delta X_{t_k})^2 \tag{13.6}$$
$$+ \sum_{k=0}^{2^n-1} \frac{\partial^2 f}{\partial t \partial x} \Delta t_k \Delta X_{t_k} + \frac{1}{2} \sum_{k=0}^{2^n-1} \frac{\partial^2 f}{\partial t^2} (\Delta t_k)^2 + \sum_{k=0}^{2^n-1} R_k. \tag{13.7}$$

where $R_k$ consists of sums of higher order partial derivatives of $f$ as a factor of $(\Delta t)^2$, $\Delta W_{t_k}(\Delta t)^2$, $(\Delta W_{t_k})^2 \Delta t$ and $\Delta W_{t_k} \Delta t$. Using the results of Lemma 13.1, we conclude that $R_k = O\Big((\Delta t)^2\Big)$ and therefore the remainder term vanish in $L^2$. Also using the results of Lemma 13.1, all terms with $(\Delta t)^2$ vanish (at least in $L^2$ if the increment of the Brownian motion appears.) Similar construction could be done for the mixed partial derivatives, which are in general factors either of $(\Delta t)^2$ or $\Delta W_{t_k} \Delta t$. Thus, all terms in (13.7) vanish in $L^2$:

$$\lim_{n \longrightarrow \infty} \left( \sum_{k=0}^{2^n-1} \frac{\partial^2 f}{\partial t \partial x} \Delta t_k \Delta X_{t_k} + \frac{1}{2} \sum_{k=0}^{2^n-1} \frac{\partial^2 f}{\partial t^2} (\Delta t_k)^2 + \sum_{k=0}^{2^n-1} R_k \right) = 0.$$

The passage to the limit in (13.6), leads to

$$f(t, X_t) = f(t_0, X_{t_0}) + \lim_{n \longrightarrow \infty} \left( \sum_{k=0}^{2^n-1} \frac{\partial f}{\partial t} \Delta t_k + \sum_{k=0}^{2^n-1} \frac{\partial f}{\partial x} \Delta X_{t_k} + \frac{1}{2} \sum_{k=0}^{2^n-1} \frac{\partial^2 f}{\partial x^2} (\Delta X_{t_k})^2 \right).$$

Since $dX_t = a_t dt + b_t dW_t$ and using the results of Lemma 13.2, the one dimensional Itô formula is proved.

*Example* For $f(t, x) = \frac{1}{2}x^2$ with $X_t = W_t$ and $a_t = 0, b_t = 1$. By applying Itôs formula, we have:

$$\begin{aligned} df &= \frac{\partial f}{\partial t}dt + a_t\frac{\partial f}{\partial x}dt + b_t\frac{\partial f}{\partial x}dW + \frac{1}{2}b_t^2\frac{\partial^2 f}{\partial x^2}dt \\ &= \frac{\partial f}{\partial t}dt + (1)\frac{\partial f}{\partial x}dW + \frac{1}{2}(1)^2\frac{\partial^2 f}{\partial x^2}dt \\ &= \frac{\partial f}{\partial t}dt + \frac{\partial f}{\partial x}dW + \frac{1}{2}\frac{\partial^2 f}{\partial x^2}dt \\ &= \frac{\partial f}{\partial x}dW + \frac{1}{2}\frac{\partial^2 f}{\partial x^2}dt \end{aligned}$$

Hence,

$$\frac{1}{2}dW_t^2 = W_t dW_t + \frac{1}{2}dt$$

and

$$\frac{1}{2}\int dW_s^2 = \int W_s dW_s + \frac{1}{2}\int dt$$

Thus,

$$I_t = \int_0^t W_s dW_s = \frac{1}{2}(W_t^2 - t), \tag{13.8}$$

Note that $W_t^2$, represents the square of the end value of the Brownian motion. Thus, $I_t$ will be considered as a time process if we change the upper bound of the integration interval. □

*Example* For $n > 1$; $f(t, x) = x^{n+1}$. By applying Itôs formula for $X_t = W_t$, we have:

$$d(W_t^{n+1}) = (n+1)W_t^n dW_t + \frac{n(n+1)}{2}W_t^{n-1}dt$$

Hence,

$$\int_0^t dW_s^n = \frac{1}{n+1}W_t^{n+1} - \frac{n}{2}\int_0^t W_s^{n-1}ds$$

It is important to note that the integral of a Brownian motion path with respect to time, represented for by $I(W_t) = \int_0^t W_s ds$ is not a stochastic integral. It represents the Area under Brownian motion path, $I(W_t)$ is a normal random variable with mean 0 and variance $\frac{t^3}{3}$: i.e $I(W_t) \sim N(0, \frac{t^3}{3})$. (The proof is similar to the constructions done in Lemma 13.1.) □

**Theorem 13.1** *Let us consider the functional* $f : [t_0, T] \times I\!R^d \to I\!R$ *with continuous partial derivatives* $\frac{\partial f}{\partial t}$, $\frac{\partial f}{\partial x^i}$ *and* $\frac{\partial^2 f}{\partial x^i \partial x^j}$ *for* $i = 1, \ldots, d$. *Moreover, consider a d-dimensional Itô-Process* $(X_t)_{t\in\mathbb{T}}$, *then we have,*

$$f(t, X_t^1, \ldots, X_t^d) = f(t_0, X_{t_0}^1, \ldots, X_{t_0}^d) + \int_{t_0}^{t} \frac{\partial f}{\partial s}(s, X_s^1, \ldots, X_s^d)ds \tag{13.9}$$

$$+\sum_{i=1}^{d} \int_{t_0}^{t} \frac{\partial f}{\partial x^i}(s, X_s^1, \ldots, X_s^d)dX_s^i$$

$$+\frac{1}{2}\sum_{i,j=1}^{d} \int_{t_0}^{t} \frac{\partial^2 f}{\partial x^i x^j}(s, X_s^1, \ldots, X_s^d)d < X^i, X^j >_s,$$

*where*

$$dX_t^i = a^i(s, X_s)ds + \sum_{j=1}^{m} b^{i,j}(s, X_s)dW_s^j \qquad \text{and}$$

$$d < X^i, X^j >_s = \sum_{k=1}^{m} b^{i,k}(s, X_s)b^{j,k}(s, X_s)ds.$$

*where* $dW_i dW_j = \delta_{ij}dt, dW_i dt = dt dW_i = dt dt = 0$. □

*Proof* Similar to the one-dimensional case, only with even more complexity.

**Theorem 13.2** (Partial integration) *Let us consider two one-dimensional Itô processes* $(X_t)_{t\in\mathbb{T}}$ *and* $(Y_t)_{t\in\mathbb{T}}$ *defined on the same probability space*

$$X_t = X_0 + \int_0^t a_s^1 ds + \int_0^t b_s^1 dW_s, \qquad Y_t = Y_0 + \int_0^t a_s^2 ds + \int_0^t b_s^2 dW_s.$$

*The stochastic partial integration formula is given by*

$$X_t Y_t = X_0 Y_0 + \int_0^t X_s dY_s + \int_0^t Y_s dX_s + \int_0^t b_s^1 b_s^2 ds. \tag{13.10}$$

*Proof* See [19].

*Example* For $X_t = Y_t = W_t$ and $a_t = 0, b_t = 1$. By applying the stochastic partial integration, we get $d(W_t W_t) = W_s dW_s + W_s dW_s + (1)(1)ds$, which is equivalent to $d(W_t^2) = 2W_s dW_s + ds$ and by integrating both sides with respect to the time, it yields $W_t^2 = 2\int_0^t W_s dW_s + \int_0^t 1ds$. Finally, it results $\int_0^t W_s dW_s = \frac{1}{2}(W_t^2 - t)$. □

*Remark 13.1* In this remark, we call the attention of the reader to the behavior of time-integral and time-differential of a Brownian motion. Since this is nowhere differentiable, we use it for the time derivative in the distributional sense of their paths. Thus, we get in both cases a Gaussian stochastic processes. Explicitly, consider a finite difference approximation of $\xi_t$ using a time interval of width $\Delta t$, $\xi_{\Delta t}(t) := \dfrac{W_{t+\Delta t} - W_t}{\Delta t}$ and consider the time integral $Z_t := \int_0^t W_s ds$, representing the area under the path of the Brownian motion $\{W_s\}_{0\leq s\leq t}$. □

## *13.3.2 Multi-indices for Stochastic Integration*

In order to be able to define the multiple stochastic integrals, we introduce the following set of multi-indices. Let us consider $m \in \mathbb{N}$ and $F = \{0, 1, \ldots, m\}$. A multi-index $\alpha$ refers to a row vector with components in $F$ such as $\alpha = (j_1, \ldots, j_l)$ where $j_i \in F$, for $1 \leq i \leq l$.

We denotes the size of $\alpha$ by $l(\alpha) := l$ and by $n(\alpha)$ the number of zero components of $\alpha$. The set of all multi-indices with respect to $F$ is represented by

$$\mathcal{M} = \bigcup_{l=1}^{\infty} F^l \cup \{v\}, \tag{13.11}$$

where $v$ refers to the empty multi-index with size zero. The following example gives more sense for the definition above:

*Example* For $\alpha = (1, 0, 2)$ it holds $(\alpha) = 3$ and $n(\alpha) = 1$ and for $\alpha = (1, 0, 0, 2, 3, 1, 0, 0)$ we have $l(\alpha) = 8$and $n(\alpha) = 4$. □

Actually, for $l, k \in \mathbb{N}$, we define the following operations on the multi-index set:

**Definition 13.2** ("$-$" *operator*). For $\alpha \in \mathcal{M}$ with $\alpha = (j_1, j_2, \ldots, j_l)$. For $l \geq 1$, we define $\alpha-$ and $-\alpha$ as follow:

$$\alpha- := (j_1, j_2, \ldots, j_{l-1}) \quad \text{and} \quad -\alpha := (j_2, \ldots, j_l).$$

If $l(\alpha) = l > 1$ then, it implies $l(-\alpha) = l(\alpha-) = l - 1$. If $l(\alpha) = l = 1$ then, it implies $-\alpha = \alpha- = v$ and $l(-\alpha) = l(\alpha-) = 0$.

**Definition 13.3** ($\star$ *operator*). Let us consider $\alpha = (j_1, j_2, \ldots, j_l)$, $\beta = (i_1, i_2, \ldots, i_k) \in \mathcal{M}$. The operator $\star$ is defined as:

$$\alpha * \beta := (j_1, j_2, \ldots, j_l, i_1, i_2, \ldots, i_k) \quad \text{and} \quad \beta * \alpha := (i_1, i_2, \ldots, i_k, j_1, j_2, \ldots, j_l).$$

**Definition 13.4** ("-[i]" *operator*). For $\alpha = (j_1, j_2, \ldots, j_l)$ and $i \in \mathbb{N}$, the Operation "$-[i]$" represents the "$i$"-times application of "$-$", where the last $i$ components should be deleted:

$$\alpha - [i] := \begin{cases} (j_1, j_2, \ldots, j_{l-i}), & \text{if } i < l; \\ v, & \text{if } i \geq l. \end{cases}$$

It yields $\alpha - [i] - [j] = \alpha - [i + j]$ for $i, j \in \mathbb{N}$. □

*Example* If $\alpha = (1, 0, 2)$, $\beta = (0, 3, 1)$, then we have

1. $-\alpha = (0, 2)$ and $\alpha- = (1, 0)$,
2. $\alpha \star \beta = (1, 0, 2, 0, 3, 1)$ and $\beta \star \alpha = (0, 3, 1, 1, 0, 2)$,
3. $\alpha - [1] = (1, 0), \alpha - [1] - [1] = \alpha - [2] = (1)$ and $(1, 0, 2) - [i] = v, \forall i \geq 3$.

□

### 13.3.3 Stochastic Multiple Itô-Integrals

Throughout the following section, all stochastic processes are defined on a probability space $(\Omega, \mathfrak{A}, P)$ with right continuous augmented filtration $\mathfrak{F} = (\mathfrak{F}_t)_{t \in \mathbb{T}}$.

**Definition 13.5** Define the set $H$ as a set of stochastic processes $(f_t)_{t \geq 0}$, which are progressively adapted to the associated filtration $\{\mathfrak{F}_t\}_{t \geq 0})$, right continuous and the left limit exists. Conceptively define the sets $H_v$, $H_{(0)}$, $H_{(1)}$ as follow

1. $H_v := \{f \in H : \forall\, t \geq t_0 \quad |f(t, w)| < \infty \quad \text{a.s.}\}$,
2. $H_{(0)} := \left\{f \in H : \forall\, t \geq t_0 \quad \int_{t_0}^{t} |f(s, w)| ds < \infty \quad \text{a.s.}\right\}$,
3. $H_{(1)} := \left\{f \in H : \forall\, t \geq t_0 \quad \int_{t_0}^{t} |f(s, w)|^2 ds < \infty \quad \text{a.s.}\right\}$.

For $j \in F \backslash \{0\}$ one sets $H_{(j)} = H_{(1)}$. □

**Definition 13.6** Let us consider $\alpha = (j_1, j_2, \ldots, j_l)$ a multi-index and $(W_t)_{t \geq 0}$ an $m$-dimensional Brownian motion. For $f \in H_{(\alpha)}$, multiple Itô-Integrals are defined per recursion as follows: □

$$I_\alpha[f(.)]_{t_0,t} := \begin{cases} f(t), & \text{if } l = 0 \\ \int_{t_0}^{t} I_{\alpha-}[f(.)]_{t_0,s} ds, & \text{if } l \geq 1 \text{ and } j_l = 0 \\ \int_{t_0}^{t} I_{\alpha-}[f(.)]_{t_0,s} dW_s^{j_l}, & \text{if } l \geq 1 \text{ and } j_l \geq 1. \end{cases}$$

here $H_{(\alpha)}$ is defined per recursion as

$$H_{(\alpha)} := \{f \in H : \quad I_{(\alpha-)}[f(.)]_{t_0,.} \in H_{(j_l)}\}, \tag{13.12}$$

for $j_l = 0, 1, \ldots, m$ and $l \geq 2$.

*Example*

$$I_{(1,2)}[f(.)]_{t_0,t} = \int_{t_0}^{t}\int_{t_0}^{s} f(z)dW_z^1 dW_s^2,$$

$$I_{(1,2,0)}[f(.)]_{t_0,t} = \int_{t_0}^{t} I_{(1,2)}[f(.)]_{0,s}ds = \int_{t_0}^{t}\int_{t_0}^{s}\int_{t_0}^{s_1} f(s_2)dW_{s_2}^1 dW_{s_1}^2 ds.$$

□

For simplification, we will use the following notation $I_{\alpha,t} = I_\alpha[1]_{0,t}$ and $W_t^0 = t$. Moreover, we will use the Kronecker symbol $\delta$ for $j_{i_1}, j_{i_2} = 0, 1, \ldots, l$. defined by $\delta_{j_{i_1}, j_{i_2}} = 1$ if $j_{i_1} = j_{i_2}$ and 0 else.

**Theorem 13.3** *Let us consider* $l \in \mathbb{N}$ *and* $\alpha = (j_1, \ldots, j_l) \in \mathcal{M}$. *For* $t \geq 0$, *we have*

$$I_{(j),t}I_{(\alpha),t} = \sum_{i=0}^{l} I_{(\alpha-[l-i])*(j,j_{i+1},\ldots,j_l),t} + \sum_{i=1}^{l} B_{jj_i} I_{(\alpha-[l-i+1])*(0,j_{i+1},\ldots,j_l),t}, \quad (13.13)$$

*where* $B_{jj_i} = \delta_{j,j_i}(1 - \delta_{0,j})$. □

*Proof* By using partial integration, we get:

$$\begin{aligned} d(I_{(j),t}I_{\alpha,t}) &= I_{(j),t}d(I_{\alpha,t}) + I_{\alpha,t}d(I_{(j),t}) + (1-\delta_{0,j})I_{\alpha-}dW_t^j dW_t^{j_l} \\ &= I_{(j),t}d(I_{\alpha,t}) + I_{\alpha,t}d(I_{(j),t}) + (1-\delta_{0,j})\delta_{jj_l}I_{\alpha-,t}dt \\ &= I_{(j),t}d(I_{\alpha,t}) + I_{\alpha,t}d(I_{(j),t})) + B_{jj_l}I_{\alpha-,t}dt \\ &= I_{(j),t)}I_{\alpha-,t}dW_t^{j_l} + I_{\alpha,t}d(I_{(j),t}) + B_{jj_l}I_{\alpha-,t}dt. \end{aligned}$$

For simplification, let us define the terms $A_{\alpha,t}^j = I_{(j),t}I_{\alpha,t}$ for $\alpha \in \mathcal{M}$, we obtain

$$\begin{aligned} A_{\alpha,t}^j &= \int_0^t I_{\alpha,s}dI_{(j),s} + \int_0^t I_{(j),s}I_{\alpha-,s}dW_s^{j_l} + B_{jj_l}\int_0^t I_{\alpha-,s}ds \\ &= \int_0^t I_{\alpha,s}dW_s^j + \int_0^t A_{(\alpha-[1]),s}^j dW_s^j + B_{jj_l}I_{(\alpha-[1])*(0),t}, \\ &= I_{\alpha*(j),t} + \int_0^t A_{(\alpha-[1]),s}^j dW_s^j + B_{jj_l}I_{(\alpha-[1])*(0),t}. \end{aligned}$$

Per induction over $l$ in $\alpha$ in $A_{\alpha-[1],t}^j$

$$\begin{aligned} A_{\alpha,t}^j &= I_{\alpha*(j),t} + \int_0^t I_{(\alpha-[1])*(j),s_l}dW_{s_l}^{j_l} + \int_0^t\int_0^{s_l} A_{(\alpha-[2]),s_{l-1}}^j dW_{s_{l-1}}^{j_{l-1}}dW_{s_l}^{j_l} \\ &\quad + B_{jj_{l-1}}\int_0^t I_{\alpha-[2]*(0),t}dW_{s_l}^{j_l} + B_{jj_l}I_{(\alpha-[1])*(0),t} \\ &= I_{\alpha*(j),t} + I_{(\alpha-[1])*(j,j_l),t} + \int_0^t\int_0^{s_l} A_{(\alpha-[2]),s_{l-1}^j} dW_{s_{l-1}}^{j_{l-1}}dW_{s_l}^{j_l} \\ &\quad + B_{jj_{l-1}}I_{(\alpha-[2])*(0,j_l),t} + B_{jj_l}I_{(\alpha-[1])*(0),t} \end{aligned}$$

Now the same procedure will be applied to $A_{(\alpha-[2]),s^j_{l-1}}$, we get:

$$A^j_{\alpha,t} = \sum_{i=1}^{l} I_{(\alpha-[l-i])*(j,j_{i+1},\cdots,j_l),t} + \int_0^t \int_0^{s_l} \cdots \int_0^{s_2} A^j_{(\alpha-[l]),s_1} dW^{j_1}_{s_1} \cdots dW^{j_l}_{s_l}$$
$$+ \sum_{i=1}^{l} B_{jj_l} I_{(\alpha-[l-i+1])*(0,j_{i+1},\cdots,j_l),t}.$$

Note that

$$A^j_{(\alpha-[l]),s_1} = I_{(j),s_1} I_{(\alpha-[l]),j_l} = I_{(j),s_1} I_{v,s_1} = I_{(j),s_l} = \int_0^{s_1} dW^j_s, \qquad (13.14)$$

hence, we have

$$\begin{aligned} I_{(\alpha-[l])*(j,j_1,\cdots,j_l),t} &= \int_0^t \int_0^{s_l} \cdots \int_0^{s_2} A^j_{(\alpha-[l]),s_1} dW^{j_1}_{s_1} \cdots dW^{j_l}_{l} \\ &= \int_0^t \int_0^{s_l} \cdots \int_0^{s_2} \int_0^{s_1} dW^j_s dW^{j_1}_{s_1} \cdots dW^{j_l}_{l}. \end{aligned} \qquad (13.15)$$

by replacing (13.14) and (13.15) in (13.14), we obtain (13.13). Thus, we achieve the proof of the theorem.

The following corollary gives a clear idea about an interesting class of multiple stochastic integrals

**Corollary 13.1** *Consider $l, j \in \mathbb{N}$ and $\alpha = (j, j, \ldots, j)$ with $l(\alpha) = l$. It holds:*

$$I_{\alpha,t} = \begin{cases} \frac{t^l}{l!} & \textit{for } j = 0, \\ \frac{1}{l}(W^j_t I_{\alpha-,t} - t I_{\alpha-[2],t}) & \textit{for } j \geq 1. \end{cases}$$

*Proof* From Theorem 13.3 ($B_{0,0} = 0$) it follows

$$\begin{aligned} t I_{\alpha,t} = I_{(0),t} I_{\alpha,t} &= \sum_{i=0}^{l} I_{(\alpha-[l-i])*(j,j_{i+1},\cdots,j_l)} \qquad (13.16) \\ &= \sum_{i=0}^{l} I_{\underbrace{(0,0,\ldots,0)}_{(l+1)-times}} \\ &= (l+1)\frac{t^{l+1}}{(l+1)!}. \end{aligned}$$

The length of the multi-index $((\alpha - [l-i]) * (j, j_{i+1}, \cdots, j_l))$ is determined by:

$$\begin{aligned} l((\alpha - [l-i]) * (j, j_{i+1}, \cdots, j_l)) &= l(\alpha - [l-i]) + l((j, j_{i+1}, \cdots, j_l)) \\ &= l(\alpha - [l-i]) + l((j)) + l(j_{i+1}, \cdots, j_l)) \\ &= l - (l-i) + 1 + (l-i) \\ &= l + 1. \end{aligned}$$

From (13.16), we get $I_{\alpha,t} = \frac{t^l}{l!}$. For $j \geq 1$ it yields $B_{jj} = 1$. Moreover,

$$\begin{aligned} I_{(j),t} I_{\alpha-,t} &= \sum_{i=0}^{l-1} I_{\underbrace{(j, \ldots, j)}_{l-times}} + \sum_{i=1}^{l-1} I_{((\alpha)-[1]-[l-i+1])*(0, j_{i+1}, \cdots, j_l)} \\ &= l I_{\underbrace{(j, \ldots, j)}_{l-times}} + \sum_{i=1}^{l-1} I_{\underbrace{((\alpha) - [1] - [l-i+1]) * (0, j, \cdots, j)}_{size=(l-1)}} \\ &= l I_{\underbrace{(j, \ldots, j)}_{l-times}} + \sum_{i=1}^{l-1} I_{\underbrace{((\alpha) - [2] - [l-i]) * (0, j, \cdots, j)}_{size=(l-1)}}. \end{aligned} \tag{13.17}$$

Using Theorem 13.3 for $j = 0$, it follows

$$I_{(0),t} I_{\alpha-[2],t} = t I_{\alpha-[2],t} = \sum_{i=1}^{l-1} I_{\underbrace{((\alpha) - [2] - [l-i]) * (0, j, \cdots, j)}_{size=(l-1)}}. \tag{13.18}$$

From (13.17) and (13.18) it follows: $I_{(j),t} I_{\alpha-,t} = l I_{\underbrace{(j, \ldots, j)}_{(l)-times}} + t I_{\alpha-[2],t}$. Thus

$$I_{\underbrace{(j, \ldots, j)}_{l-times}} = \frac{1}{l}(I_{(j),t} I_{\alpha-,t} - t I_{\alpha-[2],t})$$

**Lemma 13.4** *We have the following values of the multiple stochastic integrals for the special case* $\alpha = (j, j, \ldots, j) \in \mathcal{M}$:

$$I_{(j,j,j),t} = \frac{1}{3}\Big(I_{(j),t}\frac{1}{2}(I^2_{(j),t} - t) - t I_{(j),t}\Big) = \frac{1}{3!}\Big(I^3_{(j),t} - 3t I_{(j),t}\Big), \tag{13.19}$$

$$I_{(j,j,j,j),t} = \frac{1}{4!}\Big(I^4_{(j),t} - 6t I^2_{(j),t} + 3t^2\Big), \tag{13.20}$$

$$I_{(j,j,j,j,j),t} = \frac{1}{5!}\Big(I^5_{(j),t} - 10t I^3_{(j),t} + 15t^2 I_{(j),t}\Big), \tag{13.21}$$

$$I_{(j,j,j,j,j,j),t} = \frac{1}{6!}\Big(I^6_{(j),t} - 15t I^4_{(j),t} + 45t^2 I^2_{(j),t} - 15t^3\Big), \tag{13.22}$$

$$I_{(j,j,j,j,j,j,j),t} = \frac{1}{7!}\Big(I^7_{(j),t} - 21tI^5_{(j),t} + 105t^2 I^3_{(j),t} - 105t^3 I_{(j),t}\Big). \tag{13.23}$$

□

*Proof* Note that, since $(j, j) - [2] = v$, we have

$$I_{(j,j),t} = \frac{1}{2}(I^2_{(j),t} - t) = \frac{1}{2}\Big((W^j_t)^2 - t\Big). \tag{13.24}$$

The proof of the other multiple integrals is left to the reader (use Corollary 13.1).

To approximate numerical solutions for the SDE (13.3) we consider a generalized Milstein method. The starting point for development of the Milstein method is the stochastic Itô-Taylor expansion, compare [20–22, 26]. Thus, for a given functional $f : [t_0, T] \times I\!R^d \to I\!R$ with all its derivatives are smooth functions, the associated Itô-Taylor expansion is given by

$$f\,(\tau, \mathbf{X}_\tau) = \sum_{\alpha\in\mathcal{A}_\gamma} \mathbf{I}_\alpha\left[f_\alpha(\rho, \mathbf{X}_\rho)\right]_{\rho,\tau} + \sum_{\alpha\in\mathcal{B}_\gamma} \mathbf{I}_\alpha\left[f_\alpha(\cdot, \mathbf{X}_\cdot)\right]_{\rho,\tau}, \tag{13.25}$$

where $\rho$ and $\tau$ are two stop times processes, $\alpha$ a multi-index in the set of all multi-indices $\mathcal{M}$, $A_\gamma$ a hierarchical set and $B_\gamma$ its remainder set defined as

$$\begin{aligned}\mathcal{A}_\gamma &= \Big\{\alpha \in \mathcal{M} : \quad l(\alpha) + n(\alpha) \le 2\gamma \quad \text{or} \quad l(\alpha) = n(\alpha) = \gamma + \frac{1}{2}\Big\},\\ \mathcal{B}_\gamma &= \Big\{\alpha \in \mathcal{M}\backslash\mathcal{A}_\gamma : \quad -\alpha \in \mathcal{A}_\gamma\Big\},\end{aligned} \tag{13.26}$$

with $l(\alpha)$ and $n(\alpha)$ refer respectively, to the length and the number of zeros of the multi-index $\alpha$, and $-\alpha$ is the multi-index $\alpha$ without the first component. Note that for each construction of the sets $A_\gamma$ and $B_\gamma$ in (13.26), $\gamma$ is allowed to take the values $\gamma = 0.5, 1, 1.5, 2, \ldots$. For example, in a two-dimensional case, the corresponding hierarchical set $\mathcal{A}_1$ and its remainder set $\mathcal{B}_1$ are

$$\begin{aligned}\mathcal{A}_1 &= \Big\{v, (0), (1), (2), (1, 1), (1, 2), (2, 2), (2, 1)\Big\},\\ \mathcal{B}_1 &= \Big\{(0, 0), (0, 1), (0, 2), (1, 0), (2, 0), (0, 1, 1), (0, 1, 2), (1, 2, 2), (0, 2, 2),\\ &\quad (0, 2, 1), (1, 1, 1), (1, 1, 2), (1, 2, 1), (2, 1, 1), (2, 1, 2), (2, 2, 2), (2, 2, 1)\Big\}.\end{aligned}$$

where $v$ is the so-called empty index, see [20–22, 26, 28] among others. In the Itô expansion (13.25), $\mathbf{I}_\alpha\left[f_\alpha(\rho, \mathbf{X}_\rho)\right]$ with $\alpha = (j_1, j_2, \ldots, j_l)$, denotes the multiple Itô integrals of the function $f$ and it is defined by

$$\mathbf{I}_\alpha[f(\cdot,\mathbf{X}_\cdot)]_{t_0,t} = \begin{cases} f(t,\mathbf{X}_t), & \text{if} \quad l=0, \\ \displaystyle\int_{t_0}^{t} \mathbf{I}_{\alpha-}[f(\cdot,\mathbf{X}_\cdot)]_{t_0,s} ds, & \text{if} \quad l\geq 1 \quad \text{and} \quad j_l = 0, \\ \displaystyle\int_{t_0}^{t} \mathbf{I}_{\alpha-}[f(\cdot,\mathbf{X}_\cdot)]_{t_0,s} d\mathbf{W}_s^{j_l}, & \text{if} \quad l\geq 1 \quad \text{and} \quad j_l \geq 1, \end{cases} \tag{13.27}$$

where $\alpha-$ is the the multi-index $\alpha$ without the last component. As examples of the multiple Itô integrals (13.27), we consider

$$\begin{aligned} \mathbf{I}_{(1,2)}[f(\cdot)]_{t_0,t} &= \int_{t_0}^{t}\int_{t_0}^{s} f(z) d\mathbf{W}_z^1 d\mathbf{W}_s^2, \\ \mathbf{I}_{(1,2,0)}[f(\cdot)]_{t_0,t} &= \int_{t_0}^{t} \mathbf{I}_{(1,2)}[f(.)]_{0,s} ds, \\ &= \int_{t_0}^{t}\int_{t_0}^{s}\int_{t_0}^{s_1} f(s_2) d\mathbf{W}_{s_2}^1 d\mathbf{W}_{s_1}^2 ds. \end{aligned}$$

For the time discretization, we divide the time interval $[t_0, T]$ into equidistant subintervals $[t_n, t_{n+1}]$ of length $\Delta t$ such that $t_n = t_0 + n\Delta t$, $n = 0, 1, \ldots$. From the Itô-Taylor expansion (13.25) we construct the discrete approximation

$$f(t_{n+1}, \mathbf{Y}_{t_{n+1}}) = \underbrace{\sum_{\alpha\in\mathcal{A}_\gamma} \mathbf{I}_\alpha\left[f_\alpha(t_n,\mathbf{Y}_{t_n})\right]_{t_n,t_{n+1}}}_{\text{Main approximation}} + \underbrace{\sum_{\alpha\in\mathcal{B}_\gamma} \mathbf{I}_\alpha\left[f_\alpha(\cdot,\mathbf{Y}_\cdot)\right]_{t_n,t_{n+1}}}_{\text{Remainder}}, \tag{13.28}$$

where $\mathbf{Y}_{t_n}$ denotes the approximation of the solution $\mathbf{X}_t$ of the SDE (13.3) at the time $t = t_n$. For independent one-dimensional Wiener processes $(\mathbf{W}_t^{j_1})_{t\geq 0}$ and $(\mathbf{W}_t^{j_2})_{t\geq 0}$, with $j_1 \neq j_2$, the double Itô integrals $\mathbf{I}_{(j_1,j_2)}$ are defined as

$$\mathbf{I}_{(j_1,j_2)t_0,t} = \int_{t_0}^{t}\int_{t_0}^{s_1} d\mathbf{W}_s^{j_1} d\mathbf{W}_{s_1}^{j_2}. \tag{13.29}$$

Since this integral cannot be calculated exactly, a numerical approximation is required, see for instance [20, 22, 26]. Here, we consider the Fourier series expansion

$$\begin{aligned} \mathbf{I}^p_{(j_1,j_2)} = {} & \frac{1}{2}\Delta t \epsilon_{j_1}\epsilon_{j_2} + \Delta t\sqrt{\rho_p}(\mu_{j_1,p}\epsilon_{j_2} - \mu_{j_2,p}\epsilon_{j_1}) + \\ & \frac{\Delta t}{2\pi}\sum_{r=1}^{p}\frac{1}{r}(\zeta_{j_1,r}(\sqrt{2}\epsilon_{j_2} + \eta_{j_2,r}) - \zeta_{j_2,r}(\sqrt{2}\epsilon_{j_1} + \eta_{j_1,r})), \end{aligned} \tag{13.30}$$

where $\epsilon_{j_1}$, $\epsilon_{j_2}$, $\mu_{j_1,p}$, $\mu_{j_2,p}$, $\zeta_{j_1,r}$, $\zeta_{j_2,r}$, $\eta_{j_2,r}$ and $\eta_{j_1,r}$ are random variables pairwise independent $\mathcal{N}(0, 1)$, and $\rho_p$ is a constant defined as

$$\rho_p = \frac{1}{2\pi^2} \sum_{r=p+1}^{\infty} \frac{1}{r^2}.$$

In (13.30), $p$ is the order of the approximation on an interval. Based on a theorem in [26] that establish the relation between the order of a one-step approximation and the order of the scheme generated by such approximation, one can obtain schemes of order $p$ by means of one-step approximations of local order $p+1$. For example, the truncated Itô-Taylor expansion of order $p$ of the Itô process $\mathbf{X}_t$ (i.e., the expression obtained from the Itô-Taylor expansion removing the terms which contain multiple integrals of multiplicities equal to or greater than $p+1$) is an approximation of local order $p+1$ if the coefficients of the equation are continuous, satisfy both Lipschitz and linear growth conditions. The scheme obtained with the truncated Itô-Taylor expansion of order $p$ will be called the order $p$ weak Taylor scheme, see [20–22] for details. Not that the error estimate of the approximation $\mathbf{I}_{(j_1,j_2)^p}$ in (13.30) of the double Itô integral $\mathbf{I}_{(j_1,j_2)}$ is given in second moment by

$$\mathbf{E}\left(\left|\mathbf{I}^p_{(j_1,j_2)} - \mathbf{I}_{(j_1,j_2)}\right|^2\right) = \rho_p(\Delta t)^2, \tag{13.31}$$

where $E(w)$ denotes the expectation of a generic solution $w$. In the current study, to approximate numerical solutions to the SDE (13.3) a generalized Milstein scheme is implemented based on the Itô-Taylor expansion (13.28) as

$$\mathbf{Y}^k_{n+1} = \mathbf{Y}^k_n + \mathcal{F}^k(t_n, \mathbf{Y}_n)\Delta t + \sum_{j=1}^{N+2} \mathcal{G}^{k,j}(t_n, \mathbf{Y}_n)\Delta \mathbf{W}^j_{t_n} + \sum_{j_1,j_2=1}^{N+2} L^{j_1}\mathcal{G}^{k,j_2}(t_n, \mathbf{Y}_n)\mathbf{I}_{(j_1,j_2)}, \tag{13.32}$$

where $\Delta \mathbf{W}^1_{t_n}, \ldots, \Delta \mathbf{W}^{N+2}_{t_n}$ are independent random Gaussian variables $\mathcal{N}(0, \Delta t)$ and the differential operators $L^j$ are given as

$$L^0 = \frac{\partial}{\partial t} + \sum_{k=1}^{N+2} \mathcal{F}^k_t \frac{\partial}{\partial x^k} + \frac{1}{2} \sum_{k,i=1}^{d} \sum_{j=1}^{N+2} \mathcal{G}^{i,j} b^{k,j} \frac{\partial^2}{\partial x^i \partial x^k},$$

$$L^j = \sum_{i=1}^{N+2} \mathcal{G}^{i,j} \frac{\partial}{\partial x^i}, \qquad j = 1, 2, \ldots, N+2.$$

Note that the first-order Milstein scheme is given by the summation over all multi-index of the hierarchical set $A_1$. For the computation of the integrals $\mathbf{I}_{(j,j)}$ for $j = 0, 1, \ldots, N+2$, we have used the classical Itô calculus, we refer for example to [20, 22]. Notice that the accuracy of the Itô-Taylor expansion (13.28) depends on the number $p$ such that high accuracy is obtained for large values of $p$. However, large values of $p$ can lead to high computational cost and may limit the efficiency of the overall procedure. In the present study, all the simulations are performed with $p = 100$ which is enough to ensure an accurate representation of the Itô-Taylor expansion (13.28).

### 13.3.4 Itô-Taylor Schemes for Systems Driven by One Noise

Let $(W_t)_{t\in[t_0,T]}$ be an $m$-dimensional Brownian motion defined on a $(\Omega, \mathcal{A})^m$ with right continuous augmented filtration $\mathcal{F} = (\mathcal{F}_t)_{t\in[0,T]}$. Consider the following $d-$ dimensional Itô process $(X_t^1 \ldots, X_t^d)$, which satisfies the stochastic differential (13.33):

$$X_t^i = X_0^i + \int_0^t a_s^i ds + \sum_{j=1}^m \int_0^t b_s^{i,j} dW_s^j \tag{13.33}$$

where for all $i = 1, \ldots, d$, and $j = 1, \ldots, m$; the drift vector $(a_t^i)_{t\in[0,T]}$ and the diffusion matrix $(b_t^{i,j})_{t\in[0,T]}$ are $\mathcal{F}_t$ adapted and satisfy $\int_0^T a_s^i ds < \infty$ and $\int_0^T (b_s^{i,j})^2 ds < \infty$ a.s.

For any partition $0 = t_0 < t_1 < \cdot < t_N = T$ of the time interval $[0, T]$ with step sizes $\Delta t_n = t_{n+1} - t_n$ and maximum step-size $\Delta = \max_n \Delta t_n$, let $Y_n^\Delta$ be a numerical approximation of the exact solution $X_{t_n}$. We have to distinct between the strong and the weak convergence of $X_{t_n}$. We said that the $Y_n$ is a strong approximation of order $\gamma$ if it exists $K_{p,T} > 0$ such that

$$E_s^\gamma(Y_n^\Delta) := \left(E|Y_{N_T}^\gamma - X_T|^p\right)^{\frac{1}{p}} \leq K_{p,T}\Delta^\gamma \quad \text{with} \quad \lim_{N_T\to\infty} E_s^\gamma(Y_n^\Delta) = 0. \tag{13.34}$$

and we said that $Y_n$ is a weak approximation of order $\beta$ if it exists $K_{g,T} > 0$ such that

$$E_w^\beta(Y_n^\Delta) := \left|Eg\left(Y_{N_T}^\beta\right) - Eg(X_T)\right| \leq K_{g,T}\Delta^\beta \quad \text{with} \quad \lim_{N_T\to\infty} E_w^\beta(Y_n^\Delta) = 0, \tag{13.35}$$

where $g$ any polynomial function and $p$ is in general one or two. However, we have to note that all numerical approximation in the stochastic case are results in the mean theory in $L^2$.

*Remark 13.2* In the topic of numerical methods for SPDEs the overall convergence rate represents the scheme dependency to temporal and spatial discretization, which is usually expressed in terms of the computational cost. For the one dimensional case, if $N$ is the number of all operations needed to compute an iteration per time (arithmetical operations, random number and function evaluations) and if the constant $M$ refers the number of time steps $\Delta = \frac{T}{M}$. Suppose that the scheme has the following error bound

$$\sup_{k=0,\dots,M}\left(\left|\mathbf{v}_{t_k}-\mathbf{u}_k^{(N,M)}\right|^2_{L^2(D)}\right)^{\frac{1}{2}} \le K_T\left(\frac{1}{N^\alpha+M^\beta}\right) \tag{13.36}$$

where $\mathbf{v}_{t_k}$ is the exact solution at $t = t_k$ and $\mathbf{u}_k^{(N,M)}$ is the corresponding numerical approximation. Thus, for $\alpha, \beta > 0$, the optimal overall rate $\gamma = \frac{\alpha\beta}{\alpha+\beta}$ with respect to the computational cost is given by

$$\max_{k=0,\dots,M}\left(\left|\mathbf{v}_{t_k}-\mathbf{u}_k^{(N,M)}\right|^2_{L^2(D)}\right) \le K_T\,(NM)^{-\gamma}\,. \tag{13.37}$$

For example if $\alpha = \frac{1}{2}$ and $\beta = 1$, then $\gamma = \frac{1}{3}$. For more details we refer to [18]. □

We consider a regular function $f : I\!R^d \to I\!R$ and suppose that the assumptions of the existence of the numerical solution given in [20] are satisfied. Thus, the strong Itô-Taylor scheme of order $\gamma = 0.5,\ 1,\ 1.5,\ 2, \dots$ is given by:

$$\begin{aligned} Y_0 &= \xi_0, \\ Y_{n+1} &= \sum_{\alpha\in\mathcal{A}_\gamma} I_\alpha[f_\alpha(t_n, Y_n)]_{t_n,t_{n+1}} = Y_n + \sum_{\alpha\in\mathcal{A}_\gamma\setminus\{v\}} I_\alpha[f_\alpha(t_n, Y_n)]_{t_n,t_{n+1}}, \end{aligned} \tag{13.38}$$

where $I_\alpha$ represents the multiple Itô-Integrals and $\mathcal{A}_\gamma$ is given by

$$\mathcal{A}_\gamma = \{\alpha \in \mathcal{M}_m \mid \ell(\alpha) + n(\alpha) = 2\gamma \text{ or } \ell(\alpha) = n(\alpha) = \gamma + 0.5\}\,. \tag{13.39}$$

For the weak approximation we change the the index set $\mathcal{A}_\gamma$ by $\mathcal{A}_\beta$ such that

$$\mathcal{A}_\gamma = \{\alpha \in \mathcal{M}_m \mid \ell(\alpha) \le \beta\}\,. \tag{13.40}$$

In more detailed form, we rewrite the scheme (13.38):

$$Y_0 = \xi_0,$$

$$Y_{n+1} = Y_n + I_{(0)}[a(t, Y_n)]_{\Delta t_n} + \sum_{j=1}^m I_{(j)}[b^j(t, Y_n)]_{\Delta t_n} \tag{13.41}$$

$$+\sum_{j=1}^m I_{(j,j)}[L^j b^j(t, Y_n)]_{\Delta t_n} \tag{13.42}$$

$$+\sum_{j=1}^m I_{(j,0)}[L^j a(t, Y_n)]_{\Delta t_n} + \sum_{j=1}^m I_{(0,j)}[L^0 b^j(t, Y_n)]_{\Delta t_n} \tag{13.43}$$

$$+\sum_{j=1}^m I_{(0,0)}[L^0 a(t, Y_n)]_{\Delta t_n} + \sum_{j=1}^m I_{(j,j,j)}[L^j L^j b^j(t, Y_n)]_{\Delta t_n} \tag{13.44}$$

$$+\sum_{j=1}^m I_{(j,j,0)}[L^j L^j a(t, Y_n)]_{\Delta t_n} + \sum_{j=1}^m I_{(j,0,j)}[L^j L^0 b^j(t, Y_n)]_{\Delta t_n} \tag{13.45}$$

$$+\sum_{j=1}^m I_{(0,j,j)}[L^0 L^j b^j(t, Y_n)]_{\Delta t_n} + \sum_{j=1}^m I_{(j,j,j,j)}[L^j L^j L^j b^j(t, Y_n)]_{\Delta t_n}, \tag{13.46}$$

where Euler Maruyama (13.42), Milstein (13.42)–(13.42), Taylor of order 1.5 represented by (13.42)–(13.44) and Taylor of order 2.0 is represented by the equations (13.42)–(13.46), for $i = 1, \dots, d$ and $j = 1, \dots, m$ the differential operators $L^j$ for $j = 0, 1, \dots, m$ are given by

$$L^0 = \frac{\partial}{\partial t} + \sum_{k=1}^{d} a_t^k \frac{\partial}{\partial x^k} + \frac{1}{2} \sum_{k,i=1}^{d} \sum_{j=1}^{m} b^{i,j} b^{k,j} \frac{\partial^2}{\partial x^i \partial x^k}, \tag{13.47}$$

$$L^j = \sum_{i=1}^{d} b^{i,j} \frac{\partial}{\partial x^i}. \tag{13.48}$$

The Itô-Taylor schemes (13.42)–(13.46) correspond to the following index sets: For $\gamma = 0$ the index set

$$\mathcal{A}_{0.0} = \{v\},$$

represents the initial guess of the numerical scheme. If $\gamma = 0.5$, the construction of the index set

$$\mathcal{A}_{0.5} = \mathcal{A}_{0.0} \cup \Big\{(0), (1)\Big\},$$

leads to the Euler–Maruyama scheme. If $\gamma = 1$ then the index set

$$\mathcal{A}_{1.0} = \mathcal{A}_{0.5} \cup \Big\{(1, 1)\Big\},$$

corresponds to the first order Itô-Taylor scheme (called also Milstein scheme), and if $\gamma = 1.5$ the index-set is

$$\mathcal{A}_{1.5} = \mathcal{A}_{1.0} \cup \Big\{(0, 0), (1, 0), (0, 1), (1, 1, 1)\Big\}.$$

If $\gamma = 2.0$ the index set is

$$\mathcal{A}_{2.0} = \mathcal{A}_{1.5} \cup \Big\{(1, 1, 0), (0, 1, 1), (1, 0, 1), (1, 1, 1, 1)\Big\}.$$

The entries of the Itô-Taylor approximation are the stochastic integrals with index length less than or equal four. These stochastic integrals can be classified in four types. We present their explicit form for autonomous SDE (i.e. autonomous drift and diffusion):

$\ell(\alpha) = 1$, In this case, we define the following deterministic and stochastic integral:

$$I_{(0)}[a(t_n, X_{t_n})]_{\Delta t_n} = a(t_n, X_{t_n}) \Delta t_n. \tag{13.49}$$

$$I_{(1)}[b(t_n, X_{t_n})]_{\Delta t_n} = b(t_n, X_{t_n}) \int_{t_n}^{t_{n+1}} dW_s^1, \tag{13.50}$$

with index $\alpha \in \mathcal{M}_1$ such that $n(\alpha) \leq 1$.

$\ell(\alpha) = 2$, stochastic integral with index $\alpha \in \mathcal{M}_1$ and $\ell(\alpha) = 2$:

$$\begin{aligned} I_{(1,1)}[L^1 b(t_n, X_{t_n})]_{\Delta t_n} &= b(t_n, X_{t_n})\frac{\partial b}{\partial x}(t_n, X_{t_n}) \int_{t_n}^{t_{n+1}} \int_{t_n}^{t} dW_s^1 dW_t^1 \qquad (13.51) \\ &= b(t_n, X_{t_n})\frac{\partial b}{\partial x}(t_n, X_{t_n}) I_{(1,1),\Delta t_n}, \\ I_{(1,0)}[L^1 a(t_n, X_{t_n})]_{\Delta t_n} &= b(t_n, X_{t_n})\frac{\partial a}{\partial x}(t_n, X_n) \int_{t_n}^{t_{n+1}} \int_{t_n}^{t} dW_s^1 dt \qquad (13.52) \\ &= b(t_n, X_{t_n})\frac{\partial a}{\partial x}(t_n, X_n) I_{(1,0),\Delta t_n}, \\ I_{(0,1)}[L^0 b(t_n, X_n)]_{\Delta t_n} &= \left(a\frac{\partial b}{\partial x} + \frac{1}{2}b^2\frac{\partial^2 b}{\partial x^2}\right)(t_n, X_{t_n}) \int_{t_n}^{t_{n+1}} \int_{t_n}^{t} ds dW_t \qquad (13.53) \\ &= \left(a\frac{\partial b}{\partial x} + \frac{1}{2}b^2\frac{\partial^2 b}{\partial x^2}\right)(t_n, X_{t_n}) I_{(0,1),\Delta t_n}, \\ I_{(0,0)}[L^0 a(t_n, X_n)]_{\Delta t_n} &= \left(a\frac{\partial a}{\partial x} + \frac{1}{2}b^2\frac{\partial^2 a}{\partial x^2}\right)(t_n, X_n) \int_{t_n}^{t_{n+1}} \int_{t_n}^{t} ds dt, \qquad (13.54) \end{aligned}$$

$\ell(\alpha) = 3$, stochastic integral with index $\alpha \in \mathcal{M}_1$ and $\ell(\alpha) = 3$:

$$\begin{aligned} I_{(1,1,1)}[L^1 L^1 b(t_n, X_n)]_{\Delta t_n} &= \left(b\,(b')^2 + b^2 b''\right)(t_n, X_n) \int_{t_n}^{t_{n+1}} \int_{t_n}^{t} \int_{t_n}^{s} dW_r dW_s dW_t \qquad (13.55) \\ &= \left(b\,(b')^2 + b^2 b''\right)(t_n, X_n) I_{(1,1,1),\Delta t_n}, \\ I_{(1,1,0)}[L^1 L^1 a(t, .X_n)]_{\Delta t_n} &= (ba' + ba'')(t_n, X_n) I_{(1,1,0),\Delta t_n} \qquad (13.56) \\ I_{(1,0,1)}[L^1 L^0 b(t, .X_n)]_{\Delta t_n} &= \left(ba'b' + abb'' + b^2 b' b'' + \frac{1}{2}b^2 b'''\right)(t_n, X_n) I_{(1,0,1),\Delta t_n}, \qquad (13.57) \\ I_{(0,1,1)}[L^0 L^1 b(t, .X_n)]_{\Delta t_n} &= \left(a(bb')' + \frac{1}{2}a^2 (bb')'''\right)(t_n, X_n) I_{(0,1,1),\Delta t_n}. \qquad (13.58) \end{aligned}$$

$\ell(\alpha) = 4$, provided that $n(\alpha) = 0$, we define the multiple stochastic integral

$$I_{(1,1,1,1)}[L^1 L^1 L^1 b(t_n, X_n)]_{\Delta t_n} = b\left(b\left(b(bb')\right)'\right)' I_{(1,1,1,1),\Delta t_n}, \qquad (13.59)$$

where $a'$, $b'$ represents the spatial derivatives of the drift and the diffusion in the autonomous case. The general case needs the use of the stochastic differential operators $L^0$ and $L^1$. The integrals $I_{(1)}, \ldots, I_{(1,1,1,1)}$ are analytically formulated by the exact expressions in [10].

In the present paper, we deal with Dirichlet external boundary conditions and Neuman-like internal boundary conditions. The solutions on the common interfaces of the subdomains are effects caused by a backward step of the solutions on interiors of the subdomains. For the considered boundary-value equations, we assume non-flux boundary conditions (i.e. homogeneous Neumann conditions), which have been widely used to model practical problems from engineering and industrial applications, such as stochastic advection-diffusion equations, stochastic Burgers equation, stochastic Korteweg-de Vries equation, and stochastic Navier-Stokes equations. For more details, we refer to the works [10, 43, 47].

## 13.4 Numerical SDE and SDES Examples

In this section numerical results are presented for the reduced model of prebiotic evolution depicted in Fig. 13.1. We also illustrate the performance of the Milstein scheme for two problems in SDE with known exact solutions. In all our simulations we perform 10, 000 realizations and mean solutions are displayed. Note that equations with known analytical solutions are used to quantify the errors and to examine the convergence features of the considered method. For the sake of comparison we also consider the canonical Euler–Maruyama method widely used in the literature for solving SDE, compare for instance [20, 22, 43, 44, 46, 47].

### *13.4.1 A Stochastic Linear Equation*

We consider the stochastic Black-Scholes equation used in option pricing [22]

$$dX_t = \lambda X_t dt + \mu X_t dW_t, \qquad X_0 = x_0. \tag{13.60}$$

It is easy to verify that the analytical solution of (13.60) is given by

$$X_t = X_0 \exp\left((\lambda - 0.5\mu^2)t + \mu W_t\right). \tag{13.61}$$

The exact solution (13.61) is also used to evaluate the expected error function at time $t_n$ as

$$\mathcal{E} = \sqrt{E\Big(\sup_{0\le t_n\le 1}(X_{t_n} - Y_n)^2\Big)},$$

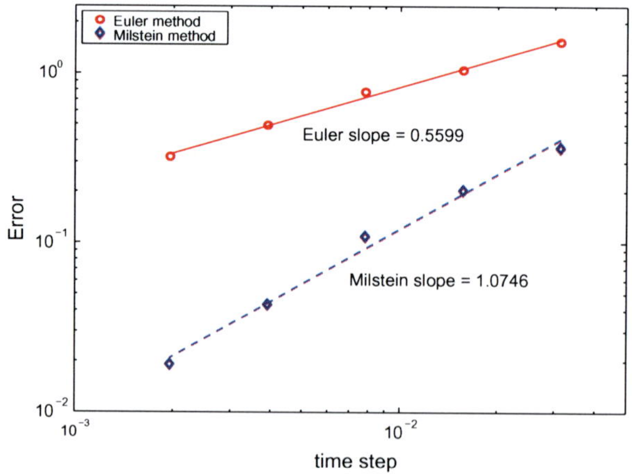


**Fig. 13.2** Error plots for the linear equation at time $t = 1$

where $X_{t_n}$ and $Y_n$ are the exact and numerical solutions at time $t_n$, respectively. In our computations we use $\lambda = -1$, $\mu = 2$, $x_0 = 1$ and simulations are stopped at time $t_n = 1$. In Fig. 13.2 we display the error norms for the Milstein and Euler schemes using five uniform step sizes $2^{-5}$, $2^{-6}$, $2^{-7}$, $2^{-8}$ and $2^{-9}$ at the considered time. A logarithmic scale is used on the $x$- and $y$-axis. It is clear that decreasing the time step size results in a decrease of errors in both schemes. As expected the Euler method shows a convergence rate of 0.5 whereas the convergence rate of the Milstein method is 1 for this linear stochastic equation.

### 13.4.2 A Stochastic Linear System

Next we solve the following two-dimensional stochastic system

$$dX_t = a(t, X_t)dt + b(t, X_t)dW_t, \tag{13.62}$$

where $X_t = \left(X_t^1, X_t^2\right)^T$ is the unknown vector. The drift vector $a(t, X_t)$ and the diffusion matrix $b(t, X_t)$ are given as

$$a(t, X_t) = \begin{pmatrix} -\lambda & \lambda \\ \lambda & -\lambda \end{pmatrix} X_t, \qquad b(t, X_t) = \begin{pmatrix} \mu & 0 \\ 0 & \mu \end{pmatrix} X_t.$$

The analytical solution of this system is given by [20]

$$X_t = P \begin{pmatrix} \exp\left(\rho^+(t)\right) & 0 \\ 0 & \exp\left(\rho^-(t)\right) \end{pmatrix} P^{-1} X_0,$$

where $\rho^{\pm}(t) = (-\lambda - 0.5\mu^2 \pm \lambda)t + \mu W_t$,

$$P = \frac{1}{\sqrt{2}} \begin{pmatrix} 1 & 1 \\ 1 & -1 \end{pmatrix} \quad \text{and} \quad X_0 = \begin{pmatrix} 1 \\ 2 \end{pmatrix}.$$

In all results presented for the system (13.62) we used $\lambda = 1$, $\mu = 2$ and different time steps. In Fig. 13.3 we display the difference between the simulated solution and analytical solution at time $t_n = 1$ using the Euler method. The obtained results for the Milstein method are depicted in Fig. 13.4. For a clear presentation a decimal logarithmic scale is used on the $y$-axis. It is evident that for both component the errors computed using the Milstein scheme show different trends than those computed using the Euler scheme. For all selected time steps, the Milstein scheme is more accurate than the Euler scheme for this linear system. To further quantify the errors in the Milstein and Euler schemes, we calculate the following errors

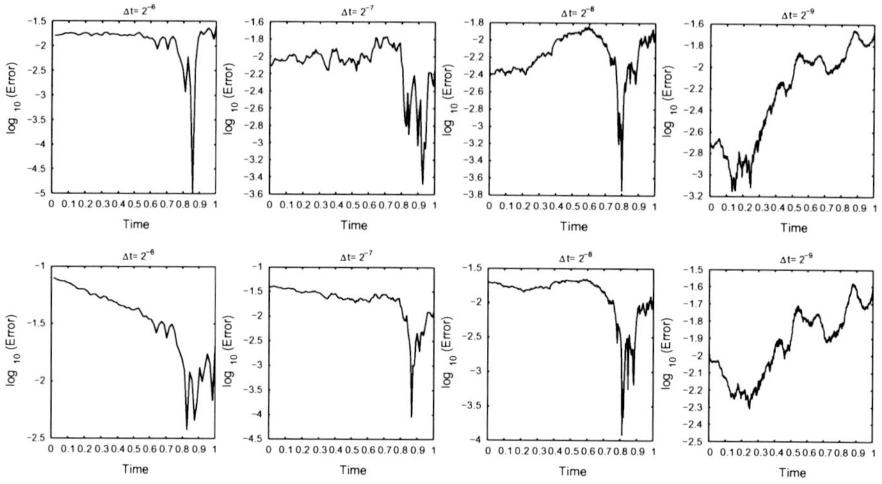


**Fig. 13.3** Errors in the solution $X_t^1$ (first row) and the solution $X_t^2$ (second row) at time $t_n = 1$ obtained using the Euler scheme

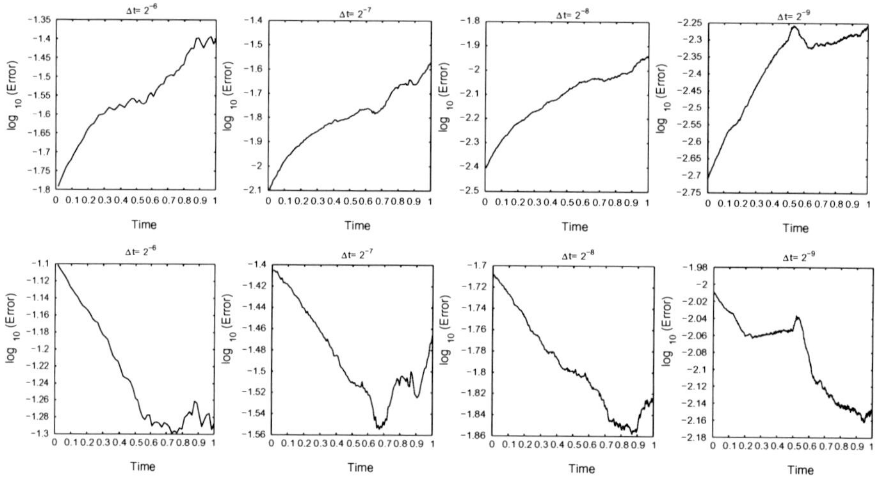


**Fig. 13.4** Errors in the solution $X_t^1$ (first row) and the solution $X_t^2$ (second row) at time $t_n = 1$ obtained using the Milstein scheme

$$\mathcal{E}_1 = \left|E(X_{t_n}^k) - E(Y_n^i)\right|, \qquad \mathcal{E}_2 = \sqrt{\left(E\left(X_{t_n}^k - Y_n^k\right)^2\right)}, \qquad k = 1, 2,$$

where $X_{t_n}^k$ and $Y_n^k$ are the exact and numerical solutions at time $t_n$, respectively.

In Table 13.1 we summarize the obtained results for different time steps. A simple inspection of this table reveals that a decay of all considered errors is achieved by decreasing the time steps for both solutions $X_t^1$ and $X_t^2$. However, a faster decay

**Table 13.1** Errors $\mathcal{E}_1$ and $\mathcal{E}_2$ for the linear system at time $t_n = 1$ using different time steps

| | Milstein method | | | | Euler method | | | |
|---|---|---|---|---|---|---|---|---|
| | $X_t^1$ | | $X_t^2$ | | $X_t^1$ | | $X_t^2$ | |
| $\Delta t$ | $\mathcal{E}_1$ | $\mathcal{E}_2$ | $\mathcal{E}_1$ | $\mathcal{E}_2$ | $\mathcal{E}_1$ | $\mathcal{E}_2$ | $\mathcal{E}_1$ | $\mathcal{E}_2$ |
| $2^{-5}$ | 0.65E-1 | 0.14E-0 | 0.13E-0 | 0.22E-0 | 0.63E-1 | 0.19E+1 | 0.63E-1 | 0.28E+1 |
| $2^{-6}$ | 0.28E-1 | 0.47E-1 | 0.59E-1 | 0.62E-1 | 0.95E-2 | 0.12E+1 | 0.95E-2 | 0.16E+1 |
| $2^{-7}$ | 0.16E-1 | 0.14E-1 | 0.32E-1 | 0.17E-1 | 0.84E-2 | 0.47E-0 | 0.84E-2 | 0.64E-0 |
| $2^{-8}$ | 0.78E-2 | 0.12E-2 | 0.16E-1 | 0.19E-2 | 0.46E-2 | 0.17E-0 | 0.46E-2 | 0.24E-0 |
| $2^{-9}$ | 0.42E-2 | 0.06E-2 | 0.82E-2 | 0.09E-2 | 0.83E-2 | 0.13E-0 | 0.83E-2 | 0.18E-0 |

has been observed in the errors computed using the Milstein scheme. Again, the Milstein method shows a first-order accuracy for this linear system. Hence, our next computations are realized with the Milstein scheme only. It should be stressed that, in our simulations the computational times required for the Milstein scheme is about 1.5 times the computational time needed for the Euler scheme. It may be noted that 10,000 realizations were sufficient for a weak convergence of the computations. The CPU times must be taken as indicative since the absolute numbers can vary with the state and configuration of the operating system.

### 13.4.3 Numerical Solution of the Stochastic Prebiotic System

Now, we turn our attention to the stochastic prebiotic system (13.2). We present numerical simulations for the prototype model sketched in Fig. 13.1. The model accounted for four catalyzed selfreplicator species along with an activated and inactivated residues. The kinetic rates $(k_{ij})_{1 \le i,j \le 4}$ are entries of the following matrix:

$$\mathbf{K} = \begin{pmatrix} K_1 \\ \\ K_2 \\ \\ K_3 \\ \\ K_4 \end{pmatrix} = \begin{pmatrix} 0.5 & 1.6 & 0.0 & 2.2 \\ \\ 1.5 & 1.0 & 2.0 & 0.0 \\ \\ 0.5 & 0.0 & 0.6 & 0.4 \\ \\ 0.1 & 0.0 & 0.0 & 0.0 \end{pmatrix}, \tag{13.63}$$

where $K_i$ for $i = 1, \dots, 4$, denote the row vectors of the matrix $\mathbf{K}$. The remaining coefficients are set to $\gamma = 1$, $\alpha_i = 1$ and $\delta_i = 0.1$ for $i = 1, \dots, 4$. Initial conditions are randomly chosen in such a way that the concentration of the sum of all the species is equal and arbitrarily fixed as 1, i.e.

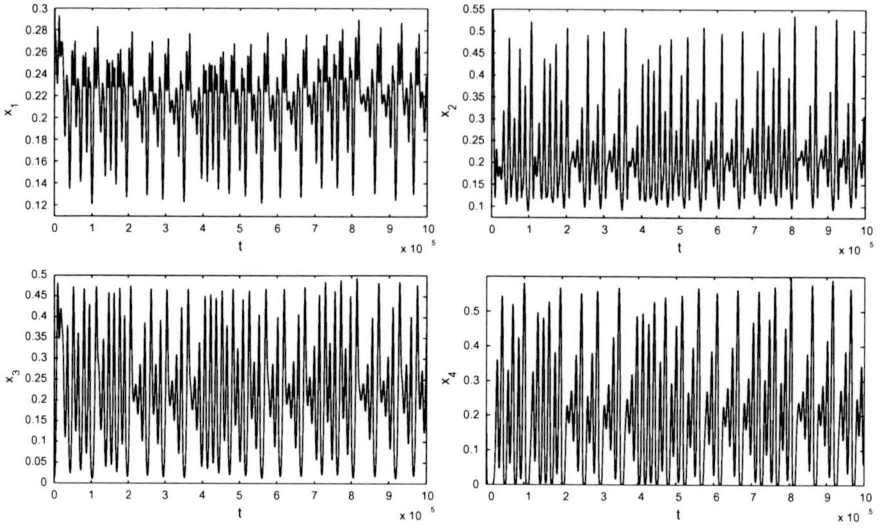


**Fig. 13.5** Time series for the four catalyzed species in the test case with additive noise

$$\sum_{i=1}^{4} x_{i,t_0} + y_{t_0} + z_{t_0} = 1.$$

Two physical stochastic excitations are used: stochastic forces driven by additive noise, that mimic a vast prebiotic scenario in which the mean effects of the medium are negligible, and stochastic forces driven by multiplicative noise, which would arise in a scenario when there is interchange of material with the surroundings. In all our simulations presented, the time step is fixed to $\Delta t = 0.1$ and the obtained results are displayed at time $t = 10^6$.

First, we consider the case with additive noise. Thus, the diffusion matrix in the system (13.3) is a $6 \times 6$-matrix given by

$$\mathcal{G}(t, \mathbf{X}(t)) = \sigma \begin{pmatrix} \mathbf{K} & \mathbf{0} \\ \mathbf{0} & \mathbf{0} \end{pmatrix}, \tag{13.64}$$

where $\mathbf{K}$ is the kinetic matrix given in (13.63) and $\sigma$ is a parameter fixed in our simulations to $\sigma = 10^{-2}$. In Fig. 13.5 we display time series for the four catalyzed selfreplicator species. Using these series, global attractors are illustrated in Fig. 13.6. From the obtained time series we see an important contribution of frequencies that correspond to high order periods. This fact is a consequence of the coexistence of different attractors such as chaos, chaotic bands and fixed points (which appear perturbed by the stochastic excitation). Note that the contribution of the stochastic perturbation to the time series and chaotic attractors is evident through the different frequencies that correspond to high order periods. It is interesting to remark that

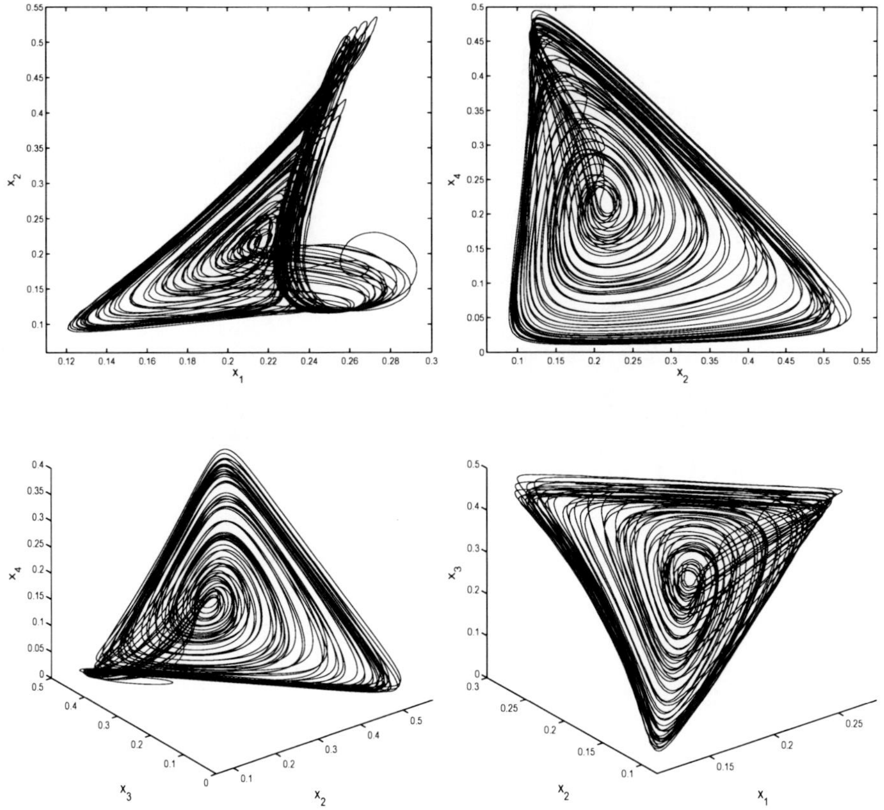

Fig. 13.6 Consecutive global attractors obtained for the four catalyzed species in the test case with additive noise

some fluctuations are present in the attractors shown in Fig. 13.6. These fluctuations are due to the presence of stochastic terms in the system (13.2) and can be reduced either by decreasing the stochastic amplitude $\sigma$ in (13.64) or increasing the number of realizations used for constructing mean solutions.

It should be pointed out that, the deterministic dynamics of this model (obtained after removing the stochastic terms by setting $\sigma = 0$) has already been analyzed in a relevant but restricted situation, a system formed by cyclically linked species (a hypercycle) in [8, 15]. Perhaps, the most relevant property of this special network is that it allows the coexistence of all species involved in the organization. Moreover, whereas for networks formed by less than four species the fixed point of coexistence is asymptotically stable, for networks larger than four, this fixed point becomes unstable appearing surrounded by a cyclic limit. This fact has special significance when the stochastic process is taken into account in the model as can be seen from the results presented in Fig. 13.6.

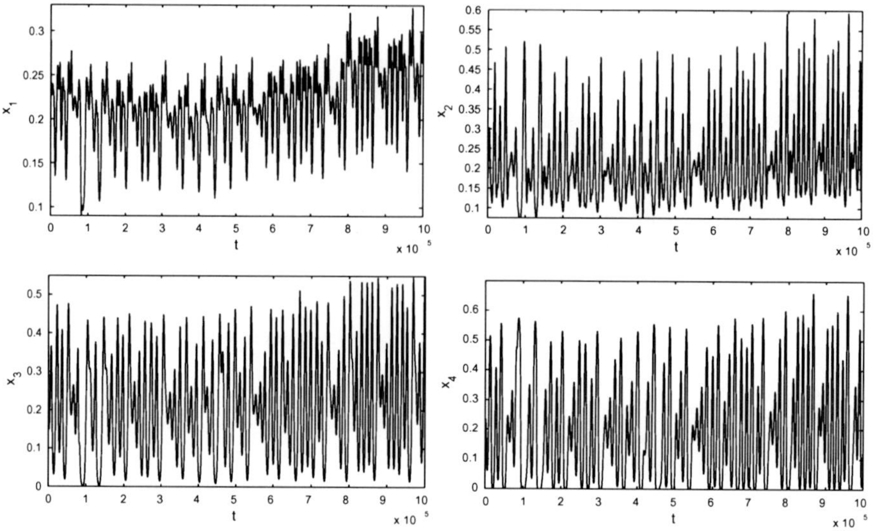


**Fig. 13.7** Time series for the four catalyzed species in the test case with multiplicative noise

Finally, we consider the case with a multiplicative noise given by the following diffusion $6 \times 6$-matrix in (13.3)

$$\mathcal{G}(t, \mathbf{X}(t)) = \sigma \begin{pmatrix} K_1\mathcal{X}(t) & 0 & 0 & 0 & 0 & 0 \\ 0 & K_2\mathcal{X}(t) & 0 & 0 & 0 & 0 \\ 0 & 0 & K_3\mathcal{X}(t) & 0 & 0 & 0 \\ 0 & 0 & 0 & K_4\mathcal{X}(t) & 0 & 0 \\ 0 & 0 & 0 & 0 & 0 & 0 \\ 0 & 0 & 0 & 0 & 0 & 0 \end{pmatrix}, \tag{13.65}$$

where $\mathcal{X}(t) = (x_1(t), x_2(t), \ldots, x_N(t))^T$ and $K_i$ is the $i$-th row of the matrix $\mathbf{K}$ in (13.63). Note that, unlike the previous test case, the considered case is a problem coupled in nature with strong stochastic perturbation and therefore, good numerical accuracy is required in order to capture the different phenomena present in its evolving solution. As a consequence, the later test case is more difficult to handle; the results shown here illustrate the robustness of the Milstein method. Note that for the diffusion matrix (13.65), the double Itô integrals $\int_{0,i \neq j, i,j=1,2}^{\Delta t} W_s^{(i)} W_s^{(j)}$ are non zero in the Milstein method resulting in more computations to be done compared to the case with additive noise (13.64).

Figure 13.7 shows the time series for the four catalyzed selfreplicator species. The associated phase-portraits for the four catalyzed species are illustrated in Fig. 13.8. Formation of complex dynamics can be clearly seen from the presented results. Starting from randomly distributed concentrations, stationary states are reached exhibiting clusters with different scales. We have also observed that the convergence to these

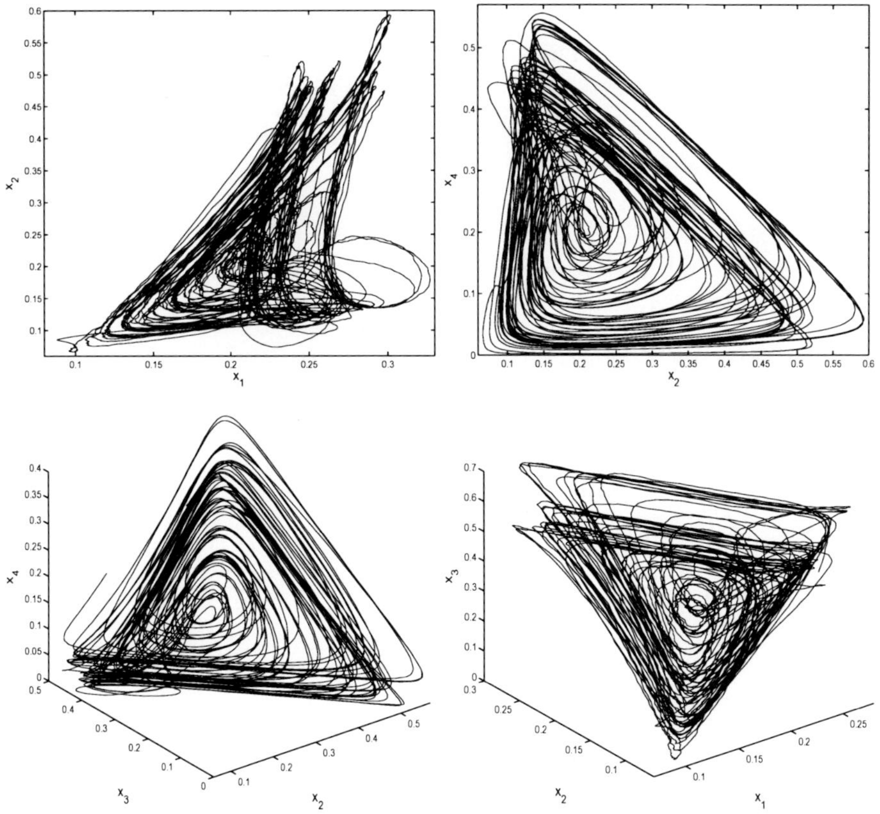


**Fig. 13.8** Consecutive global attractors obtained for the four catalyzed species in the test case with multiplicative noise

stationary states depends on the kinetic coefficients and the amplitude of stochastic excitations. We should mention that for the deterministic model, periodically distributed aggregates appear in the formed dynamics. However, for the stochastic model, this periodicity is broken and regions with a high concentration of replicators are separated from lower concentration ones, and the boundaries between the clusters remain almost constant in time. Formally, the Hop bifurcation can be investigated by analyzing the six eigenvalues of the linearization at zero as functions of the parameter $\alpha_i$. In the considered stochastic case the analysis is rather complicated. Indeed, the above mentioned eigenvalues need to be replaced by the Lyapunov exponents of the stochastic system (13.2). In this case the origin remains as a stable fixed point as long as the first Lyapunov exponent $\lambda_1$ (as a function of the bifurcation parameter $\alpha_i$) be negative. Hence, stability is lost when $\lambda_1$ becomes positive and six different qualitative behavior emerges, which depends on the sign of the other five Lyapunov exponents. Finally, the results presented in this study strengthen the hypothesis of a prebiotic scenario with stochastic reactions where all the metabolic necessities were carried out by RNA-like molecules. However, it is not clear where and when these stochastic excitations should be implemented in the kinetic reactions since no experimental information is provided regarding these issues. Further investigations are therefore, required to give an explanation to the origin of cellular structures.

## References

1. Abdulle A, Pavliotis GA (2012) Numerical methods for stochastic partial differential equations with multiple scales. J Comput Phys 231(6):2482–2497
2. Almeida RC, Oden JT (2010) Solution verification, goal-oriented adaptive methods for stochastic advection-diffusion problems. Comput Methods Appl Mech Eng 199(37–40):2472–2486
3. Angstmann CN, Donnelly IC, Henry BI, Jacobs B, Langlands TA, Nichols JA (2016) From stochastic processes to numerical methods: a new scheme for solving reaction subdiffusion fractional partial differential equations. J Comput Phys 307:508–534
4. Chacón P, Nuno J (1995) Spatial dynamics of a model for prebiotic evolution. Phys D: Nonlinear Phenom 81(4):398–410
5. Chekroun MD, Park E, Temam R (2016) The stampacchia maximum principle for stochastic partial differential equations and applications. J Differ Equ 260(3):2926–2972
6. Company R, Ponsoda E, Romero JV, Roselló MD (2009) A second order numerical method for solving advection-diffusion models. Math Comput Model 50(5–6):806–811
7. Doudna JA, Szostak JW (1989) RNA-catalysed synthesis of complementary-strand RNA. Nature 339(6225):519
8. Eigen M, Schuster P (1982) Sigmund, from biological macro-molecules to protocells: the principle of early evolution. Springer, Berlin
9. Eigen M, Schuster P (1979) The hypercycle, a principle of natural self-organization. Springer, New York
10. El-Amrani M, Seaid M, Zahri M (2012) A stabilized finite element method for stochastic incompressible navier-stokes equations. Int J Comput Math 89(18):2576–2602
11. Forst CV (1996) Chaotic interactions of self-replicating RNA. Comput Chem 20(1):69–83
12. Ghanem RG, Spanos PD (1991) Stochastic finite elements: a spectral approach. Springer, New York
13. Giletti T (2011) Traveling waves for a reaction-diffusion-advection system with interior or boundary losses. Comptes Rendus Math 349(9–10):535–539
14. Gropp W, Smith B (1993) Scalable, extensible, and portable numerical libraries. In: Proceedings of scalable parallel libraries conference. IEEE, pp 87–93
15. Hofbauer J, Schuster P (1984) Dynamics of linear and nonlinear autocatalysis and competition in stochastic phenomena and chaotic behavior in complex systems. Springer, Berlin
16. Itô K (1944) Stochastic integral. Proc Imp Acad 20(8):519–524
17. Itô K (1951) Multiple wiener integral. J Math Soc Jpn 3(1):157–169
18. Jentzen A, Kloeden PE (2011) Taylor approximations for stochastic partial differential equations, vol 83. SIAM, Philadelphia
19. Karatzas I, Shreve SE (1998) Brownian motion and stochastic calculus, 2nd edn. Graduate texts in mathematicals. Springer, New York. http://cds.cern.ch/record/396069
20. Klöden PE, Platen E (1992) Numerical solution of stochastic differential equations. Springer, Berlin
21. Kloeden P, Platen E (1999) The numerical solution of stochastic differential equations. Springer, Berlin
22. Kloeden P, Platen E, Schurz H (1994) Numerical solution of SDE through computer experiments. Springer, Berlin
23. Mai-Duy N, Tran-Cong T (2008) An efficient domain-decomposition pseudo-spectral method for solving elliptic differential equations. Commun Numer Methods Eng 24(10):795–806

24. Manouzi H, Seaı M, Zahri M et al (2007) Wick-stochastic finite element solution of reaction-diffusion problems. J Comput Appl Math 203(2):516–532
25. Mathew T (2008) Domain decomposition methods for the numerical solution of partial differential equations, vol 61. Springer Science & Business Media
26. Milstein G (1995) Numerical integration of stochastic differential equations. Kluwer Akademic Publishers, Dordrecht
27. Milstein G, Tretyakov MV (2016) Layer methods for stochastic navier-stokes equations using simplest characteristics. J Comput Appl Math 302:1–23
28. Milstein GN, Tretyakov MV (2004) Stochastic numerics for mathematical physics. Springer, Berlin
29. Mohamed K, Seaid M, Zahri M (2013) A finite volume method for scalar conservation laws with stochastic time-space dependent flux functions. J Comput Appl Math 237(1):614–632
30. Narayanan VAB, Zabaras N (2005) Variational multiscale stabilized fem formulations for transport equations: stochastic advection-diffusion and incompressible stochastic navier-stokes equations. J Comput Phys 202(1):94–133
31. Nishikawa H (2010) A first-order system approach for diffusion equation. ii: unification of advection and diffusion. J Comput Phys 229(11):3989–4016
32. Nuño JC, Chacón P, Moreno A, Morán F (1995) Compartimentation in replicator models. In: Proceedings of the 3rd European conference on advances in artificial life. Springer, London, UK, pp 116–127
33. Quarteroni A, Valli A (1999) Domain decomposition methods for partial differential equations. Oxford University Press, Oxford
34. Quarteroni A, Veneziani A, Zunino P (2002) A domain decomposition method for advection-diffusion processes with application to blood solutes. SIAM J Sci Comput 23(6):1959–1980
35. Rößler A, Seaïd M, Zahri M (2008) Method of lines for stochastic boundary-value problems with additive noise. Appl Math Comput 199(1):301–314
36. Rößler A, Seaïd M, Zahri M (2009) Numerical simulation of stochastic replicator models in catalyzed RNA-like polymers. Math Comput Simul 79(12):3577–3586
37. Schiesser W (1991) The numerical method of lines: integration of partial differential equations. Academic Press, Cambridge
38. Smith B, Bjorstad P, Gropp W (2004) Domain decomposition: parallel multilevel methods for elliptic partial differential equations. Cambridge University Press, Cambridge
39. Smith BF, Widlund OB (1990) A domain decomposition algorithm using a hierarchical basis. SIAM J Sci Stat Comput 11(6):1212–1220
40. Tveito AMBA, Bruaset AM (2006) Numerical solution of partial differential equations on parallel computers. Springer, Berlin
41. Verwer JG, Sanz-Serna JM (1984) Convergence of method of lines approximations to partial differential equations. Computing 33(3–4):297–313
42. Zafarullah A (1970) Application of the method of lines to parabolic partial differential equations with error estimates. J ACM (JACM) 17(2):294–302
43. Zahri M (2010) Numerical solution of a stochastic lorenz attractor. J Num Mat Stoch 2:1–11
44. Zahri M (2014) Multidimensional milstein scheme for solving a stochastic model for prebiotic evolution. J Taibah Univ Sci 8(2):186–198
45. Zahri M (2018) Barycentric interpolation of interface solution for solving stochastic partial differential equations on non-overlapping subdomains with additive multi-noises. Int J Comput Math 95(4):645–685
46. Zahri M, Al Madinah K (2012) On numerical schemes for solving a stochastic advection-diffusion. Int J Pure Appl Math 77(5):681–694
47. Zahri M, Seaïd M, Manouzi H, El-Amrani M (2005) Wiener-itô chaos expansions and finite-volume solution of stochastic advection equations. Finite volumes for complex applications IV. ISTE, London, pp 525–538

# Chapter 14
# A Review of Compartmental Mathematical Models Used in Diabetology

**Abdesslam Boutayeb, Mohamed E. N. Lamlili and Wiam Boutayeb**

**Abstract** This chapter is devoted to a review of compartmental mathematical models used for diabetes. Usually, compartmental models are used for communicable diseases for which dynamics is governed by the evolution of the disease based on the number of susceptible people that may become infected after a contact with infectious people. However, disease transmission is not a mandatory condition for the evolution from one compartment to another. In the case of diabetes, the main problem is not with diabetes but rather with complications of diabetes. Consequently, it is interesting to consider the evolution of diabetic people from the stage of diabetes without complication (compartment D) to the stage of diabetes with complications (compartment C) in order to see how to avoid or at least to delay as far as possible occurrence of complications. Stressing that dynamic should not be regarded in the usual way of transmitted diseases but rather as a probabilistic evolution from one stage to another, many authors have considered the evolution from pre-diabetes or diabetes without complications to diabetes with complications. Different mathematical tools were and are used, including discrete mathematics, ordinary differential equations, partial differential equations, optimal control, numerical approximations and stochastic approaches.

A. Boutayeb (✉)
Emirates Aviation University, Dubai, UAE
e-mail: x.boutayeb@gmail.com

University Mohamed Ier, Oujda, Morocco

M. E. N. Lamlili
Laboratory of Stochastic and Deterministic Modelling (LaSDM), Faculty of Sciences, University Mohamed Ier, Oujda, Morocco
e-mail: mohamed.lamlili@gmail.com

W. Boutayeb
School of High Studies in Engineering, Oujda, Morocco
e-mail: wiam.boutayeb@gmail.com



A. Boutayeb (ed.), *Disease Prevention and Health Promotion in Developing Countries*,
https://doi.org/10.1007/978-3-030-34702-4_14

## 14.1 Introduction

According to the World Health Organisation (WHO), the term diabetes mellitus describes a metabolic disorder of multiple aetiology characterised by chronic hyperglycemia with disturbances of carbohydrate, fat and protein metabolism, resulting from defect in insulin secretion, insulin action, or both. The three main types of diabetes are: (1) type1 diabetes (previously known as insulin-dependent, juvenile or childhood-onset), characterized by deficient insulin production and requires daily administration of insulin; (2) type2 diabetes (formerly called non-insulin-dependent, or adult-onset); and (3) gestational diabetes which occurs during pregnancy (blood-glucose values above normal but below those diagnosed with diabetes) [41]. Statistics released by the International Diabetes Federation (IDF) in 2017 indicate that 4 out of 5 people with diabetes live in low and middle-income countries; half of the 4 million who die from diabetes are under the age of 60 years. Prevalence of diabetes in people aged 20–79 years is expected to increase by nearly 50% globally between 2017 (425 million) and 2045 (629 million). The greatest increase will be seen in Africa (156%) and Middle East and North Africa (110%) (Table 14.1) [29].

During the last decades the number of mathematical models proposed to deal with different aspects of diabetes has grown considerably as shown by a multitude of reviews [3, 7, 8, 11, 31, 32, 34, 37]. Mathematical modelling for diabetes generally concentrates on different aspects of diabetes such as the homeostasis of glucose; glycated haemoglobin (HbA1C); computer algorithms and devices; insulin and chemical reactions; dynamical systems of populations of diabetes with and without complications; and socioeconomic burden of diabetes. However, the majority of mathematical models are dedicated to the dynamics of glucose in relation with insulin, beta-cells, alpha-cells, glucagon, free fatty acids, leptine and growth hormone. A previous review was dedicated to this part of mathematical modelling while the present review deals with the compartmental models describing, simulating and

**Table 14.1** Prevalence of diabetes in people aged 20–79 years as estimated in 2017 and expected for 2045 [29]

| Region | Prevalence 2017 (million) | Expected prevalence 2045 (million) | Increase (%) |
|---|---|---|---|
| North America and Caribbean | 46 | 62 | 35 |
| Middle East and North Africa | 39 | 82 | 110 |
| Europe | 58 | 67 | 16 |
| South and Central America | 26 | 42 | 62 |
| Africa | 16 | 41 | 156 |
| South East Asia | 82 | 151 | 84 |
| Western Pacific | 159 | 183 | 15 |
| World | 425 | 629 | 48 |

analysing the dynamics of diabetic populations with and without complications. The dynamics of populations of diabetes is relatively a new aspect of modelling developed during the last two decades.

It should be stressed that in the 1990s, journals reviewers were very reluctant to accept papers proposing compartmental models for diabetes, claiming that these kind of models are used for transmissible diseases while diabetes is a non communicable disease. It was, however, clear to see that disease transmission was not a mandatory condition for the evolution from one compartment to another. In the case of diabetes, the main problem is not with diabetes but rather with complications of diabetes. Consequently, it is wise to consider the evolution of diabetic people from the stage of diabetes without complication (compartment D) to the stage of diabetes with complications (compartment C) in order to see how to avoid or at least to delay as far as possible occurrence of complications. Moreover, other copmartments can be considered such as the pre-diabetes stage or diabetes with and without diagnosis.

## 14.2 Discrete Compartmental Models

In 2002, Boutayeb and Derouich [13] proposed an age structured discrete mathematical model for diabetes.

They assumed the following:

- Events such as birth, death and recovery occur every 15 years
- The number of males equals the number of females
- At birth there is no complication of diabetes

Then a compartmental mathematical model was proposed to monitor the size of each subpopulation as a function of age and time. Obviously, diabetes is not contagious, nor are the complications. So, the authors stressed that dynamic should not be regarded in the usual way of transmitted diseases but rather as a probabilistic evolution from one stage to another. The main purpose of the mathematical model was to show that the proportion of diabetics with complications should and can be kept as small as possible if efficient measures are taken to let people aware of the risks and also by giving them the means of regular control and diabetic education (Fig. 14.1).

The subpopulations of diabetics without complication ($D_k(t)$) and diabetics with complications ($C_k(t)$) are functions of age ($k$) and time ($t$) ( $D_k(t) + C_k(t) = n_k(t)$).

The model proposed was as follows

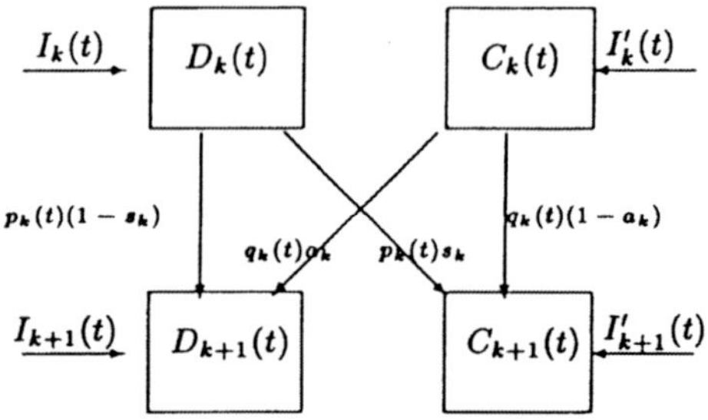


**Fig. 14.1** Dynamics of a population of diabetes with and without complications

$$D_0(t_{i+1}) = I_0(t_{i+1}) + \sum_{k=0}^{m} \frac{\theta(t_i)}{2}(\frac{1}{\gamma_k(t_i)} - 1)b_k(t_i)n_k(t_i) + \frac{\theta'(t_i)}{2}(b'_k(t_i)D_k(t_i) + b''_k(t_i)C_k(t_i)) \quad (14.1)$$

$$C_0(t_{i+1}) = 0 \quad (14.2)$$

$$D_{k+1}(t_{i+1}) = I_{k+1}(t_{i+1}) + p_k(t_i)D_k(t_i)(1 - s_k(t_{i+1})) + a_k(t_{i+1})q_k(t_i)C_k(t_i) \quad (14.3)$$

$$C_{k+1}(t_{i+1}) = I'_{k+1}(t_{i+1}) + q_k(t_i)C_k(t_i)(1 - a_k(t_{i+1})) + p_k(t_i)s_k(t_{i+1})D_k(t_i) \quad (14.4)$$

For $k = 0, 1, \ldots\ldots m-1$
with

$$I_{k+1}(t_{i+1}) = \frac{\varepsilon_k(t_i)}{\gamma'_k(t_i)}D_k(t_i) = \alpha_{k+1}(t_i)D_k(t_i) \quad (14.5)$$

$$I'_{k+1}(t_{i+1}) = \frac{\varepsilon'_k(t_i)}{\gamma''_k(t_i)}C_k(t_i) = \alpha'_{k+1}(t_i)C_k(t_i) \quad (14.6)$$

$$I_0(t_i) = \alpha_0(t_i)n_0(t_i) \quad (14.7)$$

Assuming that $b_k(t_i) = 0$, $b'_k(t_i) = 0$ and $b''_k(t_i) = 0$ for $k < A_0$ and $k > A_1$
Then a simplified model was obtained with $n_{k+1}(t_{i+1}) = D_{k+1}(t_{i+1}) + C_{k+1}(t_{i+1})$

$$n_0(t_{i+1}) = I_0(t_{i+1}) + \sum_{k=0}^{m} \frac{\theta(t_i)}{2}(\frac{1}{\gamma_k(t_i)} - 1)b_k(t_i)n_k(t_i) + \frac{\theta'(t_i)}{2}(b'_k(t_i)D_k(t_i) + b''_k(t_i)C_k(t_i)) \quad (14.8)$$

$$r_0(t_{i+1}) = 0 \quad (14.9)$$

$$n_{k+1}(t_{i+1}) = (p_k(t_i) + (q_k(t_i) - q_k(t_i))r_k(t_i)n_k(t_i) + \alpha_{k+1}(t_i)D_k(t_i) + \alpha'_{k+1}(t_i)C_k(t_i) \quad (14.10)$$

The rate $r_k(t_i)$ satisfies the recurrence relation:

$$r_{k+1}(t_{i+1}) = \frac{s_k(t_{i+1})p_k(t_i)(1 - r_k(t_i)) + (\alpha'_{k+1}(t_i) + q_k(t_i)(1 - a_k(t_{i+1})r_k(t_i)}{\alpha_{k+1}(t_i) + p_k(t_i) + (q_k(t_i)) + \alpha'_{k+1}(t_i) - \alpha_{k+1}(t_i) - p_k(t_i))r_k(t_i)} \quad (14.11)$$

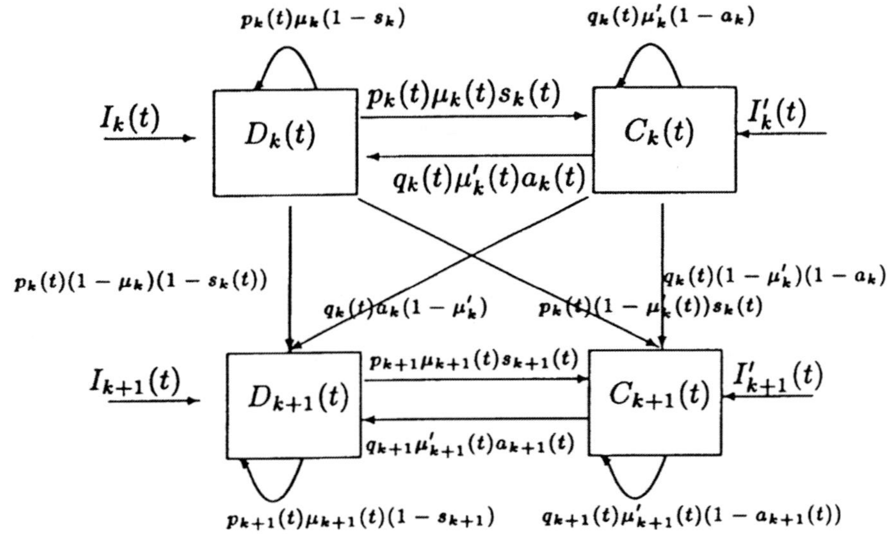


**Fig. 14.2** Dynamics of a population of diabetes with and without complications, events being registered at the beginning of the year

The authors proposed a second model in which they assumed that events such as birth, death, recovery, ...were registered at the beginning of the year while migration and immigration were neglected and the number of males equals the number of females(Fig. 14.2).

The second model was as follows

$$D_0(t_{i+1}) = \mu_0(t_i)D_0(t_i) + I_0(t_{i+1}) + \sum_{k=0}^{m} \frac{\theta(t_i)}{2}(\frac{1}{\gamma_k(t_i)} - 1)b_k(t_i)n_k(t_i)$$
$$+ \frac{\theta'(t_i)}{2}(b'_k(t_i)D_k(t_i) + b''_k(t_i)C_k(t_i)) \tag{14.12}$$
$$C_0(t_{i+1}) = 0 \tag{14.13}$$
$$D_{k+1}(t_{i+1}) = p_{k+1}(t_i)\mu_{k+1}(t_i)((1 - s_{k+1}(t_{i+1}))D_{k+1}(t_i)$$
$$+ q_{k+1}(t_i)\mu'_{k+1}(t_i)a_{k+1}(t_{i+1})C_{k+1}(t_i) + I_{k+1}(t_{i+1})$$
$$+ p_k(t_i)(1 - s_k(t_{i+1}))(1 - \mu_k(t_i))D_k(t_i)$$
$$+ a_k(t_{i+1})q_k(t_i)(1 - \mu'_{k+1}(t_i))C_k(t_i) \tag{14.14}$$
$$C_{k+1}(t_{i+1}) = q_{k+1}(t_i)\mu'_{k+1}(t_i)(1 - a_{k+1}(t_{i+1}))C_{k+1}(t_i)$$
$$+ p_{k+1}(t_i)\mu_{k+1}(t_i)s_{k+1}(t_{i+1}))D_{k+1}(t_i) + I'_{k+1}(t_{i+1})$$
$$+ q_k(t_i)(1 - a_k(t_{i+1}))(1 - \mu'_k(t_i))C_k(t_i)$$
$$+ p_k(t_i)s_k(t_{i+1})(1 - \mu_k(t_i))D_k(t_i) \tag{14.15}$$

For $k = 0, 1, \ldots\ldots m - 1$.

## 14.3 Continuous Compartmental Models Using Partial Differential Equations (Age Structure)

In 2004 Boutayeb and Twizell [14] used partial differential equations to model evolution from diabetes without complications to diabetes with complications. They proposed an age structured model as follows:

Denoting $C(a,t)$ and $D(a,t)$ the numbers of diabetics of age $a$ at time $t$, with and without complications, respectively. The size of the population of diabetics with and without complications is $n(a,t) = C(a,t) + D(a,t)$.

A schematic representation of the model is shown in Fig. 14.3.

The diagram shows that at age $a$ and time $t$, $I_2$ and $I_1$ people are diagnosed with diabetes with and without complications, respectively. The number of diabetics with complications is also increased by $psD$ (diabetics who get complications) and decreased by $d'C$ (people dying from natural mortality and mortality caused by complications). Meanwhile, the number of diabetics without complications is increased by $qeC$ (diabetics whose complications are cured) and decreased by $psD$ and $dD$.

Assuming that the number of males is equal to the number of females and that diabetes affects people of the two sexes equally, the continuous age structured model was formalized by the following partial differential equations:

$$\frac{\partial D}{\partial t} + \frac{\partial D}{\partial a} = -dD - psD + qeC + I_1 \tag{14.16}$$

$$\frac{\partial C}{\partial t} + \frac{\partial C}{\partial a} = -d'D + psD - qeC + I_2 \tag{14.17}$$

$$\frac{\partial n}{\partial t} + \frac{\partial n}{\partial a} = -dD - d'D + I_1 + I_2 \tag{14.18}$$

Replacing the death rate $d$ by $d + \delta$,the equation for $n$ becomes

$$\frac{\partial n}{\partial t} + \frac{\partial n}{\partial a} = -dn - \delta C + I_1 + I_2 \tag{14.19}$$

$$C(a,t) = r(a,t)n(a,t) \tag{14.20}$$

Differentiating with respect to $t$ and $a$ and using simple algebraic operations, the authors ended up with the following equation

$$\frac{\partial r}{\partial t} + \frac{\partial r}{\partial a} = \delta r^2 - \varepsilon r + \omega \tag{14.21}$$

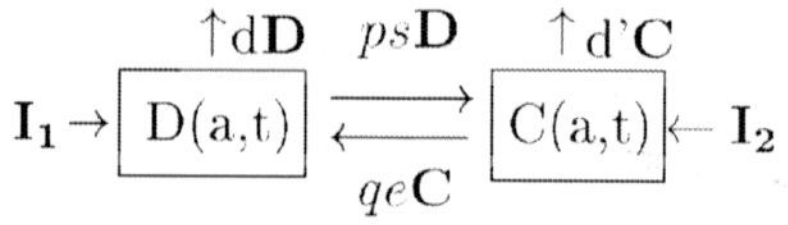


**Fig. 14.3** A schematic representation of the model

where
$\delta = \delta(a, t), \quad \varepsilon = \varepsilon(a, t) = [p(a, t)s(a, t) + e(a, t)q(a, t) + \delta(a, t) + \alpha(a, t)]$
and $\omega = \omega(a, t) = \alpha_2(a, t) + p(a, t)s(a, t)$

The boundary conditions at age zero ($a = 0$) were given by the expressions of $N(0, t)$ and $n(0, t)$,namely,

$$N(0, t) = \frac{1}{2}\int_0^A \beta_1(a, t)D(a, t) + \beta_2(a, t)C(a, t) + \beta_3(a, t)(N(a, t) - n(a, t))da \quad (14.22)$$

and

$$n(0, t)/N(0, t) = \tau(0, t) = \tau_1(0, t) + \tau_2(0, t) \quad (14.23)$$

leading to

$$r(0, t) = \frac{C(0, t)}{n(0, t)} = \frac{\tau_2(0, t)}{\tau(0, t)} \quad (14.24)$$

The initial condition was given by:

$$r(a, 0) = r_0(a) = \frac{C(a, 0)}{n(a, 0)} \quad (14.25)$$

Numerical approximations and different scenarios were proposed to estimate the following parameters:

- Natural death rate: $d_m^n = \frac{N}{N+n}(c_1 m - c_2)$
- Death rate due to complications: $\delta_m^n = c_3 \frac{N}{N+n} \exp(c_4 m)$
- Incidence of diabetes with and without complications $\alpha_m^n = c_5 m(1 - c_6 m)$
- Rate at which complications are developed:
  - Linear form for slow increase with age and decrease with time $p_m^n = c_7 + c_8 m - c_9 m$
  - Quadratic form for medium increase with age and decrease with time $p_m^n = c_{10} + c_{11} m^2 - c_{12} n$
  - Exponential form for rapid increase with age and decrease with time $p_m^n = (c_{13} + c_{14} m - c_{15} n) \exp(m)$
- Rate at which complications are developed $q_m^n = c_{16} \frac{n}{N+n} \frac{M}{M+m}$ (Table 14.2)

**Table 14.2** Values of the parameters used in the model

| Parameter | $c_1$ | $c_2$ | $c_3$ | $c_4$ | $c_5$ | $c_6$ | $c_7$ | $c_8$ |
|---|---|---|---|---|---|---|---|---|
| Value | 0.001 | 0.009 | 0.00005 | 0.448 | 0.0001 | 0.00067 | 0.00005 | 0.00004 |
| Parameter | $c_9$ | $c_{10}$ | $c_{11}$ | $c_{12}$ | $c_{13}$ | $c_{14}$ | $c_{15}$ | $c_{16}$ |
| Value | 0.00001 | 0.0001 | 0.00001 | 0.00001 | 0.006 | 0.00001 | 0.00001 | 0.001 |

## 14.4 Continuous Compartmental Models Using Ordinary Differential Equations

In 2004, Boutayeb et al. [15] proposed the following continuous model to deal with dynamics of diabetic populations with and without complications.

The numbers of diabetics with and without complications are denoted $C = C(t)$ and $D = D(t)$, respectively and $N = N(t) = C(t) + D(t)$ denotes the size of the population of diabetics at time $t$. The other variables and parameters used in the model are: the incidence of diabetes mellitus ($I = I(t)$), the natural mortality rate ($\mu$), the probability of a diabetic person developing a complication ($\lambda$), the rate at which complications are cured ($\gamma$), the rate at which diabetic patients with complications become severely disabled ($\nu$) and the mortality rate due to complications ($\delta$) (Fig. 14.4)

The diagram shows that $I = I(t)$ cases are diagnosed in a time interval of length t and are assumed to have no complications upon diagnosis. In that same time interval, the number of sufferers without complications, $D = D(t)$, is seen to decrease by the amounts $\mu D$ (natural mortality) and $\lambda D$ (sufferers who develop complications), and to increase by the amount $\gamma C$ (sufferers whose complications are cured). During this time interval, the number of diabetics with complications is increased by the aforementioned amount $\gamma C$ and by the amount $\mu C$ (natural mortality), $\nu C$ (patients who become severely disabled and whose disabilities cannot be cured) and $\delta C$ (those who die from their complications).

These rates of change are formalized by the ordinary differential equations (ODEs)

$$\frac{dD}{dt} = I(t) - (\mu + \lambda)D(t) + \gamma C(t) \; t > 0, \; D(0) = D_0 \tag{14.26}$$

$$\frac{dC}{dt} = \lambda D(t) - \theta C(t) \quad t > 0, \; C(0) = C_0 \tag{14.27}$$

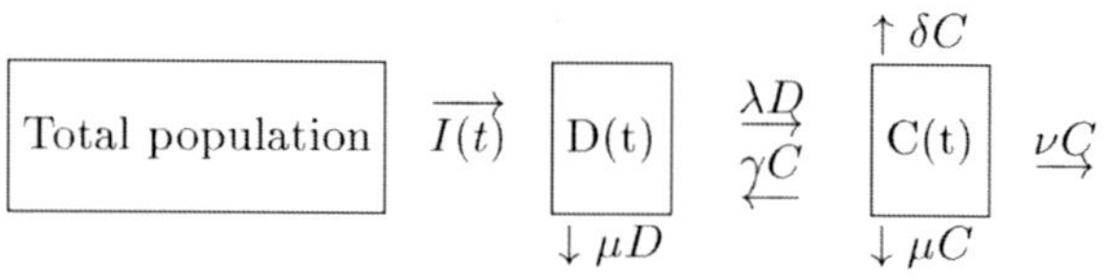


**Fig. 14.4** Dynamics of populations with and without complications

where $\theta = \gamma + \mu + \nu + \delta$, and $C_0$ , $D_0$are the initial values of $C(t)$ and $D(t)$, respectively.

Using $D(t) = N(t) - C(t)$, the previous equations give rise to the initial-value problem (IVP)

$$\frac{dC}{dt} = -(\lambda + \theta)C(t) + \lambda N(t)\ t > 0, C(0) = C_0 \tag{14.28}$$

$$\frac{dN}{dt} = I(t) - (\nu + \delta)C(t) - \mu N(t)\ t > 0, N(0) = N_0 \tag{14.29}$$

The authors used numerical approximations and numerical stability analysis to obtain and analyze numerical results, according to different scenarios. The main purpose was to stress the importance to control the incidence of diabetes and its complications and hence to convince decision makers that investment in healthcare is a cost-effective strategy.

In 2006, Boutayeb et al. [16] introduced non linearity in the model {(14.28)–(14.29)} as follows:

The authors stressed that in the case when the probability $\lambda$ of a diabetic person developing a complication, is constant, the ODEs in (14.27), (14.28) are linear in C(t) and N(t). Assuming that $\lambda$ depends on $C(t)$ and $N(t)$, gives rise to the following non-linear model

$$\lambda = \lambda(t) = \beta\frac{C(t)}{N(t)}, \qquad \beta > 0 \tag{14.30}$$

$$\frac{dC}{dt} = f_1(C, N) = (\beta - \theta)C(t) - \beta\frac{C^2}{N}\ t > 0,\ C(0) = C_0 \tag{14.31}$$

$$\frac{dN}{dt} = f_2(C, N) = I - (\nu + \delta)C(t) - \mu N(t)\ t > 0,\ N(0) = N_0 \tag{14.32}$$

They showed that this non linear model has two critical points, namely:

1. The trivial critical point: $C^* = 0,\ N^* = \dfrac{I}{\mu}$
2. The non-trivial critical point:

$$C^* = \frac{(\beta - \theta)I}{\mu\beta + (\nu + \delta)(\beta - \theta)},\quad N^* = \frac{\beta I}{\mu\beta + (\nu + \delta)(\beta - \theta)}$$

The authors carried out stability analysis to show that the trivial critical point is unstable while the non-trivial critical point is stable. Then they used an unconditionally numerical convergent method to monitor the numbers of patients in the population and, separately, those with complications.

In 2017, Rodrigues de Oliveira et al. [35] used the model {(14.30)–(14.32)} to show global stability of the system by constructing the following Liapunov function

$$V(C, N) = [(C - C^*) - C^* ln(\frac{C}{C^*})] + W[(N - N^*) - N^* ln(\frac{N}{N^*})] \tag{14.33}$$

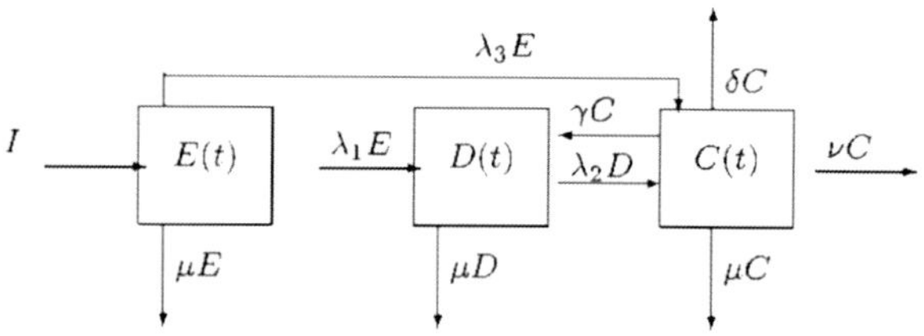


**Fig. 14.5** Dynamics of subpopulations of pre-diabetes ($E$), diabetes without complications ($D$) and diabetes with complications ($C$)

The Liapunov function satisfies $V(C^*, N^*) = 0$ and is positive for all other positive values of $C$ and $N$. The derivative of $V$ along the trajectories is given by

$$\frac{dV}{dt} = \frac{(C-C^*)}{C}\frac{dC}{dt} + W\left(1-\frac{N^*}{N}\right)\frac{dN}{dt} = (C-C^*)\left[(\beta-\theta)-\beta\frac{C}{N}\right]$$
$$+ W(1-\frac{N^*}{N})[I-(\nu+\delta)C(t)-\mu N(t) \qquad (14.34)$$

The authors also carried out numerical simulations.

In 2007, Boutayeb and Chetouani [12] considered a three compartmental model dealing with subpopulations of pre-diabetes ($E$), diabetes without complications ($D$) and diabetes with complications ($C$) (Fig. 14.5)

The model proposed was the following:

$$\frac{dE(t)}{dt} = I - (\mu+\lambda_3+\lambda_1)E(t) \qquad (14.35)$$
$$\frac{dD(t)}{dt} = \lambda_1 E(t) - (\mu+\lambda_2)D(t) + \gamma C(t) \qquad (14.36)$$
$$\frac{dC(t)}{dt} = \lambda_3 E(t) + \lambda_2 D(t) - (\mu+\gamma+\nu+\delta)C(t) \qquad (14.37)$$

where

$E = E(t)$ is the number of pre-diabetic people

$D = D(t)$ is the number of diabetics without complications

$C = C(t)$ is the number of diabetics with complications

$N = N(t) = E(t) + C(t) + D(t)$ denotes the size of the population of diabetics and pre-diabetics at time t

$I(t)$ denotes the incidence of pre-diabetes

$\mu$ : natural mortality rate,

$\beta 1$ : the probability of developing diabetes,

$\beta 2$ : the probability of a diabetic person developing a complication,

$\beta 3$ : the probability of developing diabetes at stage of complications,

$\gamma$ : rate at which complications are cured,

$\nu$ : rate at which patients with complications become severely disabled,

$\delta$ : mortality rate due to complications

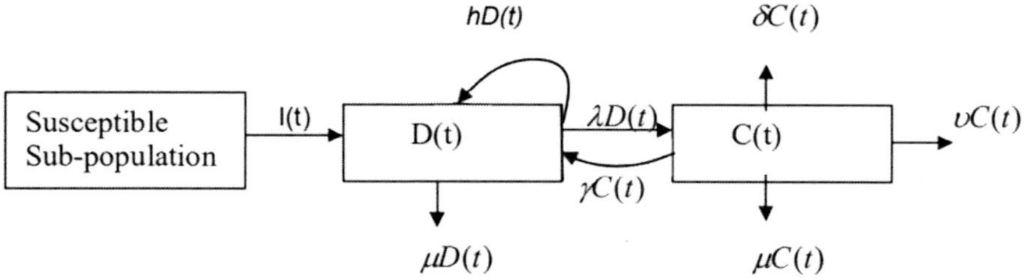


**Fig. 14.6** Dynamics of subpopulations of diabetes without complications ($D$) and diabetes with complications ($C$)

In this paper, the authors carried out stability analysis, numerical approximation and simulation.

In 2012 Adamu et al. [1] modified the model {(14.26)–(14.27)} and suggested another model defining susceptible as possessing the diabetic gene, they proposed that; a population generate non-diabetic non-susceptible sub-population, and a non-diabetic susceptible sub-population, the non-diabetic susceptible sub-population can further generate a population of diabetics without complication, who can later transit to a population with diabetic complications (Fig. 14.6).

The model proposed by these authors for the susceptible sub-population was as follows

$$\frac{dD}{dt} = I(t) - (\mu + \lambda - h)D(t) + \gamma C(t),\ D(0) = D_0 \tag{14.38}$$

$$\frac{dC}{dt} = \lambda(t))D(t) - (\gamma(t) + \mu(t) + v(t) + \delta(t))C(t),\ C(0) = 0 \tag{14.39}$$

They estimated "$h$" as $h = \frac{ex}{d}$, where " $ex$ " is the amout of calories burnt as a result of physical exercise, and "$d$" is the level of dietary calorie intake.

Assuming $I(t) = I$, they derive $\frac{dD}{dt}$ with respect to $t$ and obtain the second-order derivative $\frac{d^2D}{dt^2}$

$$\frac{d^2D}{dt^2} = (\mu + \lambda - h)^2 D(t) - (\mu + \lambda - h)\gamma C(t) - (\mu + \lambda - h)I + \gamma(\lambda(t))D(t) - \theta C(t)) \tag{14.40}$$

After some algebraic operations, they end up with the following second-order differential equation

$$\frac{d^2D}{dt^2} = -\sigma\frac{dD}{dt} + \beta D + \theta I$$

or

$$\frac{d^2D}{dt^2} + \sigma\frac{dD}{dt} - \beta D = \theta I \tag{14.41}$$

where
$\theta = \gamma + \mu + \nu + \delta$
$\sigma = \theta + \mu + \lambda - h)$
$\beta = \gamma\lambda - \lambda\theta - h\theta - \theta\mu$
The auxiliary equation of the homogeneous part is
$m^2 + \sigma m - \beta = 0$ giving roots
$m_1 = \dfrac{-\sigma + \sqrt{\sigma^2 + 4\beta}}{2}$ and $m_2 = \dfrac{-\sigma - \sqrt{\sigma^2 + 4\beta}}{2}$
With particular solution $D_p(t) = -\dfrac{\theta I}{\beta}$
The general solution of the quadratique in $D(t)$ is given by

$$D(t) = C_1 \exp(m_1)t + C_2 \exp(m_2)t - \frac{\theta I}{\beta} \tag{14.42}$$

Similarly, the solution of the quadratique in $C(t)$ is given by

$$C(t) = \frac{1}{\gamma}[C_1(-\eta_1 + \mu + \lambda - h)\exp(-\eta_1)t + C_2(-\eta_2 + \mu + \lambda - h)\exp(-\eta_2)t - \frac{(\mu + \lambda - h)\theta I}{\beta} - I] \tag{14.43}$$

where
$\eta_1 = \dfrac{\sigma + \sqrt{\sigma^2 + 4\beta}}{2}$ and $\eta_2 = \dfrac{\sigma - \sqrt{\sigma^2 + 4\beta}}{2}$
$C_1 = \dfrac{\beta D_0(-\eta_2 + \mu + \lambda - h) - \theta I \eta_2 - I\beta}{(\eta_1 - \eta_2)\beta}$
$C_2 = \dfrac{-\beta D_0(-\eta_1 + \mu + \lambda - h) + \theta I \eta_1 + I\beta}{(\eta_1 - \eta_2)\beta}$
The authors also carried out sensitivity analysis and limiting case behaviour
In 2016, Adamu et al. [2] introduced other modifications on their previous model and the model {(14.26)–(14.27)}.

The dynamics of their model was as follows: the number of diabetics without complications $DC(t)$ depletes by $\mu DC(t)$, $\beta DC(t)$ and $hDC(t)$ as a result of natural death, transition to the state of diabetes with complications and transition to the state of normalized blood sugar respectively, and increase by $\gamma C(t)$, $\rho(t)$ and $K$ as a result of recovery from complications, birth rate, and lost of normalized blood sugar respectively. The number of diabetes with complications $C(t)$ depletes by $\mu C(t)$, $\nu C(t)$, $\delta C(t)$, $\gamma C(t)$ as a result of natural death, developing disability, death from complications and recovery from complications, while it increases by $\beta DC(t)$ as a result of developing complications from $D(t)$. A further assumption concerned the subpopulation $SD(t)$ of disabled diabetic persons, excluded from the dynamics and further analysis because it is a class that cannot revert back to $DC(t)$, $DN(t)$ or $C(t)$

The model proposed was the following

$$\frac{dDC(t)}{dt} = \rho(t) - \beta I(t) - (\beta + \mu + h)DC(t) + KDN(t) + \gamma C(t) \tag{14.44}$$

$$\frac{dDN(t)}{dt} = hDC(t) - \mu DN(t) - KDN(t) \tag{14.45}$$

$$\frac{dC}{dt} = \beta DC(t) - (\gamma + \mu + \nu + \delta)C(t),\ D(0) = 0 \tag{14.46}$$

$C(0) = 0$ , $DC(0) = C_0$ and $DN(0) = D_0$

Stability analysis was carried out and the equilibrium points of the system were given by

$$DC(t) = \frac{\rho(t) + \gamma C(t)}{(\beta + \mu + h) - \dfrac{hK}{\mu + K}} \tag{14.47}$$

$$DN(t) = \frac{h(\rho(t) + \gamma C(t))}{(\mu + K)[(\beta + \mu + h) - \dfrac{hK}{\mu + K}]} \tag{14.48}$$

$$C(t) = \frac{\beta(\rho(t) + \gamma C(t))}{(\gamma + \nu + \delta))[(\beta + \mu + h) - \dfrac{hK}{\mu + K}]} \tag{14.49}$$

However, it seems that the last formula for $C(t)$ needs more algebraic calculus.

The disease free equilibrium state is given by

$$E_0 = \left( \frac{\rho(t)(\mu + K)}{[\beta + \mu + h)(\mu + K) - hK]}, \frac{h\rho(t)}{(\gamma + \nu + \delta))[(\beta + \mu + h) - \dfrac{hK}{\mu + K}]}, \right.$$

$$\left. \frac{\beta\rho(t)}{[(\gamma + \nu + \delta))[(\beta + \mu + h) - \dfrac{hK}{\mu + K}] - \gamma]} \right)$$

In 2017, Enagi et al. [26] applied the Homotopy Perturbation Method to the model {(14.26)–(14.27)} and showed that the solution of this system is given by:

$$C(t) = C_0 + \alpha t + \frac{1}{2}(\lambda\beta - \alpha q)t^2 \quad (14.50)$$

$$N(t) = N_0 + \beta t + \frac{1}{2}(-m\alpha - \mu\beta)t^2 \quad (14.51)$$

where
$\alpha = (-qC_0 + \lambda N)$
$\beta = (I - mC_0 - \mu N_0)$
$\theta = \gamma + \mu + \nu + \delta$
$q = \lambda + \theta$
$m = \nu + \delta$

The authors also used simulations with different values of the parameters and concluded that the results obtained using the Homotopy Perturbation method showed that the parameters involved played a crucial role in the size of population of diabetes at time t and the number of diabetics with complications.

In 2014, Akinsola et al. [4] modified the model of Boutayeb {(14.28)–(14.29)} just by introducing incidence $I$ in both compartments $D$ and $C$

The modified model proposed was as follows

$$\frac{dC}{dt} = I(t) - (\lambda + \theta)C(t) + \lambda N(t) \quad (14.52)$$

$$\frac{dN}{dt} = 2I(t) - (\nu + \delta)C(t) - \mu N(t) \quad (14.53)$$

The critical points were:

$$C^*(t) = \frac{(2\lambda + \mu)I(t)}{\lambda(\nu + \delta + \mu) + \theta\mu} \quad (14.54)$$

$$N^*(t) = \frac{(2(\lambda + \theta) - (\mu + \delta))I(t)}{\lambda(\nu + \delta + \mu) + \theta\mu} \quad (14.55)$$

The exact solution was obtained by deriving $\frac{dC(t)}{dt}$ and $\frac{dN(t)}{dt}$ with respect to $t$ and replacing to get second-order differential equations $\frac{d^2C(t)}{dt}$ and $\frac{d^2N(t)}{dt}$

The second-order derivatives in $C(t)$ was given by

$$\frac{d^2C(t)}{dt} + \sigma\frac{dC(t)}{dt} + \beta C(t) = \alpha I(t) \quad (14.56)$$

where
$\theta = \gamma + \mu + \nu + \delta$
$\sigma = \theta + \mu + \lambda$
$\beta = \lambda(\nu + \delta + \mu) + \theta\mu$
$\alpha = 2\lambda + \mu$

The solution was given by

$$m_1 = \frac{-\sigma + \sqrt{\sigma^2 + 4\beta}}{2} \quad \text{and } m_2 = \frac{-\sigma - \sqrt{\sigma^2 + 4\beta}}{2}$$

$$C(t) = K_1 \exp(m_1)t + K_2 \exp(m_2)t + \frac{\alpha}{\beta} I \tag{14.57}$$

$$N(t) = K_1 \exp(-m_1)t + K_2 \exp(-m_2)t + \frac{\alpha}{\beta} I + \frac{\theta}{\lambda} K_1 \exp(-m_1)t + \frac{\theta}{\lambda} K_1 \exp(-m_2)t$$
$$+ \frac{\alpha\theta}{\lambda\beta} I - \frac{I}{\lambda} - \frac{I}{\lambda}(K_1 m_1 \exp(-m_1)t + K_2 m_2 \exp(-m_2)t) \tag{14.58}$$

$$K_1 = \frac{\beta C_0(\lambda + \theta - m_2) + (\alpha m_2 - \beta)I - \lambda\beta N_0}{(\eta_1 - \eta_2)\beta} \tag{14.59}$$

$$K_2 = \frac{-\beta C_0(\lambda + \theta - m_1) - (\alpha m_1 - \beta)I + \lambda\beta N_0}{(\eta_1 - \eta_2)\beta} \tag{14.60}$$

The authors indicated that the model aided the understanding of diabetes, its complications and how it can be controlled. They investigated the stability of the equilibrium point and found it to be asymptotically stable. They affirmed also that, investigating the limiting case behaviour of each parameter in the analytic solution of the model depicts that if some measures are taken the number of diabetics with complications will be reduced to the bearest minimum.

In 2015, Akinsola et al. [5] considered again the model of Boutayeb {(14.28)–(14.29)} and presented a note on the divergence of the numerical solution of the mathematical model using Euler method. They used the exact solution obtained in their previous paper and the the Euler method

$$C_{n+1} = C_n + h(-(\theta + \lambda)C_n + \lambda C_n) \tag{14.61}$$

$$N_{n+1} = N_n + h(I - (\nu + \delta)C_n - \mu N_n) \tag{14.62}$$

In 2019, Akinsola et al. [6] used their previous model {(14.52)–(14.53)} and the exact solution obtained within and carried out numerical approximations and analysis. They concluded that "The parameter with the greatest impact was determined to be the rate at which complication are controlled ($\gamma$) using Eigenvalue Sensitivity Analysis (ESA) and Eigenvalue Elasticity Analysis(EEA). Numerical solutions of the formulated models were obtained using Euler method and Runge–Kutta method of order four. Numerical simulations of the analytic solutions were also obtained at various values".

In 2018, Widyaningsih et al. [42] proposed a mathematical model for the epidemiology of diabetes mellitus with lifestyle and genetic factors. These authors used the model {(14.28)–(14.29)} and modified it by considering that incidence is not constant but rather determined by lifestyle factors and genetic factors.

They proposed a model called susceptible diabetes complication (SDC) model, claiming that it is a mathematical model in the epidemiology of diabetes that takes into account lifestyle factors and genetic factors as causes of incidence and does not exclude disabilities from the population.

The SDC model proposed was as follows:

$$\frac{dS}{dt} = \alpha S + \alpha(1-\rho)(D+C) - \beta SD/N - \mu S \tag{14.63}$$
$$\frac{dD}{dt} = \alpha\rho(D+C) - (\lambda+\mu)D + \gamma C \tag{14.64}$$
$$\frac{dC}{dt} = \lambda D - (\gamma+\delta+\mu)C \tag{14.65}$$

with $S(0) > 0$, $D(0) > 0$, and $C(0) > 0$. The parameters $\alpha, \beta, \gamma, \delta, \lambda, \mu, \rho > 0$ and $0 \leq \rho \leq 1$ respectively denoted birth rate, interaction rate, recovery rate of complications, death rate due complications, occurrence rate of complications, natural mortality rate, and the proportion of genetic disorder's birth.

The authors used a fourth-order of Runge–Kutta algorithm to find the solution and then carried out numerical computation.

They based their model on the idea of including effect of lifestyle and genetic factors, explaining that "If the rate of interaction causing incidence is denoted by $\beta$, then the number of incidences that occur due to lifestyle factors is $\beta SD/N$". However, the way lifestyle and genetic factors are introduced in the model needs a serious discussion.

## 14.5 Compartmental Modelling with Optimal Control

In 2015, Bernard et al. [9] studied the limit cycle on the model {(14.26)–(14.27)}, their model assumed all parameters depending of time

$$\frac{dD}{dt} = I(t) - (\mu(t) + \lambda(t))D(t) + \gamma(t)C(t)\ t > 0,\ N(0) = N_0 \tag{14.66}$$
$$\frac{dC}{dt} = \lambda(t))D(t) - \theta(t)C(t)\ t > 0,\ C(0) = 0 \tag{14.67}$$

where $\theta = \gamma + \mu + \nu + \delta$

Stressing that other choices of control could be interesting, the authors choose the control $u(t) = \gamma(t)$, the rate at which complications are cured, based on the following theorem they proved:

**Theorem 15** *For all fixed control $u = \gamma$, there exists one and only one maximal solution $([0, t_m(u)], D_u(.), C_u(.))$ of the Cauchy problem {(14.66)–(14.67))} with initial conditions $D(0) = D_0 \in IR$, $C(0) = C_0 \in IR$, and $t_m(u) \in IR_+ \bigcup \{+\infty\}$.* □

Then they showed results by proving other theorems, including the following

**Theorem 16** *If* $\mu = 0, \alpha < 1 - \sigma^{-1}I$ *and* $r > I(1 - \alpha < 1 - \sigma^{-1}I \;)^{-1}$, *then there is an equilibrium state for the system*

$$\frac{dD(t)}{dt} = I(t) - (\mu(t) + \lambda(t))D(t) + \gamma(t)C(t) \tag{14.68}$$

$$\frac{dC(t)}{dt} = \lambda(t)D(t) - \theta(t)C(t) \tag{14.69}$$

$$\frac{dP_D(t)}{dt} = (r + \mu + \lambda)P_D(t) - \lambda P_C(t) - 1 \tag{14.70}$$

$$\frac{dP_C(t)}{dt} = (r + \mu + \nu + \delta)P_C(t) - (C(t))^{-1} + \gamma(P_C(t) - P_D(t)) \tag{14.71}$$

□

Beside the mathematical proofs of this theorem, it is important to stress that the assumption $\mu = 0$ is not realistic.

The authors showed existence of a control and carried out stability analysis. They concluded that by controlling the rate at which complications are cured, they could maximize the number of diabetics with complications which are cured and those without complications. Moreover, they showed that the evolution of complications of diabetics does not stabilize around the equilibrium state which is in fact a saddle point. Finally, they also stressed that it it will be interesting to see the influence of physical exercises, consumption and treatment on the number of diabetics with complications.

In 2018, Bernard et al. [10] presented another paper dedicated to unexistence of limit cycle in an optimal control problem of a population of diabetics based on the model {(14.26)–(14.27)}.

Following their previous paper in 2015, the authors stated that "Theoretically, any parameter of the model, that is $\lambda(t)$, $\mu(t)$, $\gamma(t)$, $\nu(t)$ or $\delta(t)$ can be chosen as control, but in practice, this is not possible since we cannot control the natural mortality rate for example. In this state of minds, we can control the probability of developing complications by informing the diabetic patients on a necessary good lifestyle with physical activity and healthy diet. We can also control the rate at which complications are healed or the rate at which patients with complications become severely disabled, with an increase of health expenditure. Consequently, in the following, $u$ can be chosen as $\lambda(t)$, $\gamma(t)$, $\nu(t)$"

They used a concave performance index $F(u; D; C)$, indicating, that in practice, their aim would be to minimize the complications in a population of diabetics. Consequently, $F$ can be a concave function, increasing with respect to $u = \gamma$ and/or $D$ and/or decreasing with respect to $u = \lambda$, $u = \nu$ and/or $C$.

The Hamiltonian was defined from the state equations and the concave performance index $F(u; D; C)$ as

$$H(u, D, C, P_D, P_C) = F(u, D, C) + P_D[I - (\mu + \lambda)D + \gamma C] + P_C(\lambda D - \theta C) \tag{14.72}$$

Then they showed, among others, the following two theorems

**Theorem 17** *Whatever the control u and whatever the concave performance index chosen as previously specified, there is an equilibrium state for the system*

$$\frac{dD(t)}{dt} = I(t) - (\mu(t) + \lambda(t))D(t) + \gamma(t)C(t) \tag{14.73}$$

$$\frac{dC(t)}{dt} = \lambda(t)D(t) - \theta(t)C(t) \tag{14.74}$$

$$\frac{dP_D(t)}{dt} = (r + \mu + \lambda)P_D(t) - \lambda P_C(t) - \frac{\partial F}{\partial D}(u, D, C) \tag{14.75}$$

$$\frac{dP_C(t)}{dt} = (r + \mu + \nu + \delta)P_C(t) - (C(t))^{-1} + \gamma(P_C(t) - \frac{\partial F}{\partial C}(u, D, C)) \tag{14.76}$$

□

**Theorem 18** *There is no limit cycle between the number of diabetics with complications, the one of diabetics without complications and the controlled parameter chosen as previously specified.* □

In 2014, Derouich et al. [24] added Optimal Control to the model {(14.35)–(14.37)}

$$\frac{dE(t)}{dt} = I - (\mu + \beta_3 + \beta_1)E(t) \tag{14.77}$$

$$\frac{dD(t)}{dt} = \beta_1 E(t) - (\mu + \beta_2)D(t) + \gamma C(t) \tag{14.78}$$

$$\frac{dC(t)}{dt} = \beta_3 E(t) + \beta_2 D(t) - (\mu + \gamma + \nu + \delta)C(t) \tag{14.79}$$

Where:
$E = E(t)$ is the number of pre-diabetic people
$D = D(t)$ is the number of diabetics without complications
$C = C(t)$ is the number of diabetics with complications
$N = N(t) = E(t) + C(t) + D(t)$ denotes the size of the population of diabetics and pre-diabetics at time t
$I(t)$ denotes the incidence of pre-diabetes
$\mu$ : natural mortality rate,
$\beta 1$ : the probability of developing diabetes ,
$\beta 2$ : the probability of a diabetic person developing a complication,
$\beta 3$ : the probability of developing diabetes at stage of complications,
$\gamma$ : rate at which complications are cured,
$\nu$ : rate at which patients with complications become severely disabled,
$\delta$ : mortality rate due to complications,
The controlled model is given by the following system

$$\frac{dE(t)}{dt} = I - (\mu + \beta_3 + \beta_1)(1 - u(t))E(t) \quad (14.80)$$

$$\frac{dD(t)}{dt} = \beta_1(1 - u(t))E(t) - (\mu + \beta_2)(1 - u(t))D(t) + \gamma C(t) \quad (14.81)$$

$$\frac{dC(t)}{dt} = \beta_3(1 - u(t))E(t) + \beta_2(1 - u(t))D(t) - (\mu + \gamma + \nu + \delta)C(t) \quad (14.82)$$

where $u$ is a control

The objective function is defined as

$$J(u) = \int_0^T (D(t) + C(t) + Au^2(t) + Bv^2(t))dt \quad (14.83)$$

Where $A$ is a positive weight that balances the size of the terms. $U$ is the control set defined by $U = \{u\text{measurable}, 0 \leq u(t) \leq 1, t \in [0, T]\}$

The objective is to characterize an optimal control $u^* \in U$ satisfying

$$J(u^*) = \min_{u \in U} J(u)$$

The authors proved the following results

1. Existence and Positivity of Solutions
2. The controlled system that satisfies a given initial condition $(E(0), D(0), C(0)) \in \Omega$ has a unique solution
3. There exists an optimal control $u* \in U$ such that $J(u^*) = \min_{u \in U} J(u)$
4. Given an optimal control $u^*$ and solutions $E^*$, $C^*$ and $D^*$ of the corresponding state system, there exist adjoint variables $\lambda_1$, $\lambda_2$and $\lambda_3$satisfying:

$$\frac{d\lambda_1}{dt} = (\lambda_1 - \lambda_2)(1 - u^*)\beta_1 + (\lambda_1 - \lambda_3)(1 - u^*)\beta_3 + \mu\lambda_1 \quad (14.84)$$

$$\frac{d\lambda_2}{dt} = -1 + \beta_2(1 - u^*)(\lambda_2 - \lambda_3) + \mu\lambda_2 \quad (14.85)$$

$$\frac{d\lambda_3}{dt} = -1 + (\lambda_3 - \lambda_2)\gamma + \lambda_3(\mu + \nu + \delta)\lambda_4 \quad (14.86)$$

With transversality conditions: $\lambda_1(T) = \lambda_2(T) = \lambda_3(T) = 0$

The optimal control is given by

$$u^* = \min[1, \max(0, \frac{1}{2A}[E^*\beta 1(\lambda 2 - \lambda 1) + E^*\beta 3(\lambda 3 - \lambda 1) + D^*\beta 2(\lambda 3 - \lambda 2)] \quad (14.87)$$

Numerical simulation

$$E_{i+1} = \frac{E_i + hI}{1 + h(\mu + (\beta_3 + \beta_1)(1 - u_i))} \tag{14.88}$$

$$D_{i+1} = \frac{D_i + h\beta_1(1 - u_i))E_{i+1} + h\gamma C_i}{1 + h(\mu + \beta_2(1 - u_i))} \tag{14.89}$$

$$C_{i+1} = \frac{C_i + h\beta_3(1 - u_i))E_{i+1} + h\beta_2(1 - u_i))D_{i+1}}{1 + h(\mu + \gamma + \nu + \delta)} \tag{14.90}$$

$$\lambda_1^{n-i-1} = \frac{\lambda_1^{n-i} + h\beta_1\lambda_2^{n-i}(1 - u_i) + h\beta_3\lambda_3^{n-i}(1 - u_i)}{1 + h(\mu + (\beta_3 + \beta_1)(1 - u_i))} \tag{14.91}$$

$$\lambda_2^{n-i-1} = \frac{\lambda_2^{n-i} + h\beta_2(1 - u_i))\lambda_3^{n-i-1}(\gamma + \nu_i) + h}{1 + h(\mu + \beta_2(1 - u_i))} \tag{14.92}$$

$$\lambda_3^{n-i-1} = \frac{\lambda_3^{n-i} + h\gamma\lambda_2^{n-i-1} + h}{1 + h(\mu + \gamma + \nu + \delta)} \tag{14.93}$$

$$M^{i+1} = \frac{1}{2A}[(\beta_1 E_{i+1}(\lambda_2^{n-i-1} - \lambda_1^{n-i-1}) + \beta_3 E_{i+1}(\lambda_3^{n-i-1} - \lambda_1^{n-i-1}) + \beta_2 D_{i+1}(\lambda_3^{n-i-1} - \lambda_2^{n-i-1})] \tag{14.94}$$

$$u_{i+1} = \min[1, \max(0, M^{i+1})$$

The authors recalled and stressed that the burden of diabetes can be reduced at three levels by controlling:

1. the number of people evolving from prediabetes to diabetes without complication $(\beta 1(1 - u(t)))$
2. the number of diabetic patients developing complications $(\beta 2(1 - u(t)))$
3. the number of people evolving directly from pre-diabetes to diabetes with complications due to delayed diagnosis $(\beta 3(1 - u(t)))$.

This model shows that, in a period of ten years, the population of diabetics without complications $(D(t))$ will increase by 26% and 40% with and without control respectively. More importantly, the population of diabetics with complications will increase by 104% without control while it will decrease by 74% in presence of optimal control (Table 14.3 and Fig. 14.7). This is not a mere mathematical result, pragmatic achievements can be obtained by sensitization for a healthy diet, promotion of physical activity, obesity control and smoking reduction. An optimal strategy will also need early diagnosis of diabetes and affordable treatment and healthcare in order to avoid complications or at least to delay their occurrence as far as possible.

In 2015, Boutayeb et al. [21] used optimal control on the previous model of Boutayeb et al. {(14.26)–(14.27)}

$$\frac{dD}{dt} = I - (\beta(1 - u) + \mu)D(t) + (\gamma + \nu)C(t)\ t > 0,\ N(0) = N_0 \tag{14.95}$$

$$\frac{dC}{dt} = \beta(1 - u)D(t) - (\gamma + \mu + \nu + \delta)C(t)\ t > 0,\ C(0) = C_0 \tag{14.96}$$

**Table 14.3** Simulation results and growth rates for $E(T)$, $D(T)$ and $C(T)$ with and without control

| Initial population ($10^6$) | $E(0) = 6.66$ | $D(0) = 10.20$ | $C(0) = 5.50$ |
|---|---|---|---|
| Population after 10 years without optimal control ($10^6$) | $E_1(n) = 1.96$ 70% decrease | $D_1(n) = 14.30$ 40% increase | $C_1(n) = 11.25$ 104% increase |
| Population after 10 years with optimal control ($10^6$) | $E_2(n) = 18.72$ 181% increase | $D_2(n) = 14.30$ 24% increase | $C_2(n) = 11.25$ 74% decrease |
| Difference due to optimal control ($10^6$) | $E_2(n) - E_1(n)$ $= -16.76$ | $D_2(n) - D_1(n)$ $= 1.68$ | $C_2(n) - C_1(n)$ $= 9.82$ |

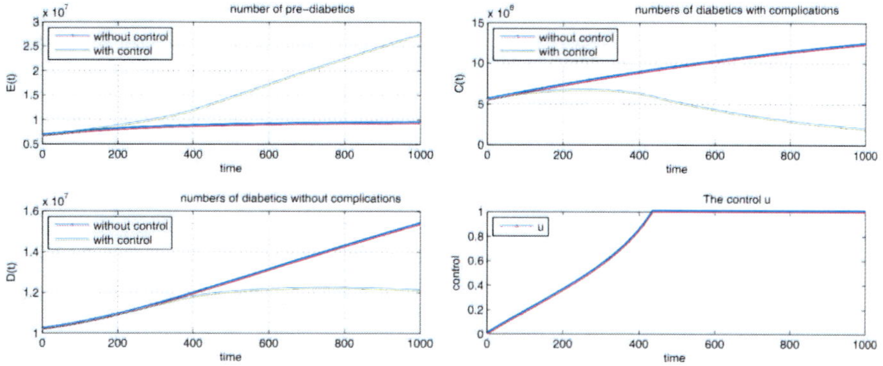


**Fig. 14.7** The effect of optimal control on the dynamics of the population of pre-diabetics and diabetics with and without complications

Where $u$ and $v$ are controls

The objective function is defined as

$$J(u, v) = \int_0^T (C(t) + Au^2(t) + Bv^2(t))dt \tag{14.97}$$

Where $A$ and $B$ are positive weights that balance the size of the terms. $U$ is the control set defined by $U = \{(u, v) \text{with} u \text{and} v \text{measurable}, 0 \leq u(t), v(t) \leq 1, t \in [0, T]\}$

The objective is to characterize an optimal control $(u^*, v^*) \in U$ satisfying:

$$J(u^*, v^*) = \min_{(u,v)\in U} J(u, v)$$

Existence of the optimal control was proved by using the results from Fleming and Rishel [27] and Pontryagin's maximum principle [38], leading to:

$$u^* = \min[1, \max(0, \frac{\lambda_2 - \lambda_1}{2A}\beta D^*(t)] \quad (14.98)$$

$$v^* = \min[1, \max(0, \frac{\lambda_2 - \lambda_1}{2B}C^*(t)] \quad (14.99)$$

For numerical simulations, the authors used the following Gauss–Seidel-like implicit finite-difference method, following Gumel et al. [28].

$$D_{i+1} = \frac{D_i + hI + h(\gamma + v_i)C_i}{1 + h(\mu + \beta(1 - u_i))} \quad (14.100)$$

$$C_{i+1} = \frac{C_i + h\beta(1 - u_i))D_{i+1}}{1 + h(\gamma + \mu + \delta + v_i)} \quad (14.101)$$

$$\lambda_1^{n-i-1} = \frac{\lambda_1^{n-i} + h\beta\lambda_2^{n-i}(1 - u_i)}{1 + h(\mu + \beta(1 - u_i))} \quad (14.102)$$

$$\lambda_2^{n-i-1} = \frac{\lambda_2^{n-i} + h\lambda_1^{n-i-1}(\gamma + v_i) + h}{1 + h(\gamma + \mu + \delta + v_i)} \quad (14.103)$$

$$M_1^{i+1} = \frac{1}{2A}(\lambda_2^{n-i-1} - \lambda_1^{n-i-1})\beta D_{i+1} \quad (14.104)$$

$$M_2^{i+1} = \frac{1}{2B}(\lambda_2^{n-i-1} - \lambda_1^{n-i-1})C_{i+1} \quad (14.105)$$

$$u_{i+1} = \min[1, \max(0, M_1^{i+1})] \quad (14.106)$$

$$v_{i+1} = \min[1, \max(0, M_2^{i+1})] \quad (14.107)$$

with $D_0 = D(0)$, $C_0 = C(0)$, $u_0 = 0$, $v_0 = 0$, $\lambda_2^n = \lambda_1^n = 0$

In summary, the model showed that without any control, diabetics having complications will represent 79% while the optimal control will lead to a total population with less than a third having complications (Figs. 14.8, 14.9). Consequently, the strategy with optimal control limits the number of diabetics with complications and hence reduces the rate of mortality caused by diabetes essentially due to complications (CVDs, kidney failure, amputations, blindness,...). Moreover, beyond mortality, the reduction of complications reduces the socio-economic burden of diabetes, including direct and indirect costs as well as intangible and not quantifiable costs such as inconvenience, anxiety, pain and more generally lower quality of life [17–19]. Concretely, achievement of optimal control can be obtained by acting on behavioral factors like healthy diet, physical activity, smoking and alcohol reduction; and metabolic risks like overweight/obesity and hypertension. Early diagnosis and efficient control of blood pressure provided by an affordable regular healthcare will also be needed.

In 2015, Yusuf [43] introduced optimal control on the model {(14.26)–(14.27)} as follows

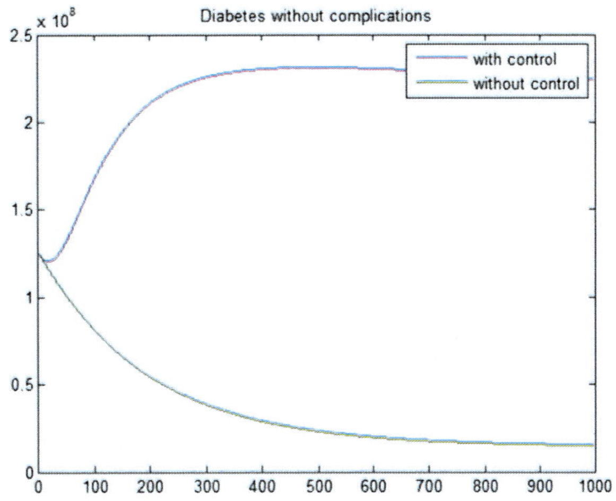


**Fig. 14.8** Evolution of the population of diabetics without complications, with and without control

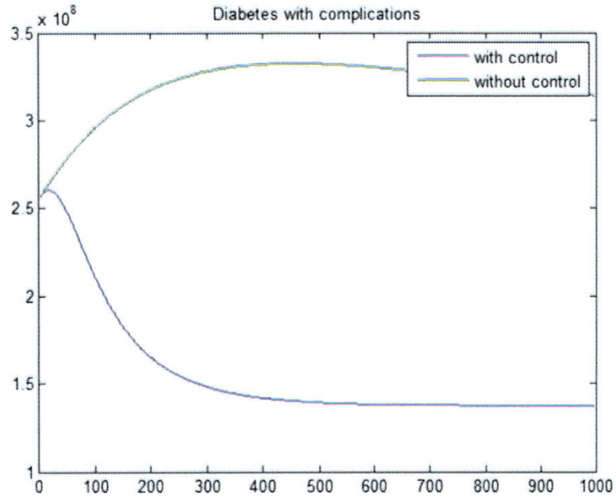


**Fig. 14.9** Evolution of the population of diabetics with complications, with and without control

$$\frac{dD}{dt} = \Lambda + u_2\gamma C - (1 - u_1)\nu D - \mu D \tag{14.108}$$

$$\frac{dC}{dt} = (1 - u_1)\nu D - u_2\gamma C - \mu C - \delta C \tag{14.109}$$

$$\frac{dN}{dt} = \Lambda - \mu N - \delta C \tag{14.110}$$

Where $u$ and $v$ are controls

The objective function is defined as:

$$Z = \min_{u_1,u_2} \int_0^{tf} (k_1 C + \frac{1}{2} k_2 u_1^2(t) + \frac{1}{2} k_3 u_2^2(t))dt \tag{14.111}$$

The authors formulated an optimal control problem subject to the model dynamics with the goal of minimizing the number of diabetic patients with complications together with the cost of managing diabetic patients with/without complications using two different control strategies. They proved the existence and uniqueness of the optimal control and characterized the controls based on Pontryagin's Maximum principle. Then they solved the resulting optimality system numerically.

Boutayeb et al. [22] introduced a new model with optimal control (see Fig. 14.10)

$$\frac{dP(t)}{dt} = n - (I_1 + I_2 + I_3 + \mu)P(t) + \gamma_1 E(t) \tag{14.112}$$

$$\frac{dE(t)}{dt} = I_1 P(t) - (\gamma_1 + \beta_1 + \beta_3 + \mu)E(t) \tag{14.113}$$

$$\frac{dD(t)}{dt} = I_2 P(t) + \beta_1 E(t) + \gamma_2 C - (\beta_2 + \mu)D(t) \tag{14.114}$$

$$\frac{dC(t)}{dt} = I_3 P(t) + \beta_2 D(t) + \beta_3 E(t) - (\gamma_2 + \mu + \delta)C(t) \tag{14.115}$$

where

$n$ : denotes the incidence of adult population
$-I_1$ : denotes the rate of healthy persons to become pre-diabetic,
$-I_2$ :denotes the rate of healthy persons to become diabetic,
$-I_3$ : denotes the rate of healthy persons developing complications,
$\mu$ : natural mortality rate,
$\beta_1$ : the probability of a pre-diabetic person to become diabetic,
$\beta_2$ : the probability of a diabetic person developing complications,
$\beta_3$ : the probability of a pre-diabetic person developing complications,
$\gamma_1$ : rate at which a pre-diabetic person becomes healthy,
$\gamma_2$ : rate at which complications are cured,

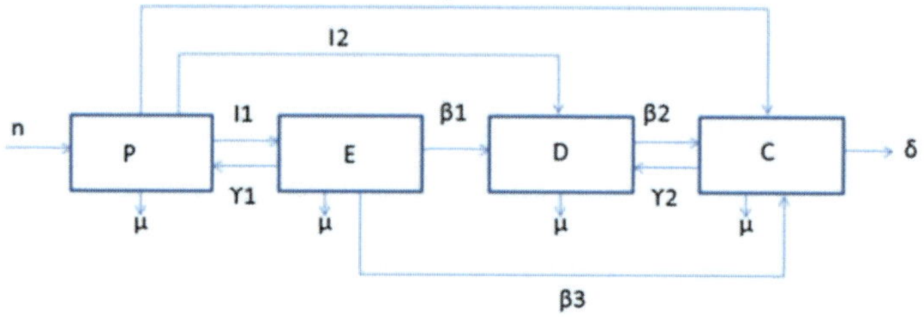


**Fig. 14.10** Dynamics of diabetes from prediabetes to diabetes with complications

$\delta$ : mortality rate due to complications,

$\mu$ : natural mortality rate

The optimal control approach is used to reduce the number of pre-diabetics in order to prevent adults from diabetes and its complications.

For the optimal control problem, authors considered the control variable $u = u(t)$ to be the percentage of healthy people being prevented from pre-diabetes per unit of time.

The controlled model based on system (1), is written as follows:

$$\frac{dP(t)}{dt} = n - I_1(1-u)P(t) - (I_2 + I_3 + \mu)P(t) + \gamma_1 E(t) \quad (14.116)$$

$$\frac{dE(t)}{dt} = I_1(1-u)P(t) - (\gamma_1 + \beta_1 + \beta_3 + \mu)E(t) \quad (14.117)$$

$$\frac{dD(t)}{dt} = I_2 P(t) + \beta_1 E(t) + \gamma_2 C - (\beta_2 + \mu)D(t) \quad (14.118)$$

$$\frac{dC(t)}{dt} = I_3 P(t) + \beta_2 D(t) + \beta_3 E(t) - (\gamma_2 + \mu + \delta)C(t) \quad (14.119)$$

The objective is to minimize the objective function defined as:

$$J(u) = \int_0^T (E(t) + Au^2(t))dt \quad (14.120)$$

Where $A$ and $B$ are positive weights that balance the size of the terms. $U$ is the control set defined by $U = \{u \text{measurable}, 0 \leq u(t) \leq 1, t \in [0, T]\}$

The optimal control $u^* \in U$ satisfies

The Hamiltonian is defined as follows:

$$H = E + Au^2 + \lambda_1 \frac{dP(t)}{dt} + \lambda_2 \frac{dE(t)}{dt} + \lambda_3 \frac{dD(t)}{dt} + \lambda_4 \frac{dC(t)}{dt} \quad (14.121)$$

Given an optimal control $u^*$ and solutions $P^*$, $E^*$, $D^*$and $C^*$ of the system, there exist adjoint variables $\lambda_1$, $\lambda_2$, $\lambda_3$ and $\lambda_4$satisfying:

$$\frac{d\lambda_1}{dt} = -\frac{dH}{dP} = \lambda_1 I_1(1-u) + \lambda_1(I_2 + I_3 + \mu) - \lambda_2(1-u) - \lambda_3 I_2 - \lambda_4 I_3 \quad (14.122)$$

$$\frac{d\lambda_2}{dt} = -\frac{dH}{dE} - 1 + \lambda_2(\gamma_1 + \beta_1 + \beta_3 + \mu) - \beta_1\lambda_3 - \beta_3\lambda_4 \quad (14.123)$$

$$\frac{d\lambda_3}{dt} = -\frac{dH}{dD} = \lambda_3(\beta_2 + \mu) - \beta_2\lambda_4 \quad (14.124)$$

$$\frac{d\lambda_4}{dt} = -\frac{dH}{dC} = -\lambda_3\gamma_2 + (\gamma_2 + \mu + \delta)\lambda_4 \quad (14.125)$$

The optimal control is obtained from the optimally condition $\frac{dH}{du} = 0$

$$u^* = \frac{1}{2A}[-PI_1(\lambda_1 - \lambda_2)]$$

For numerical simulations, the authors used the following Gauss–Seidel-like implicit finite-difference method, following Gumel et al. [37].

$$P_{i+1} = \frac{P_i + hn + h\gamma_1 E_i}{1 + hI_1(1 - u_i) + h(I_2 + I_3 + \mu)} \tag{14.126}$$

$$E_{i+1} = \frac{E_i + hI_1(1 - u_i)P_{i+1}}{1 + h(\beta_1 + \beta_3 + \gamma_1 + \mu)} \tag{14.127}$$

$$D_{i+1} = \frac{D_i + hI_2P_{i+1} + h\beta_1 E_{i+1} + h\gamma_2 C_i}{1 + h(\beta_2 + \mu)} \tag{14.128}$$

$$C_{i+1} = \frac{C_i + hI_3P_{i+1} + h\beta_2 D_{i+1} + h\beta_3 E_{i+1}}{1 + h(\gamma_2 + \mu + \delta)} \tag{14.129}$$

$$\lambda_1^{m-i-1} = \frac{\lambda_1^{m-i} + hI_1(1 - u_i)\lambda_2^{m-i} + hI_2\lambda_3^{m-i} + hI_3\lambda_4^{m-i}}{1 + hI_1(1 - u_i) + h(I_2 + I_3 + \mu)} \tag{14.130}$$

$$\lambda_2^{m-i-1} = \frac{\lambda_2^{m-i} + h\beta_1\lambda_3^{m-i} + h\beta_3\lambda_4^{m-i} + h\gamma_1\lambda_1^{m-i-1}}{1 + h(\beta_1 + \beta_3 + \gamma_1 + \mu)} \tag{14.131}$$

$$\lambda_3^{m-i-1} = \frac{\lambda_3^{m-i} + h\beta_2\lambda_4^{m-i}}{1 + h\beta_2 + h\mu} \tag{14.132}$$

$$\lambda_4^{m-i-1} = \frac{\lambda_4^{m-i} + h\gamma_2\lambda_3^{m-i}}{1 + h(\gamma_2 + \mu + \delta)} \tag{14.133}$$

$$M^{i+1} = \frac{1}{2A} I_1 P_{i+1}(\lambda_2^{m-i-1} - \lambda_1^{m-i-1}) \tag{14.134}$$

$$u_{i+1} = \min[1, \max(0, M^{i+1})] \tag{14.135}$$

Numerical results of the simulations are illustrated in Fig. 14.11.

## 14.6 Fractional-Order Model

In a recent paper, Srivastava et al. [39] extended the model (14.28)–(14.29) of Boutayeb et al. [15] to a fractional-order model. Using the following variables and parameters:

$A(t)$: The incidence of diabetes mellitus at time $t$;
$B(t)$: The number of persons having diabetics without complications at time $t$;
$C(t)$: The number of persons having diabetics with complications at time $t$;
$E(t)$: The size of the population of diabetics at time $t$;
$\delta$: The probability of a person having diabetes and developing complications;

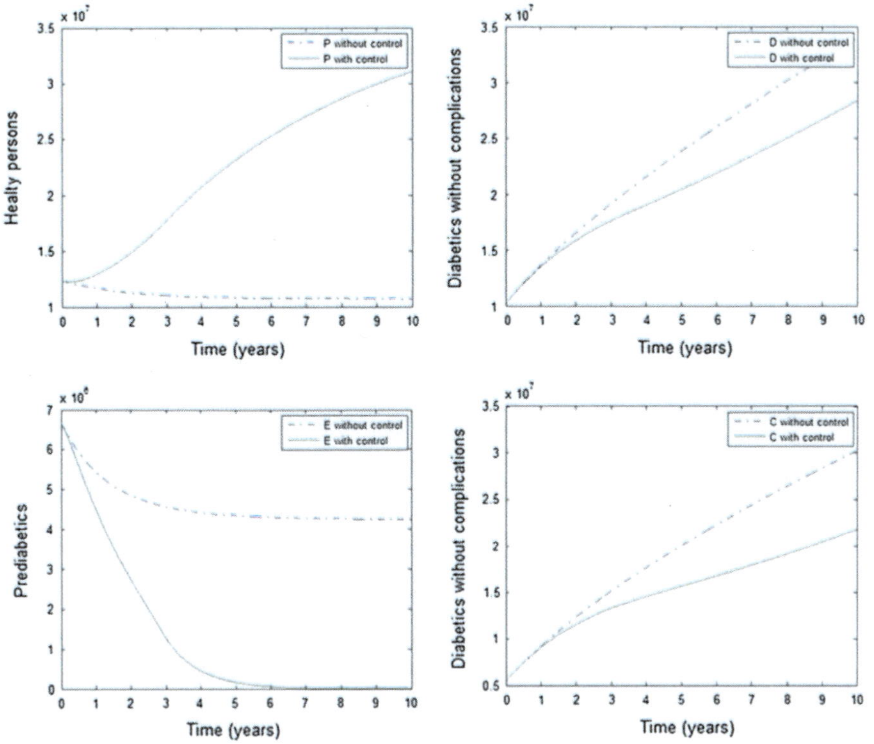


**Fig. 14.11** Evolution of healthy, pre-diabetic and diabetic with and without complications, with and without control

$\varepsilon$: natural rate of mortality;
$\lambda$: The rate of complications recovered;
$\mu$: The rate of mortality due to diabetic complications;
$v$:The rate of diabetic patients having complication and becoming severely disabled.
They started with the following mode

$$B'(t) = A(t) - (\delta + \varepsilon)B(t) + \lambda C(t) \tag{14.136}$$
$$C'(t) = A(t) - (\lambda + \mu + v + \varepsilon)C(t) + \delta B(t) \tag{14.137}$$
$$E(t) = B(t) + C(t) \tag{14.138}$$

where $E(t)$ represents the size of those persons who are diabetic at time $t$.

$$C'(t) = -(\delta + \psi)C(t) + \delta E(t) \tag{14.139}$$
$$E'(t) = A(t) - (\mu + v)C(t)) - \varepsilon E(t) \tag{14.140}$$

with $\psi = \lambda + \mu + v + \varepsilon$

They recalled that the Riemann-Liouville fractional derivative operator $D_x^\alpha$ of order $\alpha$ is defined, for a real-valued function $f(x)$ by

$$D_x^\alpha[f(x)] = \frac{1}{\Gamma(l-\alpha)}\frac{d^l}{dx^l}\int_0^x (x-\tau)^{l-\alpha-1} f(\tau)d\tau \tag{14.141}$$

$$(x > 0; l-1 < \alpha \le l; l \in IN)$$

Then they considered the Fractional-order model of diabetes and its resulting complications:

$$D_t^\alpha[B(t)] = A(t) - (\delta+\varepsilon)B(t) + \lambda C(t) \tag{14.142}$$

$$D_t^\beta[C(t)] = A(t) - (\lambda+\mu+v+\varepsilon)C(t) + \delta B(t) \tag{14.143}$$

$$E(t) = B(t) + C(t)$$

$$D_t^\alpha[C(t)] = -(\delta+\psi)C(t) + \delta E(t) \tag{14.144}$$

$$D_t^\beta[C(t)] = A(t) - (\mu+v)C(t)) - \varepsilon E(t) \tag{14.145}$$

with $\psi = \lambda + \mu + v + \varepsilon$

The authors made use of the Fixed Point Theory to determine the existence and unicity of the coupled solution. Then they carried out stability analysis and searched approximate solutions for the fractional-order mathematical model using the familiar homotopy decomposition method (HDM).

## 14.7 Stochastic Compartmental Models

In a recent paper, Zhang et al. [44] extended the model {(14.28)–(14.29)} of Boutayeb et al. [15] to a stochastic model to describe the dynamic behaviour of diabetes mellitus.

They introduced $(\Omega, F, P)$ as the canonical Wiener space, with $\{Ft\}_{t\in\mathbb{R}+}$ its natural normal filtration, and $W(t)(t \in \mathbb{R}^+)$ the standard one-dimensional Brownian motion defined on the space $(\Omega, F, P)$.

They assumed that $\Omega := \{\omega \in C(\mathbb{R}^+, \mathbb{R}) : \omega(0) = 0\}$ endowed with the compact-open topology.

Then, based on the conclusions of deterministic ordinary differential equations about diabetes mellitus, they proposed a class of Ito SDEs in the form of:

$$dC(t) = (-(\lambda(t)+\theta(t))C(t) + \lambda(t)N(t))dt + g_1(t)dW_t, \tag{14.146}$$

$$dN(t) = (I(t) - (v(t)+\delta(t))C(t) - \mu(t)N(t))dt + g_2(t)dW_t \tag{14.147}$$

where $t \in \mathbb{R}^+$;

$D(t)$ represents diabetics who have no complications in a special research region at time $t$

$C(t)$ represents diabetics who have complications in a special research region at time $t$

$N(t) = C(t) + D(t)$ is the total population with diabetes

$I(t)$ the morbidity of diabetes mellitus in a special research region at time $t$

$\mu(t)$ stands for the mortality rate, the chance of a diabetes

$\lambda(t)$ is the the chance of a diabetes mellitus person who is developing a complication

$\gamma(t)$ represents the proportion of complications which are mended

$v(t)$ represents the rate at which diabetic patients with complications become severely disabled

$\delta(t)$ represents the mortality rate due to complications

$\theta(t) = \gamma(t) + \mu(t) + v(t) + \delta(t)$

and $g_1(t)$ and $g_2(t)$ are functions with respect to t, which denote the uncertain influences.

In this paper, the authors presented theoretical results and carried out numerical experiments. They concluded that "the main result of this article is the numerical simulation of stochastic diabetes mellitus model. The results show that the methods are effective and the numerical results can match the results of theoretical analysis and reality".

## 14.8 Other Compartmental Models

In 2015, Pan et al. [36] published an important paper in the Lancet Diabetes Endocrinology. They used a mathematical model to illustrate the effect of diabetes on tuberculosis control in 13 countries with high tuberculosis, based on the following statements: (A) Diabetes increases the risk of progression from latent infection to infectious active disease, (B) diabetes increases the risk of relapse after treatment completion, (C) diabetes increases the risk of death in individuals with active tuberculosis, (D) diabetes increases the risk of death in the general population without active tuberculosis. Based on both diabetes status and TB status, including susceptible, fast latent, slow latent, infectious with active disease, recovered, and fast latent after re-infection, the model comprised six compartments:

1. **Susceptible** ($S$ and $S_{dm}$)

$$d(S)/dt = g - \beta * I * S - S * u - S * x_{dm} \tag{14.148}$$

$$d(S_{dm})/dt = x_{dm} * S - \beta * I * S_{dm} - S_{dm} * u * RR_u \tag{14.149}$$

where $S, S_{dm}, x_{dm}$ stands for diabetes free and TB free status, TB susceptible population with diabetes, and diabetes patients respectively; with parameters transmission ($\beta$), death ($u$) and diabetes-specific death ($u * RR_u$),prevalence of infectious ($I = Ip + Ip_{dm}$)

2. **Fast latent infection** ($F$ and $F_{dm}$)

$$d(F)/dt = \beta * I * S - F * j1 - F * k - F * xdm - F * u \quad (14.150)$$

$$d(F_{dm})/dt = F * x_{dm} + \beta * I * S_{dm} - F_{dm} * j1 * RR_j - F_{dm} * k - F_{dm} * u * RR_u \quad (14.151)$$

In the first few years after infection, individuals have a higher chance to progress into active TB (primary progression). They may leave the status by primary progression ($j1$), entering the stage of slow latent infection ($k$), or death ($u$).

3. **Fast latent reinfection** ($Fi$ and $Fi_{dm}$)

$$d(Fi)/dt = \beta * I * (L + R) - Fi * j1 * (1 - im) - Fi * k - Fi * x_{dm} - Fi * u \quad (14.152)$$

$$d(Fi_{dm})/dt = Fi * x_{dm} + \beta * I * (L_{dm} + R_{dm}) - Fi_{dm} * j1 * (1 - im) * RR_j - Fi_{dm} * k - F_{dm} * u * RR_u \quad (14.153)$$

4. **Slow latent infection** ($L$ and $L_{dm}$)

$$d(L)/dt = F * k + Fi * k + c * Ip - \beta * I * L - L * j2 - L * x_{dm} - L * u \quad (14.154)$$

$$d(L_{dm})/dt = L * x_{dm} + F_{dm} * k + Fi_{dm} * k + c * Ip_{dm} - \beta * I * L_{dm} - L_{dm} * RR_j - L_{dm} * u * RR_u \quad (14.155)$$

5. **Infectious pulmonary status** ($Ip$ and $Ip_{dm}$)

$$d(Ip)/dt = F * j1 + Fi * j1 * (1 - im) + L * j2 + R * q - Ip * c - CDR * INC * treat - Ip * utb - Ip * x_{dm} \quad (14.156)$$

$$d(Ip_{dm})/dt = x_{dm} * Ip + F_{dm} * j1 * RR_j + Fi_{dm} * j1 * (1 - im) * RR_j + L_{dm} * j2 * RR_j + R_{dm} * q * RR_q - c * Ip_{dm} - CDR * INC_{dm} * treat - Ip_{dm} * utb * RR_utb \quad (14.157)$$

This describe pulmonary infection, which is infectious. People in this stage may enter the status from fast latent status ($F$), fast latent status with reinfection ($Fi$), slow latent status ($L$), or relapse from recovered status ($R$). They may leave the status due to TB-specific mortality ($utb$), natural cure ($c$), or proper diagnosis ($CDR * INC$, where $CDR$ refers to the case detection rate and $INC$ refers to the incidence rate of active TB) and treatment success rate ($treat$).

6. **Recovered** ($R$ and $R_{dm}$)

$$\begin{aligned} d(R)/dt &= CDR * INC * treat - R * q - \beta * I * R - R * x_{dm} \\ &\quad - R * u \end{aligned} \tag{14.158}$$

$$\begin{aligned} d(R_{dm})/dt &= R * x_{dm} + CDR * INCdm * treat - R_{dm} * q * RR_q \\ &\quad - \beta * I * R_{dm} - R_{dm} * u * RR_u \end{aligned} \tag{14.159}$$

Recovered status is entered by people after proper diagnosis and treatment and it is left by people through reinfection ($\beta * I$), relapse ($q$), or death ($u$)

Using their model and different scenarios, the authors found, among other, that lowering the prevalence of diabetes by an absolute level of 6·6–13·8% could accelerate the decline of tuberculosis incidence by an absolute level of 11·5–25·2% and tuberculosis mortality by 8·7–19·4%. They also stated that, if interventions reduce diabetes incidence by 35% by 2025, 7·8 million tuberculosis cases and 1·5 million tuberculosis deaths could be averted by 2035.

In 2018, Dhara et al. [25] proposed a mathematical model associating diabetes with tuberculosis. They Highlighted that studies strongly support the association between these two diseases though the mechanism of association has not been clearly understood yet. The model proposed is an extension of the models {(14.28)–(14.29)} and {(14.30)–(14.32)} proposed by Boutayeb et al. in 2004 and 2006. As illustrated by Fig. 14.12, a new compartment is added to express the dynamics of tuberculosis incidence among the diabetes patients.

The governing equations are given as follows

$$D'(t) = I - (\lambda_1 + \mu_1)D(t) + \gamma_1 C(t) \tag{14.160}$$

$$C'(t) = \lambda_1 D(t) - (\gamma_1 + \mu_2 + \nu_1 + \lambda_2)C(t) + \gamma_2 T(t) \tag{14.161}$$

$$T'(t) = \lambda_2 C(t) - (\mu_3 + \gamma_2 + \xi)T(t) \tag{14.162}$$

$$\lambda_1 = \lambda_1(t) = \frac{C(t)}{D(t) + C(t)} = \frac{C(t)}{N(t)} \tag{14.163}$$

$$\lambda_2 = \lambda_2(t) = \frac{T(t)}{D(t) + C(t) + T(t)} \tag{14.164}$$

The authors carried out stability analysis and performed some numerical experiments using fourth order Adams–Bashforth–Moulton predictor corrector method.

In 2019, Danumjaya and Dhara [23] used non-standard finite difference schemes on the previous model {(14.160)–(14.164)}. They performed numerical and stability analysis.

Another model analysing the impact of diabetes on the dynamical transmission of tuberculosis was published by Moualeu et al. [33].

In 2014, Boutayeb et al. [20] proposed a mathematical model illustrating simple and efficient ways to reduce overweight/obesity in Morocco. Following a paper by Walpole et al. who estimated the adult human biomass worldwide [40], the authors proposed a Markov model that illustrates the dynamics (in time) of both human

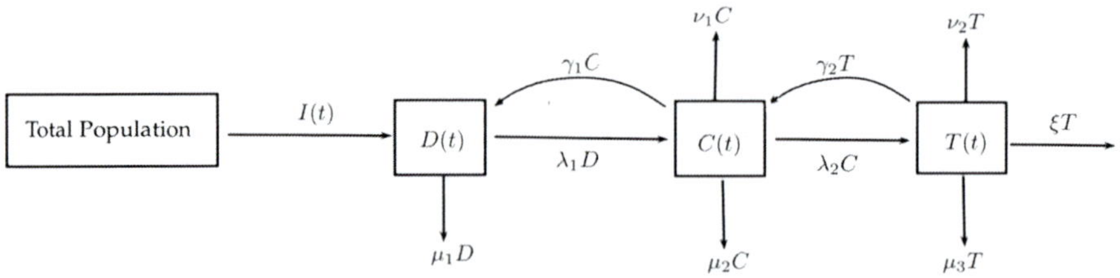


**Fig. 14.12** Population dynamics associating diabetes with and without complications with tuberculosis

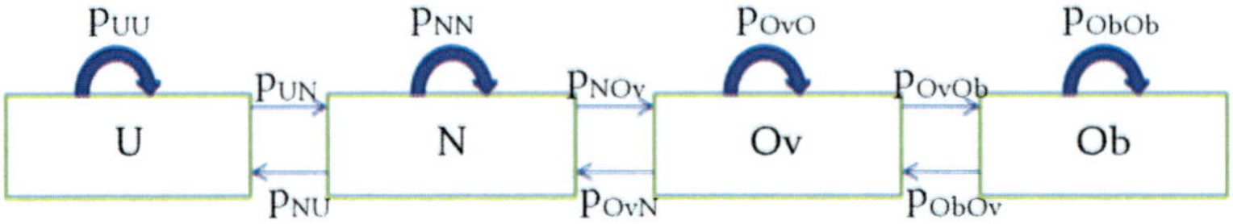


**Fig. 14.13** biomass in compartments: Underweight ($U$), Normal weight ($N$), Overweight ($Ov$) and Obesity ($Ob$)

population and human biomass in Morocco, by considering four compartments: Underweight, Normal weight, Overweight and Obese. The biomass was calculated in each category as the product of population size by the average body mass, assumed to be 45 kg, 65 kg, 85 kg and 115 kg in underweight, normal, overweight and obese category respectively.

As indicated by Fig. 14.13, the suggested Markov model was defined by the four compartments (Underweight ($U$), Normal weight ($N$), Overweight ($Ov$) and Obesity ($Ob$)), the probability $P_{ii}$ of staying in the same state $i$ and the probability $P_{ij}$ of transition from the state $i$ to the state $j$.

In 2006, Jones et al. [30] published a model explaining the growth of diabetes since 1980 and portray possible futures through 2050. The model simulations suggest characteristic dynamics of the diabetes population, including unintended increases in diabetes prevalence due to diabetes control, the inability of diabetes control efforts alone to reduce diabetes-related deaths in the long term, and significant delays between primary prevention efforts and downstream improvements in diabetes outcomes.

## References

1. Adamu I, Haruna Y, Garba E (2012) A mathematical model for attenuating the spread of diabetes and its management in a population. Glob J Math Sci 11(1–2):1–14
2. Adamu I, Momoh A, Tahir A (2016) Stability analysis of the mathematical model for the dynamics of diabetic population under the combine effect of birth rate and treatment. Int J Sci Technol 5(1):26–35
3. Ajmera I, Swat M, Laibe C, Le Novere N, Chelliah V (2013) The impact of mathematical modeling on the understanding of diabetes and related complications. CPT Pharmacomet Syst

Pharmacol 2(7):1–14
4. Akinsola V, Oluyo T (2014) Mathematical model of the complications and control of diabetes mellitus. Int J Math Comput Appl Res 4(5):1–14
5. Akinsola V, Oluyo T (2015) A note on the divergence of the numerical solution of the mathematical model for the burden of diabetes and its complications using euler method. Int J Math Comput Appl Res 5(3):93–100
6. Akinsola V, Oluyo T (2019) Mathematical analysis with numerical solutions of the mathematical model for the complications and control of diabetes mellitus. J Stat Manag Syst 1–25
7. Atanasijevic-Kunc M, Drinovec J (2011) Burden of diabetes type 2 through modelling and simulation. In: Topics in the prevention, treatment and complications of type 2 diabetes, IntechOpen
8. Balakrishnan NP, Rangaiah GP, Samavedham L (2011) Review and analysis of blood glucose (bg) models for type 1 diabetic patients. Ind Eng Chem Res 50(21):12041–12066
9. Bernard S, Nuiro SP, Pietrus A (2015) Diabetes, complications and limit cycles. Appl Math E-Notes 15:197–206
10. Bernard S, César T, Nuiro SP, Piétrus A (2018) Unexistence of limit cycle in an optimal control problem of a population of diabetics. Revista de Matemática Teoría y Aplicaciones 25(2):239–259
11. Boutayeb A, Chetouani A (2006) A critical review of mathematical models and data used in diabetology. Biomed Eng Online 5(1):43
12. Boutayeb A, Chetouani A (2007) A population model of diabetes and pre-diabetes. Int J Comput Math 84(1):57–66
13. Boutayeb A, Derouich M (2002) Age structured models for diabetes in east Morocco. Math Comput Simul 58(3):215–229
14. Boutayeb A, Twizell EH (2004) An age structured model for complications of diabetes mellitus in Morocco. Simul Model Pract Theory 12(1):77–87
15. Boutayeb A, Twizell E, Achouayb K, Chetouani A (2004) A mathematical model for the burden of diabetes and its complications. Biomed Eng Online 3(1):20
16. Boutayeb A, Chetouani A, Achouyab A, Twizell E (2006) A non-linear population model of diabetes mellitus. J Appl Math Comput 21(1–2):127–139
17. Boutayeb A, Boutayeb W, Lamlili M, Boutayeb S (2013) Indirect cost of diabetes in the arab region. Int J Diabetol Vasc Dis Res 1(4):24–28
18. Boutayeb A, Boutayeb W, Lamlili ME, Boutayeb S (2014) Estimation of the direct cost of diabetes in the arab region. Mediterr J Nutr Metablsm 7(1):21–32
19. Boutayeb W, Lamlili ME, Boutayeb A, Boutayeb S (2013) Estimation of direct and indirect cost of diabetes in Morocco. J Biomed Sci Eng 6(07):732
20. Boutayeb W, Boutayeb A, Lamlili ME, Derouich M (2014) A mathematical model of overweight/obesity in Morocco using human biomass. Int J Latest Res Sci Technol 3(6):65–67
21. Boutayeb W, Lamlili ME, Boutayeb A, Derouich M (2015) A simulation model for the dynamics of a population of diabetics with and without complications using optimal control. In: International conference on bioinformatics and biomedical engineering. Springer, pp 589–598
22. Boutayeb W, Lamlili ME, Boutayeb A, Derouich M (2016) The dynamics of a population of healthy people, pre-diabetics and diabetics with and without complications with optimal control. In: Proceedings of the mediterranean conference on information & communication technologies 2015. Springer, pp 463–471
23. Danumjaya P, Dhara M (2019) Stability preserving non-standard finite difference schemes for diabetes with tuberculosis infectious model. Lett Biomath 1–18
24. Derouich M, Boutayeb A, Boutayeb W, Lamlili M (2014) Optimal control approach to the dynamics of a population of diabetics. Appl Math Sci 8(56):2773–2782
25. Dhara M, Baths V, Danumjaya P (2018) Mathematical modeling and dynamics of tuberculosis infection among diabetic patients in India. J Anal 1–13
26. Enagi AI, Bawa M, Sani AM (2017) Mathematical study of diabetes and its complication using the homotopy perturbation method. Int J Math Comput Sci 12(1):43–63

27. Fleming WH, Rishel RW (2012) Deterministic and stochastic optimal control, vol 1. Springer Science & Business Media, Berlin
28. Gumel A, Shivakumar P, Sahai B (2001) A mathematical model for the dynamics of hiv-1 during the typical course of infection. Nonlinear Anal Theory Methods Appl 47(3):1773–1783
29. IDF (2017) Diabetes Atlas 2017. https://www.idf.org/elibrary/epidemiology-research/diabetes-atlas/134-idf-diabetesatlas-8th-edition.html
30. Jones AP, Homer JB, Murphy DL, Essien JD, Milstein B, Seville DA (2006) Understanding diabetes population dynamics through simulation modeling and experimentation. Am J Public Health 96(3):488–494
31. Li J, Johnson JD (2009) Mathematical models of subcutaneous injection of insulin analogues: a mini-review. Discret Contin Dyn Syst Ser B 12(2):401
32. Makroglou A, Li J, Kuang Y (2006) Mathematical models and software tools for the glucose-insulin regulatory system and diabetes: an overview. Appl Numer Math 56(3–4):559–573
33. Moualeu D, Bowong S, Tewa J, Emvudu Y (2012) Analysis of the impact of diabetes on the dynamical transmission of tuberculosis. Math Model Nat Phenom 7(3):117–146
34. Nucci G, Cobelli C (2000) Models of subcutaneous insulin kinetics. A critical review. Comput Methods Programs Biomed 62(3):249–257
35. de Oliveira SR, Raha S, Pal D (2017) Global asymptotic stability of a non-linear population model of diabetes mellitus. In: International conference on differential & difference equations and applications. Springer, pp 351–357
36. Pan SC, Ku CC, Kao D, Ezzati M, Fang CT, Lin HH (2015) Effect of diabetes on tuberculosis control in 13 countries with high tuberculosis: a modelling study. Lancet Diabetes Endocrinol 3(5):323–330
37. Pattaranit R, Van Den Berg HA (2008) Mathematical models of energy homeostasis. J R Soc Interface 5(27):1119–1135
38. Pontryagin LS (2018) Mathematical theory of optimal processes. Routledge, Abingdon
39. Srivastava HM, Shanker Dubey R, Jain M (2019) A study of the fractional-order mathematical model of diabetes and its resulting complications. Math Methods Appl Sci 1–14
40. Walpole SC, Prieto-Merino D, Edwards P, Cleland J, Stevens G, Roberts I (2012) The weight of nations: an estimation of adult human biomass. BMC Public Health 12(1):439
41. WHO (2018) Diabetes. http://www.who.int/news-room/factsheets/detail/diabetes
42. Widyaningsih P, Affan RC, Saputro DRS (2018) A mathematical model for the epidemiology of diabetes mellitus with lifestyle and genetic factors. In: Journal of physics: conference series, vol 1028, p 012110. IOP Publishing
43. Yusuf T (2015) Optimal control of incidence of medical complications in a diabetic's patients' population. FUTA J Res Sci 1:180–189
44. Zhang Z, Qingyi Zhan Q, Xie X (2019) Numerical study on stochastic diabetes mellitus model with additive noise. Comput Math Methods Med 1–8

# Chapter 15
# A Mathematical Model on Glucose Homeostasis in Type 1 Diabetes

**Wiam Boutayeb**

**Abstract** The aim of this chapter is to propose a mathematical model describing the interaction between Insulin, Glucose and Free Fatty Acids (FFA) while considering injected insulin bolus ($I_0$) in a type 1 diabetes person. The proposed mathematical model is governed by three ordinary differential equations representing respectively:

- The dynamics of insulin in which subcutaneous bolus injection ($I_0$) is introduced.
- The dynamics of glucose in which glucose production by liver and kidney and glucose from carbohydrate intake are separated.
- The dynamics of FFA.

Stability analysis shows that the ordinary differential system has one positive equilibrium point ($I^*$, $G^*$, $F^*$). Using numerical parameter values, the equilibrium is shown to be locally stable. Simulation was carried out for different values of the parameters, in particular according to variation in carbohydrate intake ($a_2$), insulin sensitivity ($c$) and the insulin bolus injected ($I_0$). The model shows clearly that a disorder in injected insulin, carbohydrate intake or physical activity may lead to dangerous situations of chronic hyperglycemia leading with time, to diabetes complications or hypoglycemia that may also lead to loss of consciousness or even to a sudden death.

## 15.1 Introduction

Diabetes mellitus is a metabolic disorder characterized by a defect in insulin secretion, insulin action, or both; leading to a chronic hyperglycemia. The three main types of diabetes are: (1) type 1 diabetes (previously known as insulin-dependent, juvenile or childhood-onset), characterized by deficient insulin production and requiring daily administration of insulin; (2) type 2 diabetes (formerly called non-insulin-dependent, or adult-onset) defined by insufficient insulin production/action (insulin resistance); and (3) gestational diabetes which occurs during pregnancy (blood glucose values above normal but below those diagnostic of diabetes) [13]. A good control of

W. Boutayeb (✉)
School of High Studies in Engineering, Oujda, Morocco
e-mail: wiam.boutayeb@gmail.com



A. Boutayeb (ed.), *Disease Prevention and Health Promotion in Developing Countries*,
https://doi.org/10.1007/978-3-030-34702-4_15

diabetes needs to juggle mainly with three parameters: (1) the dose of injected insulin or oral hypoglycemic drugs, (2) the quantity and quality of carbohydrates intake, and (3) the level of physical activity. Statistics released by the International Diabetes Federation (IDF) in 2017 indicate a global emergency. The number of people with diabetes (20–79 years) will increase worldwide by 48% between 2017 (425 million) and 2045 (629 million). The increase will reach 156 and 110% in the regions of Africa and Middle East and North Africa respectively. There is also over one million children and adolescents with type1 diabetes. It should be stressed that one in two adults with diabetes is undiagnosed and two thirds of people with diabetes are of working age [7].

An important number of publications were dedicated to mathematical modelling for diabetes during the last decades as indicated by the following reviews [1, 3, 4, 8–12]. In previous papers, we considered (1) mathematical modelling and simulation using $\beta$-cell mass, insulin (I) and glucose (G) under the effect of genetic predisposition to diabetes [6]; (2) the impact of obesity on predisposed people to type 2 diabetes through a mathematical model of $\beta$-cell mass, insulin (I), glucose (G), insulin receptors (R) and Free Fatty Acids (F) [5]; (3) a mathematical model on the effect of growth hormone on glucose homeostasis, governed by six ordinary differential equations associated with the variables $\beta$-cell mass, insulin (I), glucose (G), insulin receptors (R), Free Fatty Acids (F) and Growth Hormone (GH) [2]. These three models dealt with glucose homeostasis in people without diabetes, assuming that insulin was produced by beta-cells but the amount of insulin released could be insufficient or inefficient and hence could lead to diabetes. In the present paper, we propose a mathematical model studying the glucose homeostasis in a person with type 1 diabetes, based on the interaction between three variables, namely: insulin, glucose and free fatty acid (FFA). As explained earlier, this means that, due to beta-cells apoptosis, no insulin is produced by the body and, since this hormone is vital, affected people by type1 diabetes require daily administration of exogenous insulin (daily injection(s) by hand or by insulin pump). The corollary of this requirement is that a type1 diabetic person needs to control his/her glycemia regularly to avoid high levels of blood sugar that may lead to diabetes complications such as cardiovascular disease, kidney failure, blindness or amputation. Low levels of blood sugar (hypoglycemia) can also be dangerous.

## 15.2 Method

The proposed mathematical model is governed by three ordinary differential equations. It is assumed that the insulin absorption in depot is inversely proportional to the concentration of insulin in plasma. The first equation indicates that, following a subcutaneous bolus injection of $I_0$, insulin concentration $I(t)$ in the plasma increases by a rate $e\frac{I_0}{1+I(t)}$ and decreases by a rate $dI(t)$. The second equation translates how the concentration of glucose increases by the amount of glucose produced by liver and kidney ($a_1$) and glucose from carbohydrate intake ($a_2$); and the rate from FFA

$(m_1 (F(t) - F_b))$. The glucose decreases by a rate independent of insulin $(bG(t))$ and a rate $cI(t)G(t)$ representing the glucose intake due to insulin sensitivity $c$. Finally, the third equation indicates that the FFA decreases by a rate $m_2 (F(t) - F_b)$ and increases by a rate $m_3 (G(t) - G_b)$. Consequently, the mathematical model proposed is the following:

$$\frac{dI(t)}{dt} = e\frac{I_0}{1+I(t)} - dI(t) \tag{15.1}$$

$$\frac{dG(t)}{dt} = a_1 + a_2 - (b + cI(t))G(T) + m_1(F(t) - F_b) \tag{15.2}$$

$$\frac{dF(t)}{dt} = -m_2 (F(t) - F_b) + m_3 (G(t) - G_b) \tag{15.3}$$

The coefficient parameters, their interpretation and values are given in Table 15.2.

## 15.3 Results

### *15.3.1 Equilibrium Points*

The system of differential equations (15.1)–(15.3) has only one positive equilibrium point given by:

$I^* = (-d + \sqrt{}(d^2 + 4deI_0)/2d$
$G^* = (am_2 - m_1 m_3 G_b)/(m_2(b + cI^*) - m_1 m_3)$
$F^* = (m_1 F_b - a + (b + cI^*)G^*)/m_1$

**Table 15.1** Number of people with diabetes per WHO region in 2017 and 2045 (20–79 years)

| WHO region | Prevalence of diabetes in 2017 (million) | Prevalence of diabetes in 2045 (million) | Increase from 2017 to 2045 (%) |
|---|---|---|---|
| North America and Caribbean | 46 | 62 | 35 |
| Middle East 7 North Africa | 39 | 82 | 110 |
| Europe | 58 | 67 | 16 |
| South and Central America | 26 | 42 | 62 |
| Africa | 16 | 41 | 156 |
| South East Asia | 82 | 151 | 84 |
| Western Pacific | 159 | 183 | 15 |
| **World** | **425** | **629** | **48** |

*Source* IDF Diabetes Atlas 2017 http://www.diabetesatlas.org/

Using the parameter values given in Table 15.1 gives the following equilibrium point:
$P(I^* = 11.75, G^* = 87.45, F^* = 10.7)$.

### 15.3.2 Local Stability Analysis

The Jacobian of the system (15.1)–(15.3) is given by:

$$\begin{pmatrix} -\dfrac{eI_0}{(1+I)2} - d & 0 & 0 \\ -cG & -cI - b & m_1 \\ 0 & m_3 & -m_2 \end{pmatrix}$$

Replacing the parameters in the Jacobian by their values indicated in Table 15.2 shows that the three eigenvalues are negative ($\lambda_1 = -400$, $\lambda_2 = -11.4$ and $\lambda_4 = -0.004$) and hence the equilibrium point is stable.

### 15.3.3 Simulations

Simulation was carried out for different values of the parameters, in particular according to variation in carbohydrate intake ($a_2$), insulin sensitivity ($c$) and the insulin bolus injected ($I_0$).

**Table 15.2** Parameters values used in the model

| Parameter | Value | Units | Biological interpretation |
|---|---|---|---|
| $a_1$ | 585 | mg/dl.d | Glucose production rate by liver/kidney when $G = 0$ |
| $a_2$ | 415 | mg/dl.d | Glucose uptake from diet |
| $b$ | 1.44 | $d^{-1}$ | Glucose clearance rate independent of insulin |
| $c$ | 0.85 | ml/$\mu$U.d | Insulin induced glucose uptake rate (insulin sensitivity) |
| $d$ | 0.0002 | $d^{-1}$ | Insulin degradation rate |
| $e$ | 0.002 | $\mu$U/ml.d | Constant parameter |
| $I_0$ | 15 | $\mu$U/ml | Bolus (injected) insulin |
| $G_b$ | 100 | mg/dl | Basal value of glucose |
| $F_b$ | 11 | mg/dl | Basal value of Fee Fatty Acids |
| $m_1$ | 0.09 | $d^{-1}$ | Constant parameter |
| $m_2$ | 400 | $d^{-1}$ | Rate of FFA dissipation |
| $m_3$ | 10 | $d^{-1}$ | Rate of Glucose production |

#### 15.3.3.1 Simulation with Different Values of Carbohydrate Intake ($a_2$)

The value of $a_2$ was varied from 0 to 1415. Table 15.3 and Fig. 15.1 show that the values of $G^*$and $F^*$ increase with the increase of carbohydrate intake ($a_2$). It shows in particular that, for a given value of insulin bolus $I_0$, insufficient intake of carbohydrates will lead to hypoglycemia and excess of carbohydrates intake will end up with hyperglycemia. Consequently, for a good daily control of blood sugar, a person with type1 diabetes must be careful about the quantity and quality of carbohydrates he or she eats.

#### 15.3.3.2 Simulation with Different Values of Insulin Bolus $I_0$

The second kind of simulation deals with the value of insulin bolus injected. As illustrated by the values in Table 15.4 and the graphs in Fig. 15.2, it is clearly shown that insulin bolus should be adapted to each person according mainly to age, weight and physical effort. For a type 1 diabetes person, injecting a very low dose or an over dose

**Table 15.3** Simulation with different values of glucose intake ($a_2$)

| $a_2$ | $I^*$ | $G^*$ | $F^*$ |
|---|---|---|---|
| 0 | 11.75 | 51.0 | 9.8 |
| 115 | 11.75 | 61.0 | 10.0 |
| 415 | 11.75 | 87.5 | 10.7 |
| 915 | 11.75 | 131.2 | 11.8 |
| 1415 | 11.75 | 175.0 | 12.9 |

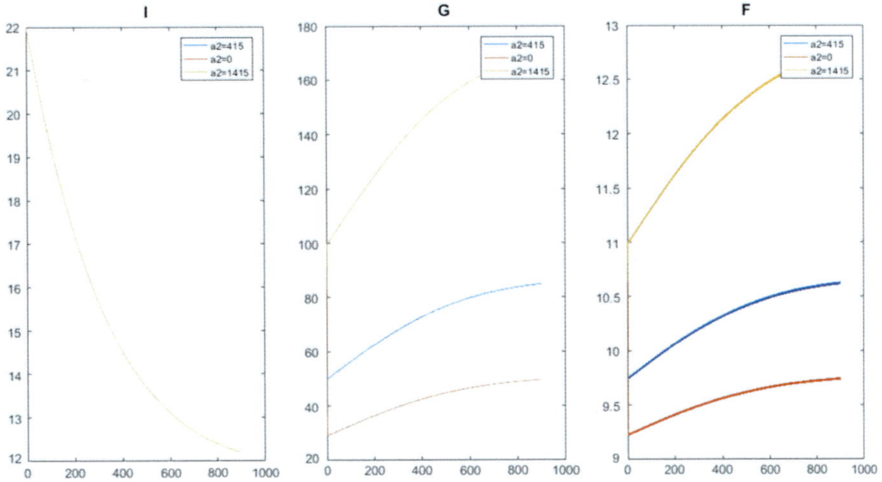


**Fig. 15.1** $I(t)$, $G(t)$ and $F(t)$ for different values of $a_2$

**Table 15.4** Simulation with different values of insulin bolus $I_0$

| $I_0$ | I* | G* | F* |
|---|---|---|---|
| 0 | 0 | 695.0 | 25.9 |
| 5 | 6.60 | 142.0 | 12.0 |
| 15 | 11.75 | 87.5 | 10.7 |
| 25 | 15.30 | 69.1 | 10.2 |
| 40 | 19.50 | 55.5 | 9.9 |

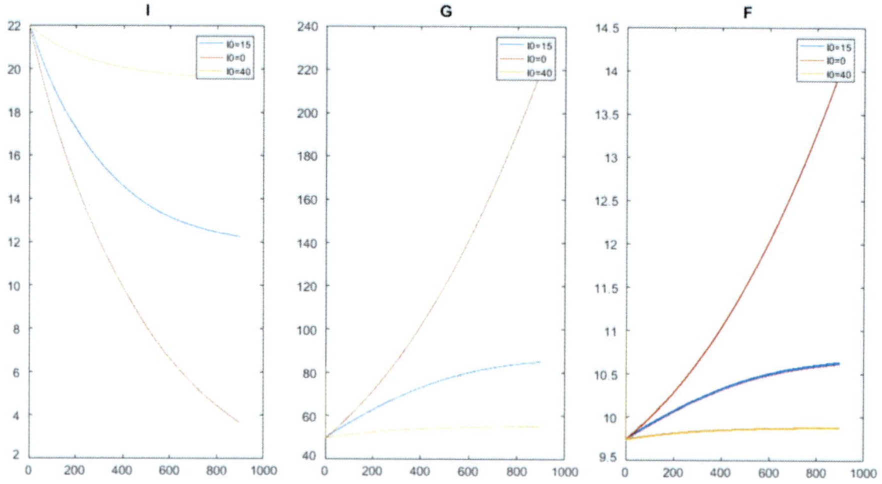


**Fig. 15.2** $I(t)$, $G(t)$ and $F(t)$ for different values of $I_0$

of insulin are both dangerous. The first case leads to a hypothetical hyperglycemic state while the second case is synonym of hypoglycemia which can lead to generalized convulsions followed by amnesia, general perturbation, unconsciousness and even sudden death.

#### 15.3.3.3 Simulation with Different Values of Insulin Sensitivity ($c$)

Another type of simulation is devoted to insulin sensitivity ($c$). Similar to the two previous simulations, decreased values of $G^*$ and $F^*$ are associated with a decrease in the value of $c$. This means for example, that for the same amount of insulin injected, obesity may reduce insulin efficiency (insulin resistance) associated with high level of glycemia. On the other hand, vigorous-intensity physical activity can foster insulin sensitivity, resulting in a hypoglycemia more or less severe (Table 15.5, Fig. 15.3).

**Table 15.5** Simulation with different values of insulin sensitivity ($c$)

| $c$ | $I^*$ | $G^*$ | $F^*$ |
|---|---|---|---|
| 0.20 | 11.75 | 263.80 | 15.0 |
| 0.42 | 11.75 | 162.80 | 12.5 |
| 0.85 | 11.75 | 87.50 | 10.7 |
| 1.00 | 11.75 | 75.76 | 10.4 |
| 1.70 | 11.75 | 52.41 | 09.8 |

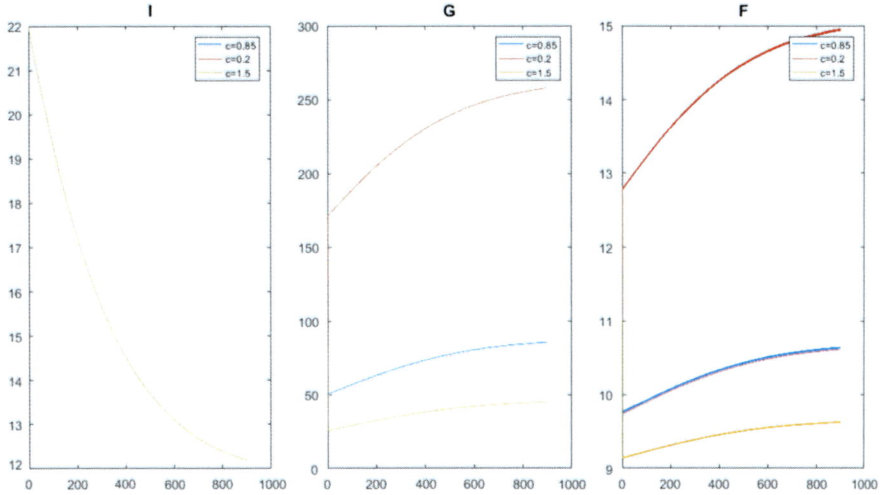


**Fig. 15.3** $I(t)$, $G(t)$ and $F(t)$ for different values of $c$

## 15.4 Conclusion

The results of different scenarios are discussed and compared to real life behavior. The model shows clearly that a disorder in injected insulin, carbohydrate intake or physical activity may lead to dangerous situations of chronic hyperglycemia leading with time, to diabetes complications or hypoglycemia that may also lead to loss of consciousness or even to a sudden death. Beside theoretical aspects, the mathematical model gives also guidelines for a pragmatic action on parameters leading to a good regular control of diabetes.

## References


1. Ajmera I, Swat M, Laibe C, Le Novere N, Chelliah V (2013) The impact of mathematical modeling on the understanding of diabetes and related complications. CPT: Pharm syst pharmacol 2(7):1–14
2. Al Ali H, Boutayeb W, Boutayeb A, Merabet N (2018) A mathematical model on the effect of growth hormone on glucose homeostasis. In: 4th CVOT Summit in cooperation with DCVD EASD study group. Munich, Germany
3. Balakrishnan NP, Rangaiah GP, Samavedham L (2011) Review and analysis of blood glucose (bg) models for type 1 diabetic patients. Ind Eng Chem Res 50(21):12041–12066
4. Boutayeb A, Chetouani A (2006) A critical review of mathematical models and data used in diabetology. Biomed. Eng. Online 5(1):43
5. Boutayeb W, Lamlili ME, Boutayeb A, Derouich M (2014) Mathematical modelling and simulation of $\beta$-cell mass, insulin and glucose dynamics: effect of genetic predisposition to diabetes. J. Biomed. Sci. Eng. 7(06):330
6. Boutayeb W, Lamlili ME, Boutayeb A, Derouich M (2015) The impact of obesity on predisposed people to type 2 diabetes: mathematical model. In: International conference on bioinformatics and biomedical engineering. Springer, pp 613–622
7. IDF (2017) Diabetes Atlas 2017. https://www.idf.org/elibrary/epidemiology-research/diabetes-atlas/134-idf-diabetesatlas-8th-edition.html
8. Li J, Johnson JD (2009) Mathematical models of subcutaneous injection of insulin analogues: a mini-review. Discret Contin Dyn Syst Ser B 12(2):401
9. Makroglou A, Li J, Kuang Y (2006) Mathematical models and software tools for the glucose-insulin regulatory system and diabetes: an overview. Appl. Numer. Math. 56(3–4):559–573
10. Nucci G, Cobelli C (2000) Models of subcutaneous insulin kinetics. a critical review. Comput Methods Prog Biomed 62(3):249–257
11. Pattaranit R, Van Den Berg HA (2008) Mathematical models of energy homeostasis. Journal of The Royal Society Interface 5(27):1119–1135
12. Smith JM, Maas JA, Garnsworthy PC, Owen MR, Coombes S, Pillay TS, Barrett DA, Symonds ME (2009) Mathematical modeling of glucose homeostasis and its relationship with energy balance and body fat. Obesity 17(4):632
13. WHO (2018) Diabetes. http://www.who.int/news-room/factsheets/detail/diabetes

# Chapter 16
# Fuzzy Logic for the Stochastic Operating Theater Optimization: A Review

**Marwa Khalfalli and Jerome Verny**

**Abstract** Aiming to increase patient satisfaction, health care centers also try to reduce their expenditures and improve their financial assets. Furthermore, surgical services receive most of the demand in hospital treatment systems. Operating room scheduling is one of the many complexities encountered in hospitals. The scheduling decision for operating room includes the assignment of surgery cases to operating rooms, and the surgery sequence in each operating room. The key objectives of the hospital authorities are to optimally utilize resources and to plan the surgery at the right time and at the right operating room. Planning and scheduling of the operating rooms present an undeniable role in providing appropriate services in hospitals. Uncertainty is one of the major problems associated with the development of accurate operating room schedules or capacity planning strategies. Two types of uncertainty that seem to be well addressed in the literature are patient arrival uncertainty and surgery duration uncertainty which is the uncertainty inherent to surgical services. In this chapter, we highlight how the fuzzy logic can be a good solution to the uncertainty problems within the operating theater.

## 16.1 Introduction

The sector of health care is continually evolving. In this specific circumstance, hospital supervisors need to make their business more beneficial. They aim to improve the performance of their organization through cost reducing and patient satisfaction while depending on given defined resources. The operating theater receives most of the patient services in the hospital centers. Its management has been widely the subject of many studies. It indicated that this area consists one of the most important sectors in the hospital which constitutes a melting pot between different units

M. Khalfalli (✉)
HF-LAB, HIGHFI, Paris, France
e-mail: marwa.khalfalli@highfi.net

J. Verny
NEOMA Business School, Mont-Saint-Aignan, France
e-mail: Jerome.verny@neoma-bs.fr



A. Boutayeb (ed.), *Disease Prevention and Health Promotion in Developing Countries*,
https://doi.org/10.1007/978-3-030-34702-4_16

and different actors. Managing the operating theater consists mainly in planning and scheduling the surgery cases to be performed.

Generally, the methodologies for scheduling surgeries at the operational level include two sub-problems: the first step allows allocating surgeries to the operating rooms. In the second step, the surgeries are sequenced within each operating room. These two sub-problems present an undeniable role in providing appropriate services in hospitals. Uncertainty is one of the major problems that can disrupt the development of accurate operating room schedules or capacity planning strategies. Two cases of uncertainty are frequently present in surgical services: uncertain patient arrival and uncertain surgery duration.

In this chapter, we are going to highlight how fuzzy logic can be a good solution to the uncertainty problems within an operating theater.

## 16.2 Fuzzy Logic

Fuzzy logic is an extension of the Boolean logic created by Lotfi Zadeh in 1965 based on his mathematical theory of fuzzy sets. By introducing the notion of the degree in the verification of a condition, we allow a condition to be in a state other than true or false. The fuzzy logic thus confers very appreciable flexibility to the reasoning that uses it, which makes it possible to take into account inaccuracies and uncertainties.

Fuzzy logic is based on the theory of fuzzy sets, which is a generalization of the theory of classical sets. That means that the latter is only a special case the theory of fuzzy sets. To make a metaphor in set language, the theory of classical sets is only a subset of the theory of fuzzy sets (Fig. 16.1).

The notation of fuzzy sets was introduced for the first time by Zadeh [29] in order to represent mathematically the inaccuracy relative to certain classes of objects. A fuzzy set is a set of values that belong to a certain class with some certainty [29]. Fuzzy logic makes it possible to make the link between numerical modeling and symbolic modeling. This allowed spectacular industrial development from very simple algorithms ensuring the transformation of symbolic knowledge into numerical entities and vice versa.

Moreover, the theory of fuzzy sets has also given birth to an original treatment of uncertainty based on the idea of order. This idea of order makes it possible to formalize

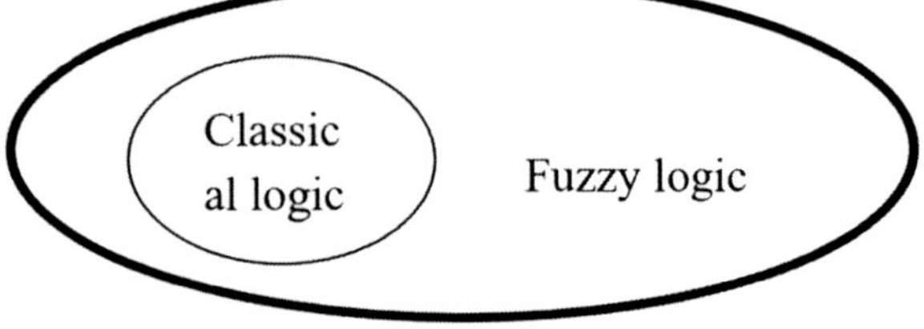


**Fig. 16.1** Relationship between classical logic and fuzzy logic

the treatment of partial ignorance and inconsistency in advanced information systems. Fuzzy sets also have an impact on automatic classification techniques and contribute to some renewal of existing approaches to decision aid.

Fuzzy logic is not really a resolution method but it represents a powerful tool and concept to take into account all the data and the uncertain parameters of the addressed problem. Fuzzy logic introduces, thanks to the concept of belonging function, a good compromise between the flexibility of the employment and the power of the representation. It thus allows the modeling of uncertainty and imprecision [2]. The role of the inference engine is to generate solutions from the knowledge base and to follow the rules.

Fuzzy sets provide us with a new mathematical tool to deal with the uncertainty of information. Since then, the theory of fuzzy sets has been promptly developed and many successful real applications of fuzzy sets in large field systems have emerged.

Decision aid models are generated to help the decision-maker to evaluate the performances of various management strategies [1, 10, 16]. In order to be most useful, the decision aid model should also include information about the uncertainties related to each of the decision options, as the certainty of the desired outcome may be a central criterion on the selection of the management policy.

In the following section, we will review the basic concepts of fuzzy logic that will be used in the rest of the chapter.

### *16.2.1 Fuzzy Variable*

Fuzzy logic is used to quantify and reason about fuzzy or vague terms of natural language. The fuzzy variable is a concept that usually has vague (or fuzzy) values for example age, temperature, height, speed.

### *16.2.2 Fuzzy Set (Value)*

Let $X$ be is a universe of the fuzzy variable discourse and $x$ are its elements One or more fuzzy sets (or values) $A$, can be defined over $X$.

Example: fuzzy variable: Age The universe of discourse: 0–120 years
Fuzzy values: Child, Young, Old

A fuzzy set $A$ is characterized by a membership function $\mu_A(x)$ that associates each element $x$ with a degree of membership value in $A$.

The value of membership is between 0 and 1 and it represents the degree to which an element $x$ belongs to the fuzzy set $A$.

### 16.2.3 Crisp Set Verus Fuzzy Set

- Crisp set A is a mapping for the elements of X to the set {0, 1}

$$A : X \rightarrow \{0, 1\}$$

$\mu_A(x) \rightarrow 1$ If x is an element of set A
$\mu_A(x) \rightarrow 0$ If x is not an element of set A
- Fuzzy set F is a mapping for the elements of X to the interval [0, 1]

$$F : X \rightarrow [0, 1]$$

Characteristic function: $0 \leq \mu_F(x) \leq 1$
For 1: full membership; for 0: no membership.
Anything between them called graded membership.

### 16.2.4 Fuzzy Relations

The fuzzy relation generalizes classical relation into one that allows partial membership. It describes a relationship that holds between two or more objects.

Example: a fuzzy relation "Friend" describes the degree of friendship between two persons, a contrast to either being a friend or not being a friend in classical relation.

It is represented as follows:

$$\mu_R = A \times B \rightarrow [0, 1]$$
$$R : \{(x, y), \mu_R(x, y) | \mu_R(x, y) \geq 0, x \in A, y \in B\}$$

A fuzzy relation is a fuzzy set defined on the Cartesian product of classical sets $\{x_1, x_2, \ldots, x_n\}$ where n-tuples $(x_1, x_2, \ldots, x_n)$ may have a varying degree of membership $\mu_{\underline{R}}(x_1, x_2, \ldots, x_n)$ within the relation.

$$R = \int_{x_1, x_2, \ldots x_n} \frac{\mu_{\underline{R}}(x_1, x_2, \ldots x_n)}{(x_1, x_2, \ldots x_n)}$$

### 16.2.5 Fuzzy Rules

Fuzzy rules are comprised of an antecedent and a consequent in the form:

IF antecedent THEN consequent = new Fuzzy Rule (antecedent, consequence)

The antecedent represents a condition and the consequent describes the consequence if that condition is satisfied.

The difference with fuzzy rules is that unlike conventional rules where the consequent either fires or not, in fuzzy systems the consequent can fire to a matter of degree.

Examples: IF temperature is very cold THEN stop air conditioner
IF temperature is normal THEN adjust the air conditioner
IF temperature is hot THEN start the air conditioner

The fuzzy rule-based inference is a generalization of a logical reasoning scheme (inferences) that combines the conclusion of multiple fuzzy rules in a manner similar to linear interpolation. For example:

Rule 1: If a person' intelligence quotient is high. Then the person is smart
Rule 2: Jack' intelligence quotient s is high
Inference: Jack is smart.

### *16.2.6 Linguistic Variables*

At the root of the fuzzy set theory lies the idea of linguistic variables. A linguistic variable is a fuzzy variable. In fuzzy expert systems, linguistic variables are used in fuzzy rules.

The description of a certain situation, phenomenon or process generally contains fuzzy qualifiers such as:

- Little, very much, enormously
- Rarely, frequently, often
- Cold, warm, hot
- Small, medium, large
- Etc....

Example: The "temperature" language variable can belong to the "cold", "warm" or "hot" fuzzy sets.

### *16.2.7 Membership Functions*

Instead of belonging to the "true" set or the "false" set of traditional binary logic, fuzzy logic admits degrees of belonging to a given set. The degree of belonging to a fuzzy set is represented by a number between 0 and 1. A precise value of the membership function linked to a value of the variable is denoted $\mu$ and called the "membership factor" (Fig. 16.2).

From this graph, it can be seen that for a value $\theta = 17°$, the factor of belonging to the "cold" set is $\mu$ cold $= 0.3$ and the factor of belonging to the "hot" set is $\mu$ hot $= 0.7$.

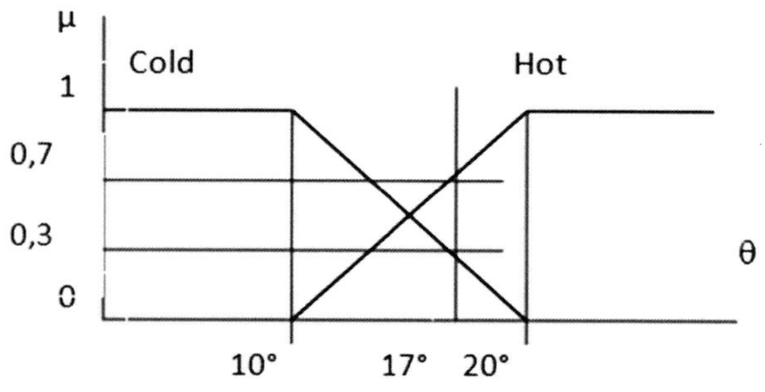


**Fig. 16.2** Membership function

The membership functions can theoretically take any form. However, they are often defined by line segments. (Very used because they are simple and contain areas where the notion is true, areas where it is false, which simplifies the collection of expertise).

*Membership Function (MF)*

- Triangular MF 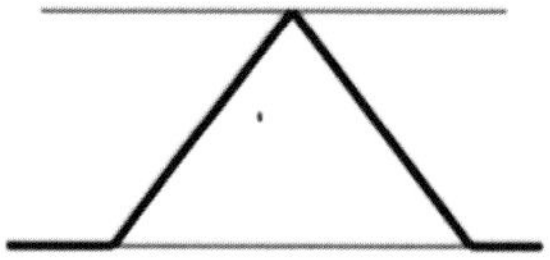
- Trapezoidal MF 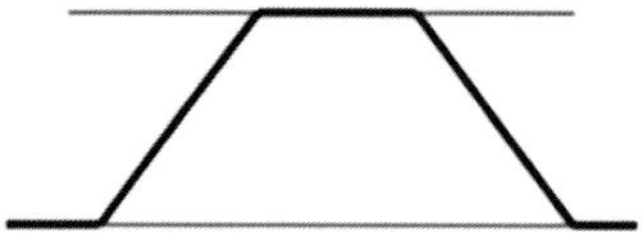
- Singleton MF 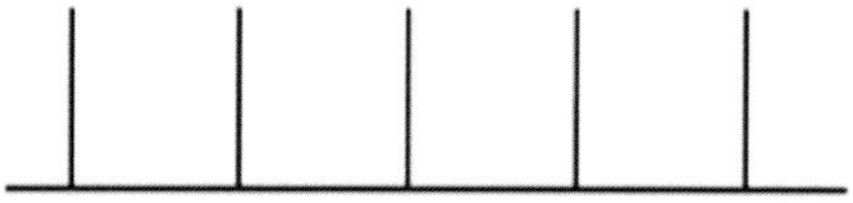

## 16.3 Fuzzy Inference System (FIS)

A Fuzzy Inference System (FIS) is designed to transform input data into output data from the evaluation of a set of rules. The inputs are derived from the fuzzification process and the set of rules normally are defined by the expertise of the expert. A FIS consists of three stages (Fig. 16.3):

**Fuzzification**: consists of characterizing the linguistic variables used in the system. It is, therefore, a transformation of the real inputs into a fuzzy part defined on a representation space linked to the input. This representation space is normally a fuzzy subset. During the fuzzification step, each input and output variable is associated with fuzzy subsets.

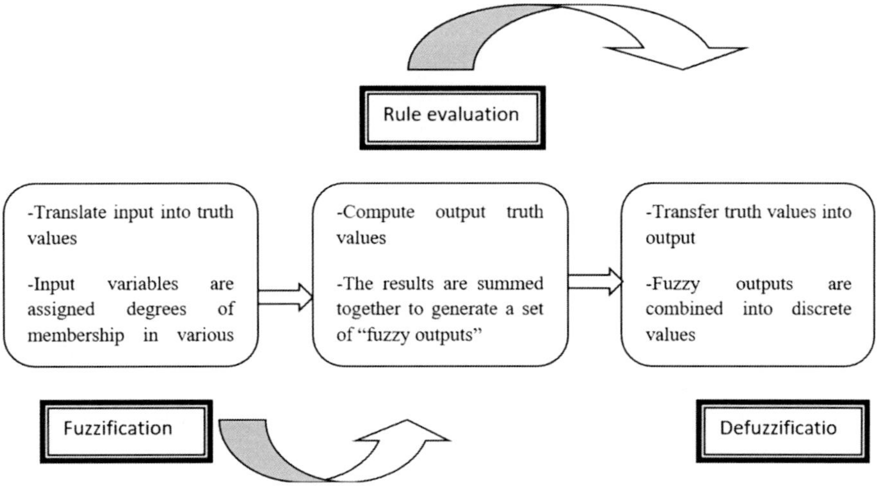


**Fig. 16.3** Fuzzy inference systems

**Inference**: consists of using the inference engine, which is a mechanism for condensing the information of a system through a set of rules defined for the representation of any problem. Each rule delivers a partial conclusion which is then aggregated to the other rules to provide a conclusion (aggregation).

**Defuzzification**: consists of characterizing the linguistic variables used in the system. It is, therefore, a transformation of the real inputs into a fuzzy part defined on a representation space linked to the input. This representation space is normally a fuzzy subset. During the fuzzification step, each input and output variable is associated with fuzzy subsets.

## 16.4 Motives to Apply Fuzzy Logic in the Operating Theater Management

Operating theater is an integrated system composed of a series of locations, generally, including surgical waiting areas, operating room, recovery room, changing rooms, prepare the room and etc. The human resources needed by operating room mainly include surgeons, nurses, and anesthetists. In addition, the operating room also requires a variety of medical equipment and supplies.

When a patient arrives, he/she is allocated to the intake area to get ready for the surgery. Then the patient is subsequently taken to surgery in an unoccupied OR, and after the surgery, the patient is sent to the recovery area for some post-anesthesia care. Surgery can last from minutes to hours, depending on the type and the complexity of the surgery, and also its assigned surgeon.

In the following, we will show the need to present some operating theater data as uncertain values.

### *16.4.1 Surgeries Duration*

The duration of a surgical procedure is subject to considerable variations depending on the type of intervention, the level of expertise of the surgeon, the patient's condition, the technique of anesthesia, etc. The duration of the intervention corresponds to the length of stay in the operating room. This duration is mainly composed of: duration of preparation for the intervention (preparation of the patient, anesthesia, etc.), duration of the surgical procedure (which varies according to its nature, the surgeon and the patient), the period of post-anesthesia care and control of the patient. This residence time, a function of multiple parameters is designated in an aggregated manner by the operating time. The variability of the operating times very often leads to modifications in the planning of the activities of the block. This leads to a deterioration in the quality of service vis-à-vis patients (waiting times, delayed intervention...) and additional operating costs (overtime...).

The estimation of the length of stay of the patient in the operating room has been the subject of some work. The duration of the surgical procedure depends on the nature of the surgical procedure, the surgeon and the patient's diagnostic results [28]. Zhou and Dexter [30] have shown that a log-normal distribution is best suited to the approximation of the duration of a surgical procedure performed by a particular surgeon. In addition, there are information systems which, by feedback, can generate an average duration for interventions.

However, few studies have focused on estimating lengths of stay in the Post-Anesthesia Care Unit (PACU). Dexter and Tinker [6] analyzed the effect of some anesthesia techniques on PACU residence time in an attempt to reduce costs in outpatient surgery. The authors, based on a statistical analysis of the data, observed that the residence time in PACU follows a log-normal law. In the same framework, the work [24] carried out within the hospital research project should lead to proposing statistical models of representation of the duration of intervention and residence time in the PACU.

Based on this work, Marcon and Kharraja [20] assumed that the duration of recovery is a function which depends mainly on the duration of the intervention. A good estimation of the per-operative durations and the duration of awakening is necessary to find operative programming that exploits the operating theater resources as well as possible.

The duration of each surgery is dependent on the surgery type and can be performed from a few minutes to hours. One of the major problems associated with the development of accurate OR planning and scheduling strategies is the uncertainty inherent to surgical services.

Since the duration of each surgery is an important parameter depending on many factors such as the skill of the surgeon or the category of the age of patients, it's possible not to have a definite or fixed value. Hence, in this work, the duration of each surgery case is considered as triangular fuzzy numbers. These fuzzy numbers are divided into 3 groups according to the conditions of the training skills of surgeons. Surgery cannot be cut off or stopped during its three stages.

Dexter et al. [8] reported that an estimate of the duration of a surgery case provided by surgeons is more accurate than that provided by the software.

### *16.4.2 Surgeries Due Dates*

A possibility distribution can be defined as the degree of occurrence of an event with imprecise data [25]. The due dates of the surgery can be modeled as fuzzy parameters. These values are to be determined by the decision maker of the considered hospital. They can be also classified into different classes such as the most pessimistic values, the most possible values, and the most optimistic values.

## 16.5 Fuzzy Operating Theater Problems Complexity

The real world is complex. This complexity generally arises from uncertainty. Humans have unconsciously been able to address complex, ambiguous, and uncertain problems thanks to the gift of thinking.

Classical logic is based on binary logic with two values of truth. In Maple, these two values true and false. On the contrary, fuzzy logic is a multi-valued logic with truth represented by a value on the closed interval [0, 1], where 0 is equated with the classical false value and 1 is equated with the classical true value. Values in [0, 1] indicate varying degrees of truth. That means that the treatment of the problem by the fuzzy aspect considers more of the number of variables than their treatment by a deterministic aspect. In addition, Lotfi Zadeh [29] suggested by his principle of incompatibility: "The closer one looks at a real-world problem, the fuzzier becomes the solution," and thus, imprecision and complexity are correlated.

## 16.6 Fuzzy Operating Theater Optimization: A Literature Review

We note that the vast majority of the work assumes that the operating rooms are dedicated only to elective surgery and that the interventions have deterministic durations. Recently, another class of scheduling problems with uncertain parameters has been developed based on fuzzy set theory, stochastic and possibility theory, which aims at dealing with cases of imprecise or vague data. The main considered sources of uncertainty are usually associated with the arrival of urgent patients, the patients' length of stay and surgery durations [11].

In the literature, few studies have considered the problem of planning with uncertainty [12, 14]. An objective that receives more and more attention nowadays is the management of uncertainty. Many studies have focused on increasing the punctuality of the realized schedule [9, 20].

Lans et al. [18] considered the problem of sequencing interventions with deterministic durations in several rooms. Operating rooms are used to carry out planned interventions as well as not programmed interventions. When an urgent patient arrives, he is operated in the first available room. Otherwise, as soon as an outstanding intervention is completed, the emergency intervention can begin and the intervention that has been scheduled will be delayed. The authors proposed to schedule the planned interventions in order to reduce the waiting time for urgent interventions.

Min and Yih [21] developed a stochastic programming model with the application of the sample average approximation method with the aim of minimizing the additional costs of the operating rooms. Denton et al. [5] described a stochastic optimization model and some practical heuristics for computing OR schedule that hedge against the uncertainty in surgery durations. They focused on the simultaneous effects of sequencing surgeries and scheduled start times.

Dexter and Traub [7] proposed a statistical method to evaluate the probability that one intervention will last more than another, allowing the sequencing of interventions so as to avoid a conflict of resources. Sier et al. [24] considered the problem of scheduling interventions with deterministic durations in several rooms while taking into account constraints related to equipment availability, patient age, duration of interventions, etc. The authors modeled the problem as a nonlinear integer program and used simulated annealing for approximate resolution.

Lebowitz [19] proposed to approximate the duration of intervention by their averages based on past information. He compared a few sequencing rules by numerical simulation and concludes that treating patients in increasing order of average durations reduces the wait time for surgeons, under and on the use of the room. Weiss [27] considered the scheduling problem with random intervention times in order to minimize the cost of under-utilization of the room and surgeons' expectations costs.

Ho and Lau [15] considered the scheduling problem in order to find a compromise between the waiting costs of patients and that of medical staff. The authors have shown that waiting times generated by any scheduling rule are influenced by three environmental factors: the no-show probability of occurrence, the coefficient of variation of the duration of interventions and the number of patients to be scheduled. They simulated the performance of nine scheduling rules (individual and per block) for different combinations of environmental factors and therefore proposed a procedure for identifying the best performing rule for each combination.

Zadeh proposed the fuzzy set theory, providing a highly effective means of handling imprecise data. In recent years, many researchers have begun to investigate the assignment problem under the fuzzy environment [29]. One of the major problems associated with the development of accurate operating room schedules or capacity planning strategies is the uncertainty inherent to surgical services [3]. Wang and Xu [26] developed a fuzzy multi-objective programming model to optimize the OR schedule. Darvish et al. [22] introduced a fuzzy model for an open shop scheduling problem with fuzzy processing times and fuzzy due dates to minimize total completion time and total weighted tardiness during the three stages of the surgery process.

Recent studies in scheduling problems have used fuzzy numbers to address the uncertainty of the data. Chanas and Kasperski [4] considered fuzzy processing times and fuzzy due dates in the case of a single machine scheduling problem. Sakawa and Kubota [23] presented a two-objective genetic algorithm to minimize maximum fuzzy completion time and maximize average agreement index. Ghrayeb [13] proposed a genetic algorithm for the fuzzy job shop scheduling problems with the objective of minimizing integral value and uncertainty of fuzzy makespan. Lahijanian et al. [17] proposed a mixed integer programming to minimize the total weighted start times. They grouped the patients based on their age into three categories and they considered the duration of the surgical elective operation as a fuzzy number. A hybrid algorithm was used for resolution.

## 16.7 Conclusion

Good management of the operating theater is strongly linked to the integration of the uncertain aspect of the operating times in the planning of the activities, in order to propose precise schedules.

The quality of an operating room scheduling is, of course, conditioned by the method used but also by the precision of the operating times estimated for each intervention. Indeed, the times corresponding to the different stages of intervention are non-deterministic. In addition, estimating operating time is not an easy task.

## References

1. Borsuk ME, Stow CA, Reckhow KH (2004) A bayesian network of eutrophication models for synthesis, prediction, and uncertainty analysis. Ecol Model 173(2–3):219–239
2. Bouchon-Meunier B, Zadeh L (1995) Fuzzy logic and its applications. Addison-Wesley, Boston
3. Cardoen B, Demeulemeester E, Beliën J (2010) Operating room planning and scheduling: a literature review. Eur J Oper Res 201(3):921–932
4. Chanas S, Kasperski A (2001) Minimizing maximum lateness in a single machine scheduling problem with fuzzy processing times and fuzzy due dates. Eng Appl Artif Intell 14(3):377–386
5. Denton B, Viapiano J, Vogl A (2007) Optimization of surgery sequencing and scheduling decisions under uncertainty. Health Care Manag Sci 10(1):13–24
6. Dexter F, Tinker JH (1995) Analysis of strategies to decrease postanesthesia care unit costs. Anesthesiol: J Am Soc Anesthesiol 82(1):94–101
7. Dexter F, Traub RD (2000) Sequencing cases in the operating room: predicting whether one surgical case will last longer than another. Anesth Analg 90(4):975–979
8. Dexter F, Macario A, Traub RD (1999) Which algorithm for scheduling add-on elective cases maximizes operating room utilization? use of bin packing algorithms and fuzzy constraints in operating room management. Anesthesiol: J Am Soc Anesthesiol 91(5):1491–1491
9. Dexter F, Blake JT, Penning DH, Sloan B, Chung P, Lubarsky DA (2002) Use of linear programming to estimate impact of changes in a hospital's operating room time allocation on perioperative variable costs. Anesthesiol: J Am Soc Anesthesiol 96(3):718–724
10. Fenton N, Neil M (2012) Risk assessment and decision analysis with Bayesian networks. CRC Press, Boca Raton

11. Fügener A (2015) An integrated strategic and tactical master surgery scheduling approach with stochastic resource demand. J Bus Logist 36(4):374–387
12. Gerchak Y, Gupta D, Henig M (1996) Reservation planning for elective surgery under uncertain demand for emergency surgery. Manag Sci 42(3):321–334
13. Ghrayeb OA (2003) A bi-criteria optimization: minimizing the integral value and spread of the fuzzy makespan of job shop scheduling problems. Appl soft Comput 2(3):197–210
14. Hans E, Wullink G, Van Houdenhoven M, Kazemier G (2008) Robust surgery loading. Eur J Oper Res 185(3):1038–1050
15. Ho CJ, Lau HS (1992) Minimizing total cost in scheduling outpatient appointments. Manag Sci 38(12):1750–1764
16. Holzkämper A, Kumar V, Surridge BW, Paetzold A, Lerner DN (2012) Bringing diverse knowledge sources together-a meta-model for supporting integrated catchment management. J Environ Manag 96(1):116–127
17. Lahijanian B, Zarandi MF, Farahani FV (2016) Proposing a model for operating room scheduling based on fuzzy surgical duration. In: 2016 annual conference of the North American fuzzy information processing society (NAFIPS). IEEE, pp 1–5
18. van der Lans M, Hans EW, Hurink JL, Wullink G, van Houdenhoven M, Kazemier G (2006) Anticipating urgent surgery in operating room departments. University of Twente, Technical Report WP-158
19. Lebowitz P (2003) Schedule the short procedure first to improve or efficiency. AORN J 78(4):651–659
20. Marcon E, Kharraja S, Simonnet G (2003) The operating theatre planning by the follow-up of the risk of no realization. Int J Prod Econ 85(1):83–90
21. Min D, Yih Y (2010) Scheduling elective surgery under uncertainty and downstream capacity constraints. Eur J Oper Res 206(3):642–652
22. Noori-Darvish S, Mahdavi I, Mahdavi-Amiri N (2012) A bi-objective possibilistic programming model for open shop scheduling problems with sequence-dependent setup times, fuzzy processing times, and fuzzy due dates. Appl Soft Comput 12(4):1399–1416
23. Sakawa M, Kubota R (2000) Fuzzy programming for multiobjective job shop scheduling with fuzzy processing time and fuzzy duedate through genetic algorithms. Eur J Oper Res 120(2):393–407
24. Sier D, Tobin P, McGurk C (1997) Scheduling surgical procedures. J Oper Res Soc 48(9):884–891
25. Torabi SA, Hassini E (2008) An interactive possibilistic programming approach for multiple objective supply chain master planning. Fuzzy Sets Syst 159(2):193–214
26. Wang D, Xu J (2008) A fuzzy multi-objective optimizing scheduling for operation room in hospital. In: 2008 IEEE international conference on industrial engineering and engineering management. IEEE, pp 614–618
27. Weiss EN (1990) Models for determining estimated start times and case orderings in hospital operating rooms. IIE Trans 22(2):143–150
28. Wright IH, Kooperberg C, Bonar BA, Bashein G (1996) Statistical modeling to predict elective surgery timecomparison with a computer scheduling system and surgeon-provided estimates. Anesthesiol: J Am Soc Anesthesiol 85(6):1235–1245
29. Zadeh LA (1965) Fuzzy sets. Inf Control 8(3):338–353
30. Zhou J, Dexter F (1998) Method to assist in the scheduling of add-on surgical cases-upper prediction bounds for surgical case durations based on the log-normal distribution. Anesthesiol: J Am Soc Anesthesiol 89(5):1228–1232

MIX
Papier aus verantwortungsvollen Quellen
Paper from responsible sources
FSC® C105338

Printed by Books on Demand, Germany